The Nutritionist

Now in an updated and expanded new edition, *The Nutritionist: Food, Nutrition, and Optimal Health, Second Edition*, provides readers with vital information about how to simply but radically improve their daily lives with the science of nutrition, balance their diets to achieve more energy, and improve health and longevity.

Complete with many informative and easy-to-read tables and charts, *The Nutritionist: Food, Nutrition, and Optimal Health, Second Edition*, utilizes the findings of the latest biological and medical studies to give experts and non-experts alike a comprehensive account of the needs of our bodies and the ways that healthy eating can improve performance in day-to-day activities.

Author Dr Robert Wildman, renowned nutrition expert, debunks myths about carbohydrates, fat, and cholesterol, elucidates the role of water in nutrition, and clearly explains the facts of human anatomy and physiognomy, the process of digestion, and vitamin supplements. Complete with a practical and comprehensive guide to the nutrition information printed on the packaging of most food items, *The Nutritionist: Food, Nutrition, and Optimal Health, Second Edition* is a necessary and extremely useful nutrition resource for anyone interested in the science and practical benefits of good nutrition.

Dr Robert E.C. Wildman is a graduate of the University of Pittsburgh, Florida State University, and Ohio State University, and is currently on the faculty at Kansas State University. Dr Wildman is also the author of *Sports and Fitness Nutrition* (2002) and editor of *The Handbook of Nutraceuticals and Functional Foods, Second Edition* (Taylor & Francis, 2007).

The Nutritionist

Food, Nutrition, and Optimal Health

Second

Dr R

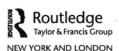
Routledge
Taylor & Francis Group

NEW YORK AND LONDON

First published 2002 by Haworth
This edition first published 2009
by Routledge
270 Madison Ave, New York NY 10016

Simultaneously published in the UK
by Routledge
2 Park Square, Milton Park, Abingdon, Oxon, OX14 4RN

*Routledge is an imprint of the Taylor & Francis Group,
an informa business*

Transferred to Digital Printing 2010

© 2002 Haworth
© 2009 Taylor & Francis

Typeset in Sabon by
RefineCatch Limited, Bungay, Suffolk

Library of Congress Cataloging in Publication Data
Wildman, Robert E. C., 1964–
    The nutritionist: food, nutrition & optimal health / by Robert E.C.
Wildman.
      p. cm.
    1. Nutrition.   I. Title
    QP141.W487 2009
    612.3—dc22
    2008029707

ISBN10: 0–7890–3423–9 (hbk)
ISBN10: 0–7890–3424–7 (pbk)
ISBN10: 0–203–88700–X (ebk)

ISBN13: 978–0–7890–3423–6 (hbk)
ISBN13: 978–0–7890–3424–3 (pbk)
ISBN13: 978–0–203–88700–4 (ebk)

For David

Contents

About the Author

Dr Robert E.C. Wildman is a graduate of the University of Pittsburgh, Florida State University, and Ohio State University, and is currently on the faculty at Kansas State University. Dr Wildman is also the author of *Sports and Fitness Nutrition* (2002) and editor of *The Handbook of Nutraceuticals and Functional Foods, Second Edition* (Taylor & Francis, 2007) as well as founder of TheNutritionDr.com (www.thenutritiondr.com) and Demeter Consultants LLC (www. demeterconsultants.com).

Preface

The seeming simplicity of our daily activities is greatly contrasted by the complexity of our true nature—quite a paradox, no doubt. It is simple in that, on the outside, the goals of our body may appear few. We internalize food, water, and oxygen while at the same time ridding ourselves of carbon dioxide and other waste materials. These operations support reproduction, growth, maintenance, and defense. Yet on the inside our body may seem very complex as various organs participate in a tremendous number of complicated processes intended to meet the simple goals previously mentioned.

Nutrition is just one part of this paradoxical relationship. The objective of nutrition is simple: to supply our body with all of the necessary nutrients, and in appropriate quantities, to promote optimal health and function. However, in practice, nutrition is far from that simple. There seem to be too many nutrients, controversial nutrients, and different conditions, such as growth, pregnancy, and exercise, to allow nutrition to be a simple topic.

Although we have long appreciated food, it has only been in the more recent years that we have really begun to understand the finer relationship between food and our body. Most nutrients have been identified within the last century or so and right now nutrition is one of the most prevalent areas of scientific research. This is to say that our understanding of nutrition is by no means complete. It continues to evolve in conjunction with the most current nutrition research. It seems that not a week goes by without hearing about yet another discovery in nutrition.

It is hard to believe that just a few decades ago the basic four food groups were pretty much all the nutrition known by most people. Today nutrition deeply penetrates into many aspects of our lives, including preventative and treatment medicine, philosophy, exercise training, and weight management. Our diet has been linked to cardiovascular health, cancer, bowel function, moods, and brain activity, along with many other health domains. We no longer eat merely to satisfy hunger. Without doubt, nutrition has become a matter of great curiosity and/or concern for most of us today.

A few problems have developed along with this most recent illumination of nutrition. One such problem is that we may have generated too much knowledge too fast. Even though we, as humans, have been eating throughout our existence, the importance of proper nutrition seems to have been thrust upon us suddenly. We did not have time to first wade into the waters of nutrition science, slowly increasing our depth. The reality is that we may be in over our heads, barely treading water to keep up with the latest recommendations. Sometimes, all we can do is try our best to follow the latest nutrition recommendations without really having the background or accessibility to proper resources truly to understand the reasons behind the recommendations.

Although nutrition has become a very complex subject many authors still try to present it in an overly simplified manner. Perhaps they believe that people are not interested in the scientific details and merely wish to be told what to do. This book attempts to break that pattern. We will spend time laying a foundation in some of the basic concepts of science and of our body in hope that it will actually make nutrition a simpler subject.

I believe that deep down a scientist lurks within all of us. Everyday we ponder the effects of certain actions before performing them. This is the so-called cause and effect relationship, the very basis of scientific experimentation. Furthermore, since most of us give at least some thought to the foods we eat, we are all a special breed of scientist. We are nutrition scientists! A nutrition scientist is one who ponders the relationship between food components and their body. You do not have to work in a laboratory to be a nutrition scientist. All you need is simple curiosity and the dedication of your time to pursue a greater understanding of nutrition. This book is written in a question and answer format to satisfy your curiosity.

Fundamental questions regarding nutrition and our body will be posed and then answered based upon the most current research. If your educational background includes a solid foundation of biology and chemistry you may wish to skip the first few chapters. However, if your science background is weak or far in the past, you may find the first few chapters of service. So, here we go. Good luck and good science!

1   The Very Basics of Humans and the World We Inhabit

Have you ever stopped and wondered why we (humans) are as we are, and why we do what we do? It is truly remarkable what our bodies are capable of doing and how our bodies operate to perform various tasks. Yet, we are just one of millions of different species inhabiting this planet, all with a unique story to tell. And, like our fellow planet-mates, we must abide by the basic objectives of life, namely to function as an independent being (self-operate), defend ourselves both externally and internally, nourish ourselves, and of course to reproduce, which is without question the ultimate objective of all life-forms.

Yet, we are special in that we have a relatively large brain and the intellectual capacity to try to understand ourselves and, in accordance, how we are to be nourished. In this chapter we will begin to explore the very basis of our being and the world we live in. This will begin to set the stage for understanding what it will take to nourish our body for optimal health and longevity. We will answer questions about basic concepts such as elements, atoms, molecules, oxidation, chemical reactions, water solubility, and acids and bases. If you have a science background this chapter might seem too rudimentary and you might consider moving on to the next chapter.

What Is Nutrition?

We will start out as simply as possible. The shortest definition of *nutrition* is the science pertaining to the factors involved in nourishing our body. Nutrition hinges upon the special relationship that exists between our body and the world we live in. From the moment of conception to the waning hours of advanced age, we live in a continuum to nourish our body. More specifically, we strive on a daily basis to bring nourishing substances into our body. These nourishing substances are called *nutrients*, which are chemicals that are used by our body for energy or other human processes. Proper nourishment supports body businesses such as growth, movement, immunity, injury recovery, and disease prevention, and, of course, the ultimate business at hand for all life-forms, reproduction.

All that we (our body) are, ever were, or are going to be is borrowed from the environment that we inhabit. This unique state of indebtedness is primarily attributed to our nutrition intake. We must be grateful to the earth's crust for lending us minerals that strengthen our bones and teeth and allow us to have electrical operations that drives nerve and muscle function. We must also pay homage to plants for the carbohydrate forms that power our operations and for the amino acids that make the protein in our muscle.

Nutrition refers to the science of nourishing our body.

All too often we do not truly appreciate the relevance of nutrition to our basic being. But again, please keep in mind that nearly everything we are and are able to do is either a direct or indirect reflection of our past and current nutrition intake. No matter how oversimplified nutrition may seem in television commercials and on cereal boxes, it is without a doubt one of the most complex and interesting sciences out there. One of the major tasks of this book is to provide an understandable overview of nutrition as it applies to optimal health and longevity.

How Do We Begin to Understand Nutrition?

Certainly any great building must be constructed upon a solid foundation. So let us go ahead and commit ourselves to building a solid scientific foundation to explore nutrition. So, before we begin to learn how to nourish our body, we need to have a better understanding of what needs to be nourished. Our body is the product of nature and as such it must adhere to the basic laws of nature. In fact, you can think of nutrition as the scientific offspring of more basic sciences such as chemistry and biology. Therefore, understanding the *what's*, *why's*, and *how's* of nutrition will be a lot easier once a few basic areas of chemistry and biology are appreciated. What follows are some fundamental principles of chemistry and biology and a description of their relevance to nutrition and the body.

It's Atoms and Molecules That Make the Man, Not Clothes

What Is the Most Basic Composition of Our Body?

Let's say that we had access to fancy laboratory equipment capable of determining the most fundamental composition of an object. If we used this equipment to assess a man or woman it would spit out some interesting data on our most basic level of composition—*elements*. Elements are substances that cannot be broken down into other substances. Scientists have determined that there are one hundred or so of these elements in nature. Some of the more recognizable elements include carbon, oxygen, hydrogen, nitrogen, iron, zinc, copper, potassium, and calcium. All of the elements known to exist can be found on the periodic table of elements, which we have all come across at one point or another in our schooling. (the periodic table of elements is included as Appendix A in case you feel the need for another peek.) Now, imagine that everything that you can think of is merely a skillful combination of these same elements. This includes cars, boats, buildings, clouds, oceans, trees, and of course our body. In fact, our body employs about twenty-seven of the elements as displayed in Table 1.1 and Appendix A.

What Is the Element Composition of Our Body?

The late, great Carl Sagan in his personal exploration of the cosmos said that we are made up of "star stuff." What he meant was that our body is made up of many of the very same elements that make up planets and other celestial bodies in the universe. We humans, as well as other life-forms on our planet, have simply borrowed these elements. Interestingly, four of these elements, namely oxygen, carbon, hydrogen, and nitrogen, make up greater than 90 percent of our body weight. Since the majority of these elements are found in our body as part of substances such as water, proteins, carbohydrates, fats, and nucleic acids (DNA and RNA), it only makes sense that these substances must be the major chemicals of

Table 1.1 Elements of Our Bodies

Major Elements (>0.1% Body Weight)	Percentage of Body Weight	Minor Elements (<0.1% Body Weight)	Percentage of Body Weight
Oxygen (O)	63	Iron (Fe)	<0.1
Carbon (C)	18.0	Selenium (Se)	<0.1
Hydrogen (H)	9.0	Copper (Cu)	<0.1
Nitrogen (N)	3.0	Cobalt (Co)	<0.1
Calcium (Ca)	1.5	Fluoride (F)	<0.1
Phosphorus (P)	1.0	Iodine (I)	<0.1
Potassium (K)	0.4	Molybdenum (Mo)	<0.1
Sulfur (S)	0.3	Manganese (Mn)	<0.1
Sodium (Na)	0.2	Vanadium (V)	<0.1
Chloride (Cl)	0.2	Chromium (Cr)	<0.1
Magnesium (Mg)	0.1	Boron (B)	<0.1
		Zinc (Zn)	<0.1
		Aluminum (Al)	<0.1
		Tin (Sn)	<0.1
		Silicon (Si)	<0.1
		Arsenic (As)	<0.1

our body. For example, a lean, young adult male's body weight may be approximately 62 percent water, 16 percent protein, 16 percent fat, and less than 1 percent carbohydrate. Most of his remaining weight (about 5 percent) would be attributed to minerals. We will spend a lot more time talking about the finer details of body composition in later chapters.

> Our body is mostly made of water, fats, protein, carbohydrate, minerals, DNA, and other special molecules.

What Is the Relationship Between Elements and Atoms?

Atoms are the building blocks of everything that exists. From the clothes on your back to the car you drive to the food you eat—everything is composed of atoms. Each individual atom belongs to only one element. This is to say that even though there are an incomprehensible number of atoms on this planet and the universe making up everything we know and are yet to know, all of these atoms belong to only one of a hundred or so elements (see Appendix A). This is similar to each one of the billions of people living on this planet being native to only one of a hundred or so countries.

In a world where size is judged relative to the size of humans, the atom is indeed minuscule. It has been said that if we could line up a million atoms end to end they would barely cover the distance across the period at the end of this sentence. However, they do indeed exist even though you cannot see them with the naked eye.

All atoms have a similar blueprint to the image displayed in Figure 1.1. There are three principal particles called *neutrons, protons*, and *electrons*. Because they are smaller than the atom that they come together to form, they are often called *subatomic* particles. Protons bear a positive charge (+) while electrons have a negative charge (−) and neutrons do not bear any charge at all. By design an element has the same number of electrons as protons and is said to be neutral. However, as we'll see next that isn't how many atoms exist naturally.

Can Certain Atoms Have a Charge?

Atoms of certain elements naturally exist in a charged state, which means that they have either lost or gained electrons. It really is a matter of simple algebra. If an atom exists without an electron, it will have a single positive charge (1^+) and if it exists without two electrons it will develop a double positive charge (2^+). On the contrary, if an atom has an extra electron, it

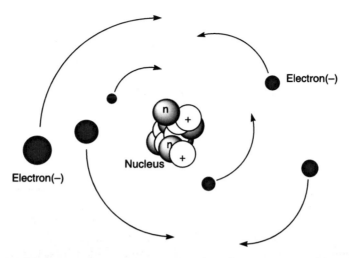

Figure 1.1 This is a carbon atom. Protons (white) have a positive charge (+) and neutrons (shaded) are electrically neutral (n) are found in the nucleus. Electrons (black) have a negative charge (−) and orbit the nucleus at the speed of light!

will have a single negative charge (1^-) and if an atom has two additional electrons it will have a double negative charge (2^-). It is important to keep in mind that this isn't random; some atoms are simply more stable in a charged state. Charged atoms are often called *electrolytes* because their charge gives them electrical properties as discussed further below.

The processes of losing and gaining electrons are interrelated, as displayed in Figure 1.2. So, if one atom gains an electron, it is actually removing the electron from another atom which wants to give it up to become more stable. This activity is referred to as *oxidation* and *reduction*, whereby oxidation refers to the loss of an electron while reduction refers to the gain of an electron. You might be thinking that this may have

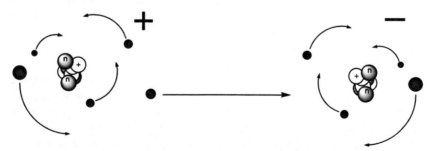

Figure 1.2 An electron is lost by the atom on the left (yielding a positive charge) and gained by the atom on the right (yielding a negative charge).

something to do with anti*oxidant* nutrients, such as vitamins C and E and a whole host of others such as β-carotene and lycopene. If you were, then you are right and have the mind of a scientist. Furthermore, you may have heard the term oxidation used in reference to energy operations in our body (for example, oxidation of fat). Again, you would be on the right track—but we are getting ahead of ourselves.

Oxidation refers to when an atom or molecule loses an electron.

Many elements important to nutrition and the proper functioning of our body exist naturally in a charged state. These elements include sodium, chlorine, potassium, iodine, magnesium, and calcium. The charge associated with an atom is often displayed in superscript next to the element's symbol from the Periodic Table of Elements. For instance, sodium is written as Na^+, potassium as K^+ (both of which have given up an electron, while calcium is written as Ca^{2+} and magnesium as Mg^{2+} as they have given up two electrons. On the contrary, chlorine is written as Cl^-, fluorine as F^- and iodine as I^- as they have gained an electron and thus a negative charge. Actually, we tend to refer to chlorine, fluorine, and iodine as chloride, fluoride, and iodide with respect to this electrical state.

How Do Atoms Combine with Each Other?

A couple of millennia ago, the Greeks believed that water was one of the four elements of nature, along with fire, air, and earth, and that all things were made from combinations of these elements. Today, we of course know that there are more than a hundred elements. And, in fact, water is not a single element but a combination of atoms of two elements, namely hydrogen (H) and oxygen (O). When two or more atoms of the same or different elements combine together, *molecules* are formed. Therefore, water is a molecule. The chemical formula for a water molecule (H_2O) is probably the most widely quoted of all *chemical formulas*. A chemical formula is merely a molecule's atomic recipe. Thus, for each molecule of water, two hydrogen atoms (subscript 2 behind H) are bound to one oxygen atom (no subscript, so 1 is implied).

From our previous description of the size of atoms you can imagine then that an ordinary glass of water must contain millions of water molecules. In fact, we can use water to tidy up our understanding of elements, atoms, and molecules. If we have an 8 ounce (oz) glass of pure water, we can say that the container is accommodating millions of molecules of water, and thus millions of atoms; however, only two elements are present, oxygen and hydrogen.

Atoms can link together or *bond* by two means. First, charged atoms can interact with oppositely charged atoms. Remember, as in so many aspects of life, opposites attract. Perhaps the best example of this kind of bonding is sodium chloride (NaCl) or common table salt. Here, the negatively charged chloride ions (Cl$^-$) are attracted and electrically stick to positively charged sodium ions (Na$^+$). You can also check your toothpaste for sodium fluoride (NaF) or toothpaste salt. By the way, the term *salt* is a general term that describes these types of electrical interactions.

Na$^{+\nearrow}$ Cl$^-$ sodium chloride (table salt)
Na$^{+\nearrow}$ F$^-$ sodium fluoride (toothpaste salt)

Another way that atoms can bond with each other is by sharing electrons. This is a fascinating event whereby atoms share electrons between them to form a stable union. In Figure 1.3 and throughout this book you will see a straight line connecting atoms that are bonded in this manner. Probably the best examples of this type of bonding are the so-called *organic* molecules, which refers to those molecules that contain carbon atoms. Organic also refers to that which is living. Therefore, the most important molecules of life must be carbon based. In fact, a large portion of this book discusses organic molecules, such as proteins, carbohydrates, fats, cholesterol, nucleic acids, and vitamins.

What Is the Design of Molecules?

One limitation of an ink-and-paper representation of molecules is that it often fails to truly capture the three-dimensional beauty of molecules. For example, DNA molecules exist in a spiral staircase design, while many protein molecules appear to be all bunched (or "globbed") up. The three-dimensional design of a molecule helps determine what that molecule can do (its properties). Furthermore, we will see that many of the important molecules in our body are actually combinations of smaller molecules. For instance, proteins are made from amino acids, and fat molecules are made from fatty acids and glycerol.

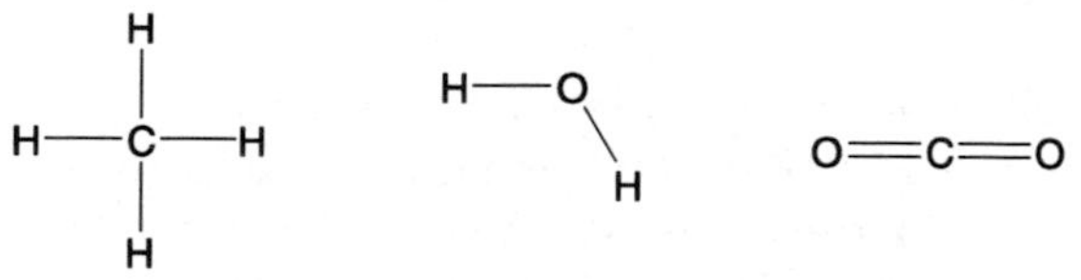

Methane (CH$_4$)   Water (H$_2$O)   Carbon dioxide (CO$_2$)

Figure 1.3 Methane (CH$_4$) and carbon dioxide (CO$_2$) are organic molecules while water (H$_2$O) is not.

How Do Molecules Interact with One Another?

Molecules in our body, or anywhere else in nature, mingle among one another. And, if things are right, they can interact. When molecules interact the process is called a *chemical reaction*. For instance, in the reaction below, A and B are substances that react and are called *reactants*. As a result of this chemical reaction, different substances are produced and are called *products*. In the chemical reaction below the products are C and D.

$$A + B \rightarrow C + D$$

or

$$6CO_2 + 6H_2O \rightarrow C_6H_{12}O_6 + 6O_2$$

In a more realistic reaction, carbon dioxide (CO_2) reacts with water to form carbohydrate ($C_6H_{12}O_6$) and oxygen (O_2). Look familiar? It might, since it is photosynthesis, the process whereby plants make carbohydrates.

The reaction arrow ($\rightarrow$) separating the reactants and products merely shows which way the chemical reaction will proceed. A reaction may proceed in only one direction or it may be reversible, whereby the reaction will proceed in either direction. A reversible-reaction arrow looks like you might expect ($\leftrightarrow$). If there is a number (coefficient) in front of reacting or produced substances this merely tells us how many molecules of a substance must react or be produced in order for the chemical reaction to make sense or to be "balanced."

In chemical reactions, molecules can react to form new molecules.

What Are Enzymes?

You may remember from a high school or college chemistry lab that when you performed an experiment using two or more chemicals, another chemical was often added to help the reaction to take place or to speed it up. That chemical was an *enzyme*. Enzymes are proteins and it is their job to regulate and accelerate most chemical reactions that occur in living things. Life itself would be impossible without *enzymes*.

Enzymes are called *catalysts*, meaning they speed up the rate of a reaction between two or more chemicals. A given chemical reaction between two chemicals may take place without an enzyme, but the rate of the reaction may be incredibly slow. It might take hours, days, weeks, or even years to happen. This would be simply unacceptable, as the proper functioning of our body may require that same chemical reaction to take place numerous times in a fraction of a second. Enzymes speed up the rate at which chemical reactions occur. Another important feature of enzymes is that they are extremely specific. Most enzymes will work on only one reaction, just as a key will fit into one lock.

Enzymes are special proteins that speed up and regulate chemical reactions.

Is It Possible for Chemical Reactions to Be Linked Together?

In various situations in our body, many chemical reactions actually occur in series. Here, the product(s) of one chemical reaction become reactants in the next chemical reaction and so on. These reaction series are more commonly referred to as *pathways*, as depicted in Figure 1.4. We will discuss many pathways throughout our exploration.

Energy Is Everything

What Is Energy?

Energy may be best understood as a potential or presence that allows for some type of work to be performed. Some of energy's more recognizable forms are heat, light, mechanical, chemical, and electrical energy. Without energy we simply would not exist. The universe, if it existed at all, would be a frigid, barren, motionless void.

Energy is neither created nor destroyed, however it can be converted from one form to another. This means that while the total amount of energy in the universe remains constant, the quantity of the different forms can change relative to one another. For instance, you are probably reading this book by the light of a nearby lamp. The light bulb has a thin filament inside, which transforms the electrical energy running from the wall socket and through the cord to the filament in the bulb where it is converted into two other forms of energy—light and heat. As the filament illuminates, there is a reduction in electrical energy and an increase in light and heat energies. So energy is not lost but transformed to other forms.

A little bit closer to nutrition, food contains chemical energy in the form of carbohydrates, proteins, fats, and alcohol. Once inside our body the

$$A + B \longrightarrow C + D \longleftrightarrow E + F \longrightarrow G + H$$

Figure 1.4 Here A and B are the initial reactants and G and H are the end products of the pathway.

chemical energy of these substances can be transformed into mechanical energy to power muscular movement and other activities as well as heat to maintain our body temperature. Furthermore, we can store these energy molecules when we cannot immediately use them.

Do Chemical Reactions Involve Energy?

Molecules house energy in the bonds between atoms. So, when a chemical reaction takes place and the molecules are broken at their bonds and bonds are formed for the new (product) molecules, energy has to be involved. Generally speaking there are two types of chemical reactions— those that release energy (*energy releasing*) and those that require the input of energy (*energy demanding*). If a chemical reaction is said to be energy releasing, it means that more energy will be released in the disruption of the bonds of the reacting molecule than is needed to form the new bonds in the product molecule(s), as shown in Figure 1.5.

Said differently, if the energy within the bonds of the products is less than the energy associated with the initial energy in the bonds of the reactants, then the reaction can proceed without a need for an input of outside energy. In this situation, there is leftover energy. On the other hand, if the energy that is required to form the bonds of a new molecule(s) is greater than the energy that will be released by disrupting the reacting molecule(s), then an outside energy source will be needed. This is often the case when complex molecules are being built in our body. To do so, the energy released from energy-releasing reactions is used to "drive" the energy-demanding reactions.

Beyond those chemical reactions that either release or require appreciable amounts of energy, there are many chemical reactions that take place without a release or demand for energy. Here the energy associated with the bonds of the reactants and products of chemical reactions is the same. These would be the reversible reactions we discussed earlier, where one enzyme catalyzes the reaction in both directions.

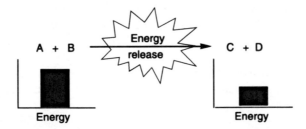

Figure 1.5 Energy is released from a chemical reaction. The bar graphs below the reactants and products show the energy in the bonds. There is less energy in the products thus energy was released in this reaction.

How Does Food Energy Become Our Body's Energy?

On a daily basis we acquire energy from foods in the form of carbohydrates, protein, fat, and alcohol. However, we cannot use these molecules for energy directly. These substances must first engage in chemical reaction pathways that break them down and allow for us to capture much of their energy in a form that we can use directly. With the exception of alcohol, these food energy molecules are also stored in our body to be used as needed.

To be more specific, when these energy molecules are broken down some of their energy is captured in so-called "high-energy molecules." By far the most important high-energy molecule is *adenosine triphosphate* or, more commonly, ATP. Figure 1.6 displays a simplified version of ATP. When energy is needed to power an event in our body it is ATP that is used directly. So, the energy in carbohydrate is used to generate ATP, which in turn can directly power an energy-requiring event or operation in our body. As you might expect, the release of the energy from these little molecular powerhouses is controlled. Specific enzymes are employed to couple ATP with an energy-requiring chemical reaction or event and the transfer of energy.

> Adenosine triphosphate (ATP) is the principal energy molecule to power body activities.

Interestingly, not all of the energy released in the breakdown of carbohydrates, protein, fat, and alcohol is incorporated in ATP. It seems that we are able to capture only about 40 to 45 percent of the energy available in those molecules in the formation of ATP. The remaining 55 to 60 percent of the energy is converted to heat, which helps us maintain our body temperature (Figure 1.7). The final product of the chemical reaction pathways that breakdown carbohydrates, proteins, fat, and alcohol is primarily carbon dioxide (CO_2), which we then must exhale, and water (H_2O), which helps keep our body hydrated.

Looking at the ATP molecule, we notice what looks like a *phosphate*

High-energy bonds

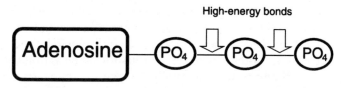

Figure 1.6 Adenosine triphosphate (ATP) is the most significant "high-energy molecule" in our body. A lot of energy is harnessed in the bonds (arrows) between the phosphates (PO_4).

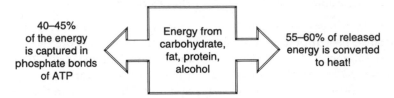

Figure 1.7 Only about 40 to 45 percent of the energy released from carbohydrate, protein, fat, and alcohol is captured in the phosphate bonds
of ATP and other high-energy molecules; the remaining energy is converted to heat.

tail (see Figure 1.6). Phosphate is made up of phosphorus (P) bonded to
oxygen (O) and, as indicated in its name, ATP contains three phosphates.
The energy liberated during the breakdown of energy nutrients is used to
link phosphates together to make ATP. These phosphate links are thus
little storehouses of energy. When energy is needed, special enzymes in
our cells are able to break the links between adjacent phosphate groups.
This releases the energy stored within that link, which can be harnessed to
drive a nearby energy-requiring reaction or process.

Water Solubility Determines How Chemicals Are Treated in Our Body

Why Do Some Things Dissolve in Water While Others Do Not?

On the average, adults will maintain about 60 percent of their body
weight as water. Since water is the predominant substance in the body, it
is important to understand how other substances interact with it. What
we are really talking about is a substance's ability or inability to dissolve
into water.

If a substance dissolves easily into water it is said to be *water soluble*.
On the other hand, if a substance does not dissolve into water it is said to
be *water insoluble*. As a general rule, water-insoluble substances will
dissolve in lipid substances, such as oil (fat). Therefore, we can call these
substances either water insoluble, lipid soluble, or fat soluble.

Examples of water insolubility are often obvious. Some of us have been
frustrated by the inability of traditional salad dressings, such as vinegar
(water-based) and oil, to stay together and not separate into two layers.
Meanwhile, others have witnessed oil tanker spills whereby the oil does
not dissolve into the body of water but rather forms a layer on top of the
water, posing a threat to the aquatic life. As with many water-insoluble
substances, the oil from the tanker or in the salad dressing is less
dense than water, allowing it to float on top of the water or water-based
fluid.

Some elements and molecules easily dissolve in water while others (for example, lipids) do not.

The key to understanding water solubility requires a closer look at the bonds between hydrogen and oxygen atoms in a water molecule. As Figure 1.8 shows, two hydrogen atoms share electrons with one oxygen atom. Hydrogen atoms are the smallest atom (element) and contain only one proton (positive charge); meanwhile the larger oxygen atom has eight protons. As a result, oxygen tends to pull the shared electrons (negative charge) in the bond closer to it because it has a greater positive charge in its nucleus. This leads to a partial negative charge associated with oxygen atoms and a partial positive charge associated with hydrogen atoms. It is an electron tug-of-war, with hydrogen atoms having a weaker pulling force. It is important to see that even though the electrons in the bond spend more time closer to oxygen, they still some spend time closer to hydrogen. So, the charge associated with hydrogen and oxygen is not a full charge, but partial charges. This is like having extra money 25 percent of the time and owing money the remaining 75 percent of the time or vice versa. Partial charge will be displayed with the Greek lowercase letter delta in superscript (δ^+ or δ^-).

The partial charges associated with hydrogen and oxygen in a water molecule allows it to be somewhat electrical. And, partially charged water molecule atoms can then interact with other water molecules because of opposite charge attraction as displayed in Figure 1.8. This is the glue that holds water together. This glue helps us understand how you can fill a glass up with water and briefly exceed the rim of the glass before the water begins to spill over. The water molecules at the top of the

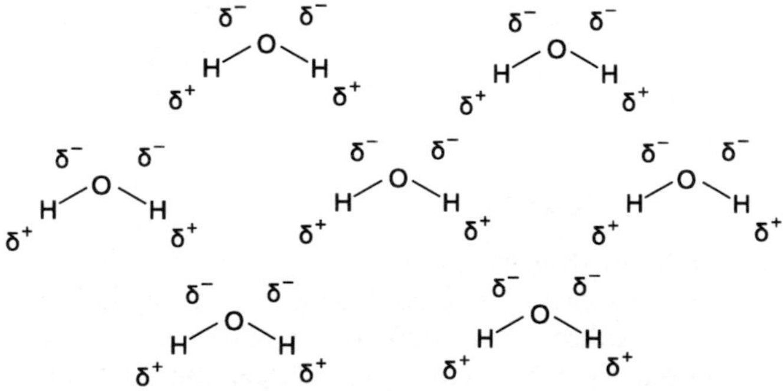

Figure 1.8 Water molecules are attracted to one another and other charged chemicals because of the partial positive charges on the H atoms and negative charges on the O atoms.

glass are attracted to the other water molecules beneath them and they "hold on" electrically, which keeps the too-full glass from overflowing, to a point.

Since atoms in a water molecule bear partial charges it only makes sense that they can interact with other substances that have a charge. This includes sodium (Na^+), potassium (K^+), and chloride (Cl^-). When these atoms (and other charged chemicals) are dissolved in water, the resulting fluid becomes even more electrical and can carry an electric current. This is why scientists often refer to charged atoms and some molecules as *electrolytes*, which means "electricity loving." Sodium and chloride are the main electrolytes in sports drinks. These beverages are often called fluid and electrolyte replacements, because they are water based and contain electrolytes such as sodium, chloride, potassium, calcium, and magnesium.

Certain elements (atoms), such as sodium, can have a charge and are called electrolytes.

On the other hand, lipids, such as fats and cholesterol, do not have a significant charge and as a result they are water insoluble. In general, the partial charges of water atoms do not find lipid molecules electrically attractive. Therefore, the two substances do not mix. Or, from another perspective, the partial charges of water molecules are more attracted to water and other charged substances and as a result lipid substances get pushed aside.

Since lipid molecules fail to dissolve into water, they tend to clump together. As mentioned previously, because lipids are generally less dense than water, they tend to sit on top of water. This explains why some salad dressings separate with the oil on top. It also explains why oil spills lay on top of water and can be cleaned up by using a corralling device called a boom.

Acids and Bases Contribute to the Chemistry Lab of Our Body

What Are Acids and Bases?

The world is filled with *acids* and their counterparts, *bases*. These substances are in our foods and beverages, as well as throughout nature. An acid is any molecule that has the potential to release a hydrogen ion (H^+) when mixed into a water-based fluid. A hydrogen ion is a hydrogen atom that breaks away from a molecule but in the process leaves an electron behind. Because it has lost an electron, it will have a positive charge and because it has a positive charge, it easily dissolves into water.

When an acid is added to water, the hydrogen-ion content of the water will increase. On the other hand, a base is any substance that when dissolved in water will take up hydrogen ions from the fluid. Simply stated, an acid will increase the hydrogen ion content of a water-based fluid whereas a base will decrease it. Therefore, acids and bases are opposites.

We often indicate the level of *acidity* or *alkalinity* (basicity) to refer to the amount of hydrogen ions dissolved in water or a water-based fluid. Our body can be considered a container of water-based fluid, and, as will soon become more obvious, the concentration of hydrogen ions in our body fluid will greatly influence function and health.

How Do We Measure Acidity or Alkalinity?

Acidity and alkalinity indicates the level of hydrogen ions in a water-based fluid and we use the *pH scale* to assess a fluid. The pH scale ranges from 0 to 14, with 0 being the most acidic and 14 being the most basic as shown in Figure 1.9. Thus, a pH of 7 is said to be neutral because it splits the two extremes. A pH lower that 7 means a higher hydrogen ion concentration and thus greater acidity. On the other hand, an alkaline solution has a pH greater than 7 and has a lower level of hydrogen ions.

The pH scale was conceived by Sören Sörensen who was a pretty good biochemist and an excellent brewer of beer! Back in the days before sophisticated pH meters, one could speculate as to whether a fluid was acidic or basic based on taste. Acidic substances tend to have a sour taste (lemon juice, orange juice), while more alkaline substances taste bitter.

So what is the big deal about pH? Our body has but a narrow pH range

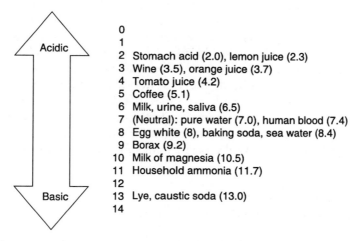

0	
1	
2	Stomach acid (2.0), lemon juice (2.3)
3	Wine (3.5), orange juice (3.7)
4	Tomato juice (4.2)
5	Coffee (5.1)
6	Milk, urine, saliva (6.5)
7	(Neutral): pure water (7.0), human blood (7.4)
8	Egg white (8), baking soda, sea water (8.4)
9	Borax (9.2)
10	Milk of magnesia (10.5)
11	Household ammonia (11.7)
12	
13	Lye, caustic soda (13.0)
14	

Figure 1.9 The pH of common substances, including our blood which has a pH of about 7.4.

at which it can function appropriately. As noted on the scale in Figure 1.9, the pH of our blood is about 7.4. This means that the pH of our body is slightly basic. If the pH falls below or above 7.4 these conditions are referred to as *acidosis* and *alkalosis*, respectively. Nearly all chemical reactions in our body are controlled by enzymes, most of which function in our best interest at a pH around 7.4. Thus, when our pH falls or climbs, the efficiency of many enzymes is significantly affected. Some enzymes will work harder and others will work less hard, thus impacting key chemical reactions in our body. This can compromise normal function and possibly our vitality.

Inherent to our body are systems that help us maintain the pH of our body fluid (for example, blood) around 7.4. These systems are called *buffering* systems and they act either to soak up excessive hydrogen ions or to release them when our body pH begins to change. Thus pH can be maintained at the 7.4 ideal despite changing internal factors.

Free Radicals Are Biological Bullies; Antioxidants Are Cellular Superheroes

What Are Free Radicals and Antioxidants?

Over the past decade or so, more and more attention has focused upon *free radicals* or *oxidants* and their counterparts, *antioxidants*. Once we understand free radicals, it is easy to appreciate the importance of nutrients associated with antioxidant activities of vitamins and minerals such as vitamins C and E and selenium, copper, iron, manganese, and zinc as well as other nutrients such as lycopene, lutein, and zeaxanthin.

A free radical is a substance that interacts with other molecules by taking an electron from them or by forcing an electron upon them. In most cases it is the former event. You will remember that earlier we called the process of losing an electron *oxidation* and the process of gaining an electron *reduction*. The major difference between proper oxidation and reduction and the damaging activity of free radicals is a matter of acceptability and stability of the molecules that free radicals interact with. Since free radicals often interact with molecules that do not want to give up an electron, free radicals can be viewed as biological bullies. They will interact with other molecules without regard for the stability of these molecules. Typically, free-radical substances include oxygen, for example:

- superoxide (O_2^-)
- hydrogen peroxide (H_2O_2)
- hydroxyl radicals (OH^-)

One obvious feature of the free radicals just listed is that they closely resemble the oxygen (O_2) we breathe—so how abnormal could they be?

The presence of free radicals in our body is not necessarily a disease and seems to be unavoidable. That's because free radicals are normally produced when we breakdown carbohydrates, protein, and fat for energy. Furthermore, certain immune processes purposely generate free-radical substances to attack foreign entities or debris in our body. However, free radicals can certainly lead to disease if their presence becomes too great and they are left to their own devices. This tends to happen when we allow free radicals access to our body via the foods we eat and the substances we breathe. Cigarette smoke is loaded with free-radical substances, probably more than one hundred different kinds.

> Free radicals are molecules that can take electrons from other molecules thereby causing damage.

Free radicals can cause damage within the human body by attacking extremely important molecules such as DNA, proteins, and special fatty acids. If these or other molecules are attacked by free radicals and have an electron removed from their structure (oxidation) it is like pulling a bottom card from a house of cards. The victimized molecule is rendered weak and unstable and subject to breakdown. An example of this oxidative damage can be demonstrated by leaving vegetable oil out in an open container exposed to sunlight. The presence of oxygen and energy from sunlight leads to the formation of oxygen-based free radicals, which attack the fat causing them to break down in smaller molecules. Some of these molecules can produce an offensive odor and taste.

Throughout time we have accepted the presence of free radicals, and our body has evolved to meet the challenge. We are armed with a battery of antioxidants to keep the free radicals in check. The term *antioxidant* implies that these molecules will prevent free radicals from pulling electrons (oxidation) from other molecules. They may do so by donating their own electrons to a free radical. This pacifies a free radical and spares other molecules. Antioxidants are unique because they remain relatively stable after giving up an electron. They are designed to handle this process.

Congratulations for making it through Chapter 1. For many people these concepts may seem easy; however, for others, they may present more of a challenge. One thing is certain: if you have at least a general comprehension of these concepts, nutrition becomes a lot easier to understand. In Chapter 2 we discuss some of the finer aspects of the structure and function of our body.

2   How Our Body Works

It is obvious that humans are not the only life-form or *organism* residing on this planet. In fact, we are only one of several million different species of organisms. Organisms include everything from mammals, birds, reptiles, and insects, to plants, bacteria, fungi, and yeast. But bear in mind that even though organisms such as a tomato plant and an octopus may seem completely different, they have numerous similarities which strongly suggest a common ancestry for all life-forms co-habilitating Earth, which includes humans. On the other hand, we humans have numerous features that are shared with only a few other species, namely apes, and further still we enjoy other features that no other species enjoys. In this chapter we will answer basic questions about the human body and how it works. This is critical because before you can know how to nourish the body, you need to know what it is and how it functions.

Cells Are Little Life Units

What Are Cells?

Among the millions of species on this planet, the *cell* is the common denominator. Cells are the most basic living unit. In many species, such as bacteria and amoeba, the entire organism consists of a single isolated cell. But for plants and animals, including us, the organism exists as a compilation of many cells working together. In fact, every adult human is a compilation of some 60 to 100 trillion cells.

As a rule of nature life begets other life and thus all cells must come from existing cells. This is to say that in order to create a new cell, an existing cell has to divide into two cells. It also suggests that all life-forms on Earth may be derived from the same cell or type of cell. The process of cell division is tightly regulated and, as we will discuss in later chapters, when this regulation is lost and cells divide out of control, cancer can arise.

When you and I were conceived, an egg (ovum) from our mother was penetrated by our father's sperm. This resulted in the formation of the first cell of a new life. Therefore, everyone you know was only a single cell at first. That cell had to then develop and divide in two cells, which themselves divided to create four cells, and so on.

> Our body is composed of 60 to 100 trillion cells, each of which contributes to overall health and well-being.

The term *cell* implies the concept of separation. Each cell has the ability to function on its own. In living things composed of numerous cells, such as humans, individual cells are also sensitive and responsive to what is going on in the organism as a whole. Therefore, these cells survive as independent living units and also cooperatively participate in the vitality of the organism to which they belong.

What Do Cells Look Like?

Human cells can differ in size and function. Some are bigger and some longer, some will make hormones while others will help our body move. In fact, there are roughly two hundred different types of cells in our body. Although these cells may seem unrelated, most of the general features will be the same from one cell to the next. Therefore, we can discuss cells by describing the features of a single cell. The unique characteristics of different types of cells such red blood cells, muscle cells, and fat cells will be described as they become relevant later in this chapter and book.

Let's begin by examining the outer wall, or more scientifically the *plasma membrane* of cells. As shown in Figure 2.1, the plasma membrane separates the inside of the cell from the outside of the cell. The watery environment inside the cell is called the *intracellular fluid*. Meanwhile, the watery medium outside of cells is called the *extracellular fluid*. Previously, it was noted that our body is about 60 percent water. Of this 60 percent, roughly two-thirds of the water is intracellular fluid while the remaining one-third is extracellular fluid, which would include the plasma of our blood.

What Types of Substances Are Found in the Intracellular and Extracellular Fluids?

In our body fluids we would find small dissolved substances such as ions, amino acids, and the carbohydrate glucose, as well as larger proteins. The

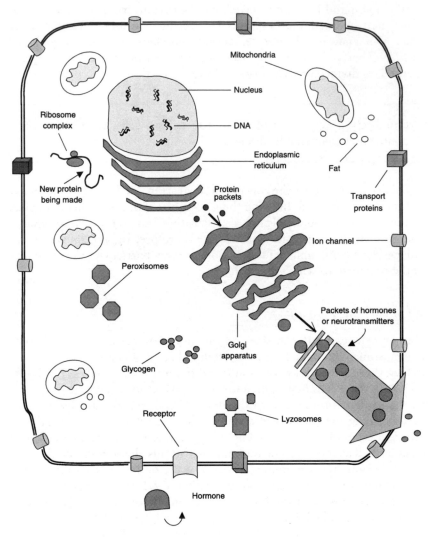

Figure 2.1 Basic cell structure and functions.

major ions (or electrolytes) would include potassium (K^+), sodium (Na^+), chloride (Cl^-), calcium (Ca^{2+}), magnesium (Mg^{2+}), phosphate (PO_4^{3-}), and bicarbonate (HCO_3^-). As demonstrated in Figure 2.2, all of these and other substances will be found in both the intracellular and extracellular fluids. However, the concentration of substances dissolved in either fluid varies and the plasma membrane is bestowed with the awesome responsibility of functioning as a barrier between the two mediums.

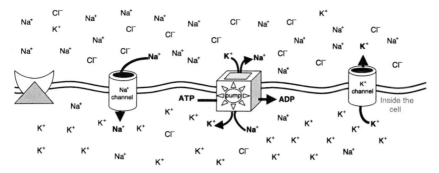

Figure 2.2 The concentration of sodium (Na⁺) and chloride (Cl⁻) is more abundant in the extracellular fluid while potassium (K⁺) is more concentrated in the intracellular fluid. These electrolytes move down their concentration gradients through channels and are pumped against their concentration gradient by energy (ATP) requiring pumps.

What Would We Expect to Find Inside of Our Cells?

Immersed in and bathed by the intracellular fluid are small compartments called *organelles*. The word organelle means "little organ." Two of the more recognizable organelles are the *nucleus* and *mitochondria*. Other organelles include *endoplasmic reticulum, Golgi apparatus, lysosomes,* and *peroxisomes* (see Figure 2.1). The various organelles are little operation centers within cells. Each type of organelle performs a different and specialized job (Table 2.1). Each organelle has its own membrane with many similarities to the plasma membrane. Therefore, as we discuss the nature of the plasma membrane below you can keep in mind that some of these features also pertain to organelle membranes as well.

Table 2.1 Overview of Organelle Function

Organelle	Function and Specialized Features
Nucleus	Houses almost all of our DNA
Mitochondria	Is the site of most ATP manufacturing in cells; houses some DNA
Lysosomes	Involved in breaking down unnecessary or foreign substances; contains acidic environment and digestive enzymes
Endoplasmic reticulum	Involved in making proteins and lipid substances destined to be exported from cell
Peroxisomes	Like lysosomes but with different assortment of enzymes; site of detoxification
Golgi apparatus	The final packaging site for substances ready to be exported from a cell

Cells contain special compartments called organelles, which have special functions to support total cell function.

Also within the intracellular fluid of certain cells we would expect to find some energy reserves in the form of *fat droplets* and *glycogen* (carbohydrate) (see Figure 2.1). The amount of glycogen and fat will vary depending on the type of cell. Another important component of cells is *ribosomes*. Ribosomes are the actual site where proteins are constructed.

Do Individual Cells and Our Body as a Whole Attempt to Maintain an Optimal Working Environment?

Just as you clean your apartment or house and determine what kind of stuff is found within your living area, so too will our cells clean and regulate the contents in their intracellular fluid. This allows each cell to maintain an optimal operating environment. Scientists often use the term *homeostasis* to describe the efforts associated with the maintenance of this optimal environment. Furthermore, just as it is the responsibility of each cell to maintain its own ideal internal environment; at the same time many of our organs work in concert to regulate the environment within our body as a whole. These organs include the kidneys, lungs, skin, and liver. Many of our most basic functions, such as breathing, sweating, urinating, digesting, and the pumping of our heart, are actually functions dedicated to homeostasis (Table 2.2). Therefore, homeostasis is the housekeeping efforts of all our cells working individually as well as together to provide an environment conducive to optimal function.

What Is the Composition of the Plasma Membrane?

Each cell is enveloped by a very thin membrane measuring only about 10 nanometers (nm) thick. A nanometer is one-billionth of a meter— pretty thin indeed. The makeup of the plasma membrane is a very clever

Table 2.2 General Mechanisms of Homeostasis

- Regulation of the ion (electrolyte) concentrations inside and outside of cells
- Blood pressure regulation
- Regulation of optimal levels of blood gases (O_2 and CO_2)
- Maintaining optimal body temperature
- Regulating blood glucose and calcium levels
- Maintaining an optimal pH level

combination of lipids and proteins with just a touch of carbohydrate and other molecules. Interestingly, plasma membranes use the basic principle of water solubility to allow for its barrier properties and it is the lipid that provides this character. Molecules that are somewhat similar to triglycerides (fat) called *phospholipids* are arranged to provide a water-insoluble capsule surrounding cells. What that means is that water-soluble substances such as sodium, potassium, and chloride, carbohydrates, proteins, and amino acids are not able to move freely through the membrane whereas some lipid substances and gases move more freely. The plasma membrane will also contain the lipid substance cholesterol. Cholesterol appears to increase the stability of the plasma membranes.

Since the plasma membrane functions as a barrier between the outside and inside of the cell, there must be a means (or doorways) whereby many water-soluble substances can either enter or exit a cell. One of the roles of proteins in the plasma membrane is to function as doors, thereby allowing substances such as sodium, potassium, chloride, glucose, and amino acids to enter or exit a cell. This is shown in Figures 2.1 and 2.2.

Do Proteins in the Plasma Membrane Have Special Roles?

If we were to weigh all of the components of the plasma membrane we would find that about half the weight of the membrane is protein. However, this is a bit misleading as the much smaller lipid molecules of the plasma membrane tend to outnumber protein molecules by about fifty to one. This means that the proteins tend to be larger and complex, which implies that they have important functions while phospholipids and cholesterol provide more structural support.

Are Some Membrane Proteins Involved in the Movement of Substances In and Out?

Let us go into a little more detail about just how some of the proteins function as doorways in our plasma membranes. Some of these proteins function as channels or pores that will allow the passage of only one specific substance across the membrane. This is like opening the stadium doors for fans before a game. The concentration of fans outside the stadium is much higher than within and the natural flow is for the general movement of people into the stadium, an area of lower concentration.

Proteins in the plasma membrane act as receptors, transporters, channels, pumps, and enzymes.

Plasma membrane channels allow the passage of ions such as sodium, potassium, chloride, and calcium down their concentration gradient. The movement can be in massive amounts resulting in a sudden and significant change in a cell's environment. As an example, *ion channels* are especially important in nerve and muscle cells, and drugs often prescribed for people with cardiovascular concerns are calcium-channel blockers, which will be discussed more in just a bit and also in Chapter 13.

We should stop for a moment and emphasize a very important concept. In nature, when provided the opportunity, things tend to move from an area of higher concentration to an area of lower concentration. This is referred to as *diffusion*. The movement of substances across our plasma membranes is an excellent example of diffusion. For example, skeletal muscle cells are told to contract by calcium (Ca^{2+}). Thus for a muscle cell to be relaxed (not contracted) calcium must be pumped out of the intracellular fluid into the extracellular fluid as well as into a special organelle in muscle cells. In fact, the calcium concentration outside the muscle cell will be greater than ten times that inside when a muscle cell is relaxed. Then, when that muscle cell is told to contract, calcium channels on the plasma membrane and the organelle open and calcium diffuses into the intracellular fluid thereby allowing contraction to occur.

Let's use calcium-channel blocker drugs, which are used to treat high blood pressure and angina, as an example. Calcium-channel blockers (also called calcium blockers or CCBs) inhibit the opening of calcium channels (pores) on heart muscle cells and muscle cells lining certain blood vessels. This reduces contraction of the muscle cells and as a result the heart pumps less vigorously and blood vessels relax, both contributing to a lowering of blood pressure and reduced stress on the heart.

Channels or pores are not the only types of proteins found in our plasma membranes. Other proteins can function as *carriers* that can "transport" substances across the membrane. Here again substances would be moving down their concentration gradient. These carrier proteins tend to transport larger substances such as carbohydrates and amino acids. Perhaps the most famous example of a carrier protein is the glucose transport protein (GluT), which is the primary concern in diabetes mellitus. We will spend much more time on glucose transporters later on.

Not all substances move across the plasma membrane by moving down their concentration gradient. Since this type of movement seems to go against the natural flow of nature, to make this happen certain membrane proteins must function as *pumps*. Quite simply, pumps will move substances across a membrane against their concentration gradient or from an area of lower concentration to higher concentration. Pumps need energy which is derived from ATP. In fact, a very respectable portion of the energy that humans expend every day is attributed to pumping substances across cell membranes. We will go into much more detail about this later on in this chapter and other chapters.

Are Some Cell Membrane Proteins Receptors?

Last, but certainly not least, not all proteins in the plasma membrane function in transport operations. Some proteins function as *receptors* for special communicating substances in our body such as *hormones* and *neurotransmitters*. Typically, receptors will interact with only one specific molecule and ignore all other substances. In a way, then, these proteins can also be viewed as being involved in transport processes; however what's being transported isn't ions or molecules but information.

What Is DNA?

DNA (deoxyribonucleic acid) is found in almost all the cells of our body. Within those cells DNA is mostly housed in the nucleus, while a much smaller amount of DNA can be found in mitochondria. DNA contains the instructions (blueprints) for putting specific amino acids together to make proteins. You see, the human body contains thousands of different proteins, all of which our cells have to build using amino acids as the building blocks. Without the DNA's instructions, our cells would not know how to perform such a task.

DNA is long and strand-like and organized into large structures called *chromosomes*. Normally we have twenty-three pairs of chromosomes in our nuclei. If we were to take a chromosome and find the end points of the DNA, we could theoretically straighten it out like thread from a spool. If we did so we would find thousands of small stretches called *genes* on the DNA. We have thousands of genes, which contain the actual instructions for building specific proteins.

> Human DNA contains around twenty-five thousand genes, which code for proteins. Each person has a unique gene profile.

To oversimplify one of the most amazing events in nature, when a cell wants to make a specific protein, it makes a copy of its DNA gene in the form of *RNA* (ribonucleic acid). You see, DNA and RNA are virtually the same thing. However, one of the most important differences is that the RNA can leave the nucleus and travel to where proteins are made in cells—the ribosomes (see Figure 2.1). At this point both the blueprint instructions (RNA) and the amino acids are available and it's the job of the ribosomes to link (bond) amino acids together in the correct sequence.

What Does "Tissue" Mean, and Do the Tissues Throughout Our Body Work as a Team?

Humans are truly a complex array of organs and other tissues designed to support the basic functions and vitality of our body. We are able to process inhaled air and ingested food and regulate body content. We selectively take what we need from the external environment and eliminate what we do not need. We think, move about, and reproduce. Many of these operations occur without us even being aware of them (see Tables 2.2 and 2.3). One other term we should be familiar with is *tissue*. Quite simply, tissue is composed of similar or cooperating cells performing similar or cooperative tasks. These cells may be grouped together to form fascinating tissues such as bone, skin, muscle, nerves, and blood.

Cells Produce Energy

Where Is ATP Made in Cells?

ATP is made in our cells by capturing some of the energy released from energy molecules when they are broken down in energy pathways. Most of the ATP made in our body is made in mitochondria (singular: mitochondrion). For this reason mitochondria are often referred to as the "powerhouses" of our cells. A relatively small portion of the ATP generated in our cells each day will be made in the intracellular fluid outside the mitochondria. As you might expect, cells with higher energy demands will have more mitochondria. This is certainly true for heart and skeletal muscle cells and cells within our liver.

What Does the Term Metabolism Mean?

Each and every second of every day our cells are engaged in the operations that help keep them alive and well. At the same time the efforts of each cell also contribute to the proper functioning of our body as a whole. To do so each cell must perform an incredible number of chemical reactions every second. The term *metabolism* refers to those chemical reactions collectively.

The term metabolism is somewhat general. For instance, total body metabolism refers to all the energy released from all the chemical reactions and associated processes in our body. Said differently, total body metabolism is the total of all reactions taking place in each cell added together. However, if we wanted to describe just those chemical reactions within a specific tissue, such as muscle or bone, we would say "muscle metabolism" or "bone metabolism." We can be even more focused and use the term metabolism to describe only those reactions associated with a single nutrient or nutrient class. For example, if we were discussing the

Table 2.3 Primary Functions of the Major Tissue and Organs in Our Body

Bone	Provides structure and the basis of movement of limbs and our entire body. Also serves as a mineral storage. Primarily composed of minerals and protein and smaller amount of cells, nerves and blood vessels.
Skeletal muscle	We have three kinds of muscle (skeletal, cardiac (heart) and smooth), which is largely water and protein and to a lesser degree carbohydrate and fat. Contraction of muscle results in movement of some type. Skeletal muscle is connected to bone and provides movement of our limbs and body.
Heart and blood	Our heart is mostly muscle (cardiac). Contraction of cardiac muscle establishes the blood pressure in our heart, which drives blood through our blood vessels. We have about 100,000 miles of blood vessels and our blood is, for the most part, a delivery medium!
Smooth muscle	Smooth muscle lines tubes in our body such as airways, blood vessels, digestive tract, reproductive tract, etc.) Smooth muscle is responsible for regulating the flow of content (gases, fluids, semi-solids) through those tubes.
Lungs	Serves as the site of oxygen and carbon dioxide exchange between our body and the air around us.
Liver	Perhaps the "hub" of nutrition. Our liver is involved in maintain blood glucose, regulating blood lipid levels, processing amino acids, making plasma proteins (e.g., clotting factors, transport proteins), and bile and metabolizing and storing many vitamins, minerals, and other nutrients.
Kidneys	Regulate the composition of our body fluid. They do this by filtering and regulating the composition of our blood, which in turn regulates the composition of the fluid in-between our cells and inside of our cells.
Adrenal glands	Our adrenals are steroid hormone producing factories. They produce cortisol (stress hormone), aldosterone, a lot of DHEA and lesser amount of androstenedione, testosterone, and estrogens.
Thyroid gland	Produces the hormones thyroid hormone and calcitonin. Thyroid hormone is one of the most influential hormones in regulating our energy expenditure.
Brain and spinal cord	Our brain is an information processing center and the spinal cord is the conduit for signals to leave (or be carried to) our brain to the rest of our body. Our brain initiates and regulates muscle activity, processes sensory information and controls body temperature and appetite.
Skin	Site of heat removal and protective coating. Some vitamin D is produced in our skin.
Pancreas	Produces the hormones insulin and glucagon and digestive enzymes.
Pituitary gland	Produces a slew of hormones including thyroid stimulating hormone (TSH) and adrenocorticotrophic hormone (ACTH).

chemical reactions that involve only proteins or carbohydrates, we would be discussing protein or carbohydrate metabolism, respectively.

In general, chemical reactions and/or pathways will release energy. Ultimately, this extra energy will be converted to heat. Since body temperature remains fairly constant, the heat produced in metabolism must be removed from our body. Therefore, our total body metabolism can be estimated by measuring how much heat is lost from our body. Researchers can do this in specialized laboratories as discussed in a later chapter.

The Skeleton Provides the Framework of Our Body

What Is the Skeleton?

The exquisite appearance of the human body is founded upon our skeleton. Our skeleton is a combination of 206 separate bones and supporting ligaments and cartilage. The bones of our skeleton are attached to muscles, which allow us to move about. Bones also provide protection. For instance, the skull and the vertebrae enclose the brain and spinal cord, respectively, thereby protecting the invaluable central nervous system (CNS). Twelve pairs of ribs extend from our vertebrae and protect the organs of our chest. Bone also serves as a storage site for several minerals, such as calcium and phosphorus, and is the site of formation for many of our blood cells.

By approximately 6 weeks of pregnancy the skeleton is rapidly developing and is visible in a sonogram. Bones continue to grow until early adulthood, complementing the growth of other body tissue. Up until this point, bones grow in both length and diameter. Around this time the longer bones of our body, such as the femur, humerus, tibia, and fibula, begin to lose the ability to grow lengthwise and our adult height is realized. Some of the bones of the lower jaw and nose continue to grow throughout our lives, although the rate of growth slows dramatically.

As you may expect, the longest, heaviest, and strongest bone in our body is the femur or thigh bone. These bones extend nearly two feet in some of us, and provide much of the support we need against the force of gravity. Meanwhile, the three small bones in the inner ear are the smallest bones in our body. In addition, the tiny pisiform bone of the wrist is also very small, having the approximate size of a pea.

What Is Bone?

Our fascination with the fossil remains of dinosaurs and other ancient creatures may lead us to believe that bone is a hard, nonliving part of our body and part of the bodies of other animals, including those from long ago. Although bone is indeed solid and strong, allowing form, movement, and organ protection, it is living tissue and constantly changing.

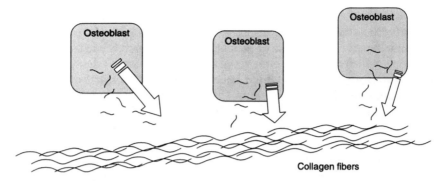

Figure 2.3 These bone cells (osteoblasts) are making collagen proteins which form into collagen fibers that are like rope in the matrix of bone. Mineral complexes then adhere to the collagen. Collagen makes bone strong and minerals make it hard.

Bone contains several different types of cells, which are supported by a thick fluid called the *matrix*. As oversimplified in Figure 2.3, within the matrix reside proteins, primarily collagen, and to a much lesser degree other related substances, such as some really unique carbohydrates. Also in the matrix are mineral deposits, largely a calcium- and phosphate-based crystal called *hydroxyapatite,* as well as calcium phosphate. Bone is roughly 60 to 70 percent mineral complexes and the remainder is largely protein (also see Figure 10.1), primarily collagen. Hydroxyapatites are like tiny, long, and flat sheets of minerals that actually lie on top and along longer collagen fibers. These mineral deposits provide the hard and compression-resisting properties to bone. For the most part, it is also these mineral complexes along with some proteins that exist as fossils long after the death of an animal.

> Bone is composed of minerals such as calcium, phosphate, and magnesium and protein such as collagen.

In addition to some cells, proteins, carbohydrates, and minerals, other tissue can be found in bone. For instance, small blood vessels run throughout bone and deliver substances to and away from bone. Some nerves can be found in bone as well.

Is Bone Constantly Changing?

Bone is constantly being *turned over*. Specific cells within bone are constantly breaking down bone components such as proteins and mineral complexes. Meanwhile, other cells are constantly building bone. Although this may seem counterproductive its merit lies in the ability of bone to adapt or be remodeled according to the demands placed upon it. For example, one of the benefits of weightlifting is an increased stress placed on bone, which causes the bone to adapt by increasing its density. In this case, the efforts of cells that build bone will exceed the efforts of cells that will break down bone components. On the contrary, prolonged exposure to zero gravity (weightlessness) in outer space will decrease the stress placed upon bone resulting in a loss of bone density. In this situation, the efforts of cells that break down bone will exceed those efforts of cells that build bone components.

Nervous Tissue Is Electrical and "Excitable"

What Is Nervous Tissue?

Nervous tissue is composed mostly of nerve cells or *neurons*, which serve as the basis for an extremely rapid communication system in our body. It also provides the basis for thinking. The central nervous system includes the brain and spinal cord and represents the thinking and responsive portion of our nervous tissue. Links of neurons extend from the central nervous system to various organs and tissues in our body, thus allowing the central nervous system to regulate their function. In addition, links of neurons extend to our skeletal muscle thereby allowing the central nervous system to initiate and control our movement. Special neurons function as sensory receptors and are located in the skin and sensory organs (tongue, nose, ears, eyes) as well as deeper in tissue inside our body. These receptors keep the brain informed as to what is going on inside and outside our body. They register pain and sensation (sight, hearing, taste, smell, and touch) and relay that information to the brain where it is interpreted.

How Do Neurons Work?

Neurons are often referred to as *excitable* cells. Excitable cells are able to respond to a stimulus by changing the electrical properties of their plasma membrane. Only muscle and nerve cells are excitable and the basis for excitability lies in the electrolytes (ions) that are dissolved into our extracellular and intracellular fluids. As mentioned before, the concentrations of the different electrolytes are not the same across the plasma membrane (Figure 2.4). In general the concentrations of sodium (Na^+), chloride (Cl^-), and calcium (Ca^{2+}) are much greater in the extracellular fluid, while the concentration of potassium (K^+) is greater in the intracellular fluid. This means that these electrolytes have the potential to move across the plasma membrane, down their concentration gradient, when their respective ion channels open up.

When an excitable cell is stimulated, ion channels open in a specific and

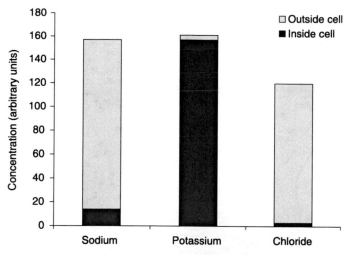

Figure 2.4 Relative difference in the concentrations of sodium, potassium, and chloride dissolved in the fluid inside and outside of our cells. Cells use a lot of energy (ATP) to maintain these concentration differences by pumping sodium and potassium across the plasma membrane.

timely fashion. This allows electrolytes to move either into or out of the cell depending on the direction of their concentration gradient. The movement of the charged electrolytes changes the electrical nature of the plasma membrane at the site of the stimulus. Furthermore, when the cell is stimulated at one point on its plasma membrane, the excitability or impulse then moves along the plasma membrane like a ripple on a pond. Thus the excitability spreads and is often called a *nerve impulse*, as shown in Figure 2.5.

How Do Neurons Become Excited?

Neurons become excited in response to a stimulus. Sensory neurons are sensitive to specific stimuli in their surrounding environment. For example, sensory neurons found in human skin are sensitive to touch, pain, and change in temperature outside of the body. Meanwhile, sensory neurons located inside the body are sensitive to pain and changes in temperature inside the body. Sensory receptors in the ears, eyes, nose, and mouth register sound, light, smell, and taste, respectively. Once these neurons are excited by a stimulus, the excitability or impulse moves along that neuron toward the brain, where it is interpreted. Our brain initiates impulses as well. Some of these impulses travel throughout the brain for thinking processes and memory recall. Or these impulses may travel away from the brain toward destinations outside the central nervous system such as skeletal muscle, the heart, and other organs.

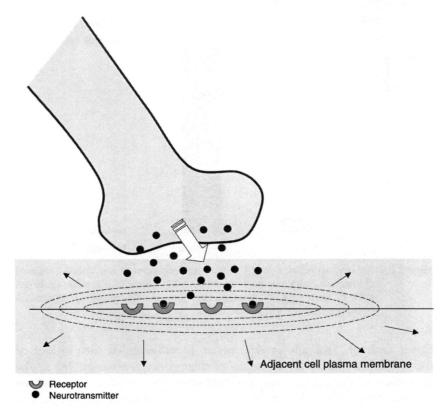

Figure 2.5 Neurotransmitters released at the end of the neuron will interact with
receptors on the adjacent cell (muscle or nerve). This can result in
excitability of that cell, which may stimulate muscle contraction or
transmit a nervous impulse.

How Do Neurons Communicate?

Although some neurons are very long and may extend several feet or so,
the trek of an impulse traveling either from a sensory neuron to the brain
or from the brain to other parts of the body requires several neurons
linked together. These neurons are lined up end to end, but they do not
actually touch. An impulse reaching the end of one neuron is transferred
to the next neuron by way of special communicating chemicals called
neurotransmitters (see Figure 2.5.)

Nerves provide rapid communication system within our brain and
spinal cord and to various areas of our body.

Many different neurotransmitters are employed by our nervous tissue, including serotonin, norepinephrine, dopamine, histamine, and acetylcholine. Many of these will be discussed in later chapters, as either they are derived from nutrients or nutrients play an important role in putting them together. In fact, most neurotransmitters are made of amino acids. Furthermore, some neurotransmitters are very important in regulating how much and what types of foods we eat.

What Is the Brain?

As an adult, the human brain weighs about three and a half pounds and is protected by the skull. The brain is designed to interpret sensory input and decipher other incoming information, to develop both short- and long-term memory, to originate and coordinate most muscular movement, and to regulate the function of many of our organs. With all that it does, it is easy to conclude that our brain is densely packed with neurons. And, with so many neuron operations taking place within the brain, the electrical activity can be measured by placing sensors on the skin of the head. The recorded output of this measurement is called an electroencephalogram or simply EEG.

No other animal on this planet has such a developed brain relative to its body size. In fact, the human brain is so big that during pregnancy the size of the baby's head is a primary factor dictating the timing of birth. If babies were not born until the 10th or 11th month of pregnancy, it would be extremely difficult for the head to fit through the mother's birth canal.

What Is the Spinal Cord?

The spinal cord extends from the brain and serves mostly as a relay station connecting the brain to the rest of the body. For protection, the human spinal cord is encased by bony vertebrae. The region of the spinal cord closest to the brain connects the brain to regions of the body in that proximity. This would include the chest and arms. Moving further down the spinal cord and away from the brain, you begin to find the interconnections between the central nervous system and the lower portions of our body, such as our legs. However, because the nerve links extending from the lower extremities must move through the upper regions of the spinal cord in order to connect with the brain, damage to the upper region of the spinal cord will affect the lower as well as the upper areas of our body. Thus, if damage occurs lower in the spinal cord it may result in temporary or permanent paralysis of only the lower extremities. However, if the spinal cord is damaged higher up, it can result in paralysis of both lower and upper extremities.

When you would like to move a particular body part, the process (idea) originates in the brain in a region called the *motor cortex*. Motor means movement! Once initiated, the impulse is carried along a linkage of nerve cells to the skeletal muscle responsible for moving the limb or body part that is to move. Incredibly the whole process only requires a couple neurons linked in series connecting the motor cortex of the brain to the muscle and occurs in a fraction of a second.

While the motor cortex of our brain is busy sending signals to our skeletal muscle, signaling it to move, another region of our brain is evaluating and refining the movement. This region is called the *cerebellum*, which is behind and lower than the more recognizable parts of the brain. It is also this region of the brain that is particularly sensitive to the effects of alcohol and explains why movement becomes less refined when we are intoxicated.

Skeletal Muscle Allows Movement

What Is Skeletal Muscle?

Skeletal muscle is made up of very specialized cells that have the ability to shorten when they are stimulated. With the exception of reflex mechanisms, such as the knee tap by a physician, movement of our skeletal muscle is under the command of our brain, as mentioned earlier. Because muscle cells are very long they are often referred to as *muscle fibers* (see Figure 2.6). The fibers are bundled up like a box of dry spaghetti or

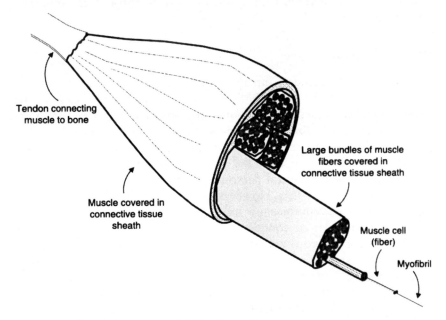

Tendon connecting
muscle to bone

Large bundles of muscle
fibers covered in
connective tissue sheath

Muscle covered in
connective tissue
sheath

Muscle cell
(fiber)

Myofibril

Figure 2.6 General structure of skeletal muscle.

straight wires in a cable. The muscle fiber bundles are themselves bundled up and are part of larger collection of similar bundles which make up a particular muscle. Skeletal muscle is so named because it is generally anchored at both ends to different bones of our skeleton by tendons. When muscle contracts, it pulls on a specific bone, which moves the bone, thus moving a body part.

How Does Skeletal Muscle Work?

Like neurons, skeletal muscle fibers are also excitable. In fact, the excitability process of muscle cells is very similar to that of neurons, while the end result is different. Excitability in muscle fibers leads to the contraction of the muscle cell while neurons merely carry the electrical nerve impulse to another neuron or to skeletal muscle or to other tissue and organs.

The inside of skeletal muscle fibers appears very different from other cells because of the contractile apparatus it contains. Each muscle fiber contains a tremendous amount of small fibrous units called *myofibrils*, as shown in Figures 2.6 and 2.7. The prefix *myo* refers to muscle and *fibril* means little fiber. Each myofibril is a stalk-like collection of proteins. The predominant proteins are *actin* and *myosin*, which are referred to as the thin and thick filaments, respectively. They are organized into a series of tiny contraction regions called a *sarcomere* (Figure 2.7). Myofibrils are composed of thousands of sarcomeres situated side by side.

When skeletal muscle fibers become excited, calcium (Ca^{2+}) channels open and calcium floods in and around the myofibrils and bathes the sarcomeres. Calcium then interacts with specific proteins associated with

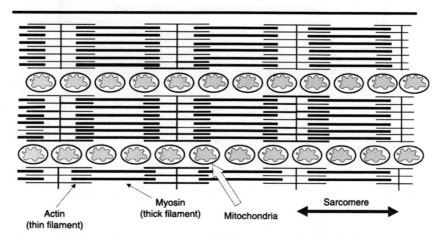

Figure 2.7 Inside a skeletal muscle cell are proteins involved in contraction. These are myosin (thick filaments) and actin (thin filaments). Mitochondria are the site of aerobic energy (ATP) formation.

actin and induces sarcomere contraction. The contraction of one muscle fiber is really the net result of the shortening of all the tiny sarcomeres in each myofibril within that cell. Further, the contraction of the muscle itself is the net result of contraction and shortening of muscle fibers that make up that muscle.

Skeletal muscle cells have another unique characteristic. They contain an organelle called the *sarcoplasmic reticulum* which is actually a modified version of the endoplasmic reticulum found in other cells. This organelle stores large quantities of calcium. In fact, when a skeletal muscle cell is stimulated, most of the calcium that bathes the sarcomeres actually comes from the sarcoplasmic reticulum.

What Powers Muscle Contraction?

In order for muscle fibers to contract, a lot of ATP must be used (Figure 2.8). Some of the energy released from ATP is used to power the contraction. Interestingly, ATP is also necessary for a contracted muscle cell to "relax" as well. When the muscle is no longer being stimulated, ATP helps the thick and thin filaments to dissociate from each other so

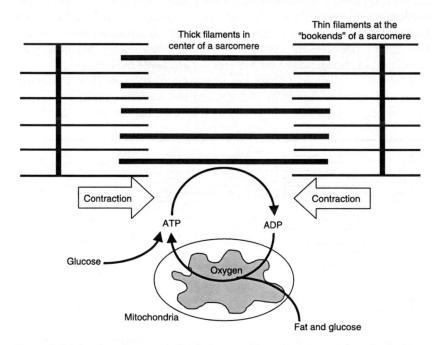

Figure 2.8 Muscle cell contraction is powered by adenosine triphosphate (ATP). The energy released by ATP allows myosin to pull actin filaments towards the center of the sarcomere. The net effect of all the sarcomere contraction is a shortening of the entire muscle cell. Carbohydrate and fat are mostly used to regenerate the ATP as it is being used.

that each sarcomere can return to a relaxed (or unstimulated) position. In addition, ATP is necessary to pump calcium out of intracellular fluid of the muscle fiber. Calcium is either pumped out of the cell or more likely into sarcoplasmic reticulum organelles.

If ATP is deficient, muscle fibers become locked in a contracted state called *rigor*. *Rigor mortis* occurs when the human body dies as the integrity of muscle cell membranes decrease. This allows calcium to leak into the contracting regions of muscle fibers from the extracellular fluid and from within the sarcoplasmic reticulum. As a result, calcium bathes myofibrils and contraction is invoked. Usually there is enough ATP in these dying cells to power the contraction. The dying cell then remains locked in a contracted state.

The Heart and Circulation Are a Delivery System

What Is the Heart and Circulation?

Some ancient philosophers believed that the heart was the foundation of our soul. Today we recognize the heart for its true function, that of a muscular pump. The adult heart is about the size of its carrier's fist and weighs about one-half pound (Figure 2.9). It serves to pump blood through thousands of miles of blood vessels to all regions of our body. Blood leaves the heart through *arteries* on route to tissue throughout the

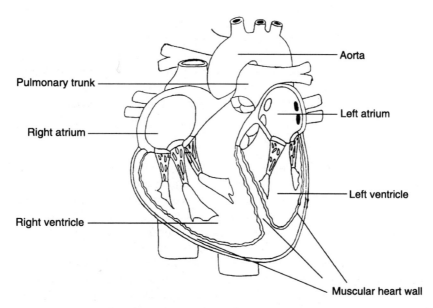

Figure 2.9 The anatomy of our heart. There are four chambers (right and left atria and ventricles).

body. Arteries feed into smaller *arterioles* and subsequently tiny *capillaries*, which then thoroughly infiltrate tissue. Most blood vessel mileage is attributable to capillaries. These blood vessels are so numerous in tissue that nearly every cell in our body will have a capillary right next to it or very close. This is like having one river (artery) flowing into town that branches to the extent whereby every house has its own little stream (capillary).

> Our heart is made up of muscle, nerves, and connective tissue and can beat more than two billion times during a lifetime.

As blood reaches the end of the capillaries and the tissue has been properly served, the blood will then drain into larger *venules*. The venules will eventually drain into larger *veins*, which ultimately return blood to the heart. This is like the streams draining into larger steams, which then drain back into the larger river. Quite simply, our blood serves as a delivery system. It delivers oxygen, nutrients, and other substances to cells throughout our body. At the same time, blood also serves to remove the waste products of cell metabolism, such as carbon dioxide and heat from our tissue. Capillaries are the actual sites of exchange of substances between our cells and the blood.

Our heart consists of four chambers (two atria and two ventricles), left and right. The left half, consisting of the left atrium and ventricle, serves to receive oxygen-rich blood returning from the lungs and to pump it to all the tissues throughout the body. The right half of the heart, consisting of the right atrium and ventricle, serves to receive oxygen-poor blood returning from tissue throughout our body and to pump it to the lungs. Therefore, our heart functions as a relay station for moving blood throughout our body in one large loop, hence the term *circulation*.

How Does Our Heart Work?

Our heart is composed mostly of muscle cells that are somewhat similar to skeletal muscle cells yet retain certain fundamental differences. Although most of the events involved in contraction of heart (cardiac) muscle are the same as skeletal muscle, the heart is not attached to bone. Furthermore, our heart does not require the brain to tell it when to contract (beat). However, the brain certainly can play both a direct and indirect role in regulating the beating of our heart. The stimulus that invokes excitability in the heart comes from a specialized pacemaker region within our heart, called the sinoatrial node (SA node). The human heart may beat in excess of two billion times throughout a person's life.

Unlike skeletal muscle, which pulls on bone when it contracts, the heart constricts in a wringing fashion when it contracts. As the heart contracts, the pressure of the blood inside the heart (ventricles) increases. This serves to propel blood out of the heart into the arteries. This increase in pressure also provides the driving force that forces blood to surge through our blood vessels. The dynamics of blood flow will be discussed in more detail in the final chapter.

What Is the Composition of Blood?

The blood is composed of two main parts, the *hematocrit* and the *plasma*, which can be assessed clinically (Figure 2.10). *Red blood cells* (RBCs) are the sole component of the hematocrit and function primarily as a shuttle for oxygen. Hematocrit is the percentage of our blood that is RBCs, which is typically 40 to 45 percent for an adult.

Plasma is about 55 percent of our blood. Of the plasma, about 92 percent is water while the remaining 8 percent includes over 100 different dissolved or suspended substances such as nutrients, gases, electrolytes, hormones, and proteins such as albumin and clotting factors. The remaining components of our blood are the *white blood cells* (WBCs) and *platelets*, which collectively make up about 1 percent of blood. WBCs are the principal components of the human immune system and provide a line of defense against bacteria, viruses, and other intruders. Some WBCs attack foreign invaders and useless materials while others manufacture antibodies and other immune factors. Last, but certainly not least, platelets participate in the clotting of blood.

What Are Red Blood Cells?

Red blood cells (RBCs) have the responsibility of transporting oxygen throughout the body. About 33 percent of the weight of an RBC is attributed to a specialized protein called *hemoglobin* and thus RBCs are often referred to as "bags of hemoglobin." Hemoglobin is a large and complex

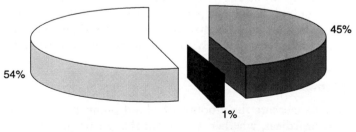

□ Hematocrit   ■ White blood cells and platelets   □ Plasma

Figure 2.10 The components of our blood. The hematocrit is composed of red blood cells. Roughly 90 percent of the plasma is water and the remaining 10 percent is largely proteins, electrolytes, and lipoproteins.

protein that contains four atoms of iron. Hemoglobin's job is to bind to oxygen so that it can be transported in the blood. There are about 42 to 52 million RBCs per milliliter (or cc) of blood; and each RBC contains about 250 million hemoglobin molecules. Since each hemoglobin molecule can carry four oxygen molecules, the potential exists to transport one billion molecules of oxygen in each RBC.

There are two reasons for the need for such a large amount of hemoglobin in our blood. First, oxygen does not dissolve very well into our blood. Second, the demand for oxygen is extremely high in our body. Therefore, hemoglobin increases the ability of the blood to carry oxygen tremendously. Any situation that significantly decreases either the number of RBCs or the level of hemoglobin they carry can compromise oxygen delivery to our tissues and potentially compromise function and health.

How Do We Bring Oxygen into Our Body and Get Rid of Carbon Dioxide?

When the heart pumps, blood is propelled from the right ventricle into the *pulmonary arteries* for transport to the lungs. Pulmonary means lungs. Upon reaching the lungs and the pulmonary capillaries, carbon dioxide exits the blood and enters into the airways of our lungs. It is then removed from our body when we exhale. At the same time, oxygen enters the blood from the airways of our lungs and binds with hemoglobin in RBCs. The oxygen-containing blood leaves the lungs and travels back to the heart as part of circulation. Thus every breath you take serves to exchange gases, bringing needed oxygen into your body while removing carbon dioxide.

How Does the Heart Supply Blood Throughout Our Body?

As our heart contracts, blood is pumped from the left ventricle into the *aorta*. Blood moves from the aorta into the arteries, then arterioles, and finally tiny capillaries in our tissue. The blood leaving our left ventricle is rich with oxygen while the blood returning to our heart from tissue throughout our body has given up oxygen to working cells while acquiring carbon dioxide. This blood is then pumped by the right ventricle to the lungs to reload the hemoglobin with oxygen and release carbon dioxide.

What Is Cardiac Output?

If we were to measure the amount of blood pumped out of our heart during one heartbeat, whether it be from the left or right ventricle, we would know our *stroke volume*. Then, if we multiply the stroke volume by our heart rate (heartbeats per minute) we would know the *cardiac output*:

cardiac output = stroke volume (milliliters) × heart rate (beats/min).

Cardiac output is the volume of blood pumped out of the heart, either to the lungs or toward body tissue, in 1 minute. It should not matter which of the two destinations we consider, as they occur simultaneously and will have a similar stroke volume of about 5 to 6 liters (or quarts) per minute.

During exercise both heart rate and stroke volume increase, which consequently increases cardiac output. For some of us, cardiac output may increase as much as five to six times during heavy exercise. This allows for more oxygen-rich blood to be delivered to working skeletal muscle.

Where Does the Cardiac Output Go?

If referring to the cardiac output of the right ventricle, there is only one place for it to go: the lungs. Said another way, 100 percent of the cardiac output from the right ventricle is destined for our lungs. However, the blood pumped out of the left ventricle has many destinations. Under resting and comfortable environmental conditions about 13 percent of the left ventricle's cardiac output goes to our brain, 4 percent goes to our heart, 20 to 25 percent goes to our kidneys, and 10 percent goes to our skin. The remaining cardiac output from the left ventricle (48 to 53 percent) will then go to the remaining tissue in our body, such as the digestive tract, liver, and pancreas.

During exercise, a greater proportion of this cardiac output is routed to working skeletal muscle. This requires some redistribution or stealing of blood routed to other less active areas at that time, such as our digestive tract. Contrarily, during a big meal and for a few hours afterward, a greater proportion of this cardiac output is routed to the digestive tract, which steals a portion of the blood directed to areas having no immediate need, such as skeletal muscle.

What Is Blood Pressure?

Whether blood is in the heart or in blood vessels, it has a certain pressure associated with it. In fact, blood moves through circulation from an area of greater blood pressure to an area of lower blood pressure. As mentioned earlier, when the heart contracts the pressure of the blood in the ventricles increases. This establishes a blood pressure gradient that drives the movement of blood through the blood vessels. This is somewhat like turning on a garden hose. When you turn on a garden hose, the water pressure is greatest close to the faucet (versus toward the open end of the hose). The result is that water moves from the area of greater water pressure toward the area of lesser water pressure and out the end of the hose.

We define *pressure* as a force exerted upon a surface and can measure it in millimeters of mercury (mmHg). If we apply this definition to our blood, we can say that blood pressure is the force exerted by blood upon the walls of a blood vessel. When blood pressure is measured, two numbers are provided, for instance 120/80 or "120 over 80." What this means is that the pressure exerted by the blood is 120 mmHg during heart contraction and 80 mmHg when the heart is relaxing between beats. The first number is the *systolic* or blood pressure when our heart contracts. The second number is the *diastolic* pressure and it is blood pressure when our heart is relaxing. Blood pressure is typically measured in the large artery of the arm because of its accessibility.

Our Kidneys Are Filtering Systems

What Do Our Kidneys Do?

Typically understated in function, our kidneys regulate the composition and volume of the blood. Our two kidneys, along with their corresponding *ureters*, the *bladder*, and the *urethra*, make up our urinary or *renal* system. Although our kidneys are only about 1 percent of our total body weight, they receive about 20 to 25 percent of our left ventricle's cardiac output. Amazingly, our kidneys will filter and process approximately 47 gallons (180 liters) of blood-derived fluid daily.

Each one of our two kidneys is home to about one million tiny blood processing units called *nephrons*. Each nephron will engage in two basic operations. First, they filter plasma into a series of tubes; second, they will process the filtered fluid. As you might expect, the filtered plasma-derived fluid not only contains water but also small substances dissolved within, such as electrolytes, amino acids, and glucose. Cells (e.g., RBCs, WBCs) and most proteins in our blood are too large and are not filtered out of the blood.

There are two possible fates for the components of the filtered fluid. They can either be returned to the blood or not and ultimately become a component of urine. Normally, the reuptake of substances such as glucose and amino acids back to the blood is extremely efficient. Contrarily, the reuptake of water and electrolytes is more regulated. For example, if the concentration of sodium is too high in the blood, then less sodium will be returned to the blood and more will go into urine so that an optimal blood level is achieved. On the other hand, if the level of sodium in the blood is low, then more of the filtered sodium is returned to the blood and less is lost in the urine. As you might expect, the processes engaged in reabsorbing glucose, amino acids, electrolytes, and other desired substances require a lot of energy (ATP). Because of this normal kidney operations make a significant contribution to our total daily energy use.

Our kidneys filter our blood, collecting excessive substances and cell waste materials in urine for removal.

What Is the Composition of Urine?

Of the forty-seven gallons of fluid filtered and processed by the nephrons daily, less than 1 percent actually becomes urine. Our urine is generally composed of things our body has no need for, such as some by-products of cell metabolism, and also excessive quantities of things we normally need such as water and electrolytes. About 95 percent of urine is water, while the remaining 5 percent is substances dissolved within.

Do Our Kidneys Do Anything Else?

Beyond regulating the composition of our blood, the kidneys engage in other operations involved in homeostasis. For instance, our kidneys are very sensitive to the amount of oxygen being transported in the blood. If they detect that the level of oxygen in our blood is too low, they will release a substance (hormone) into the blood that tells bones to make more RBCs. If there are more RBCs, then logically more oxygen can be transported in the blood. Furthermore, the kidneys are vital in the normal metabolism of vitamin D, which will be discussed in Chapter 9.

Digestion Makes Nutrients Available to Our Body

What Does "Digestion" Mean and What Is It All About?

The term *digest* means to break down or disintegrate. Therefore, digestion serves to break down the food we eat into smaller substances that are suitable for absorption into our body. All of the activities of digestion take place in our digestive or gastrointestinal tract. The digestive tract is a tube 22 to 28 feet long that actually passes through our body as shown in Figure 2.11. As food moves through the length of the digestive tract, it is really on the outside of the body. Only when a substance crosses the cell lining of the digestive tract and enters into our circulation is it actually inside our body, which is called *absorption.*

Digestion requires both physical and chemical operations. The teeth, along with the musculature of the mouth, stomach, and small intestine, work to physically grind, knead, and mix food with digestive juices. At the same time, the muscular lining of our digestive tract serves to propel the digestive mixture forward.

Chemical digestion involves the activities of *digestive enzymes* that will break down large complex food molecules into smaller substances appropriate for absorption. Proteins, carbohydrates, and lipids must be split into simpler molecules for absorption. Furthermore, the vitamins and minerals found in foods must be liberated from other food molecules

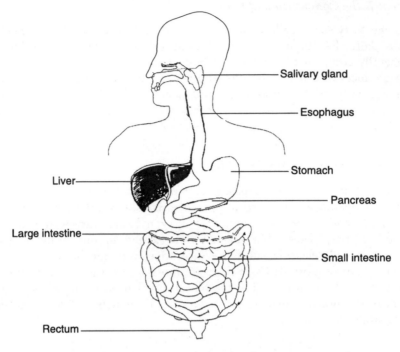

Figure 2.11 The digestive system includes the digestive tract and supporting organs including our liver, pancreas, and gall bladder.

and complexes in order to be absorbed as well. *Bile* is also involved in chemical digestion; however, it functions not as an enzyme but more as a detergent. Bile is pivotal in the digestion and absorption of lipid substances.

What Happens to Food in the Mouth?

Once food is in the mouth it is bathed in saliva. Saliva adds moisture to the food that is being chewed. This will improve the ease of swallowing. Each day we will produce about 1 to 1.5 quarts (liters) of saliva. Furthermore, saliva also contains both a carbohydrate and lipid digestive enzyme that begins the chemical digestive process. Once we swallow, food travels through the esophagus and depots in the stomach.

Our digestive tract is over 20 feet long and serves to chemically and physically breakdown food and absorb nutrients.

What Is the Stomach and What Does It Do?

The stomach, typically a bit less than a foot in length, functions as a reservoir for swallowed food. The volume of our stomach depends on the quantity of food therein. An empty stomach may have a volume of only 1 to 3 ounces (approximately 50 to 75 milliliters) whereas a full stomach can expand to volumes of 2 to 3 quarts (approximately 2 to 3 liters).

The stomach is a very muscular organ. It churns food and mixes it with stomach juice. Stomach juice contains hydrochloric acid (HCl), which renders the stomach a very acidic environment (pH 1.5 to 2.5). A protein-digesting enzyme is also found in stomach juices. The presence of this enzyme, along with the acidic environment, will begin protein digestion. On the average, our stomach may produce about 2 to 3 quarts (approximately 2 to 3 liters) of stomach juice daily. Beyond protein digestion, the acidic stomach juice also kills most bacteria in foods.

Our stomach is sealed at both ends by tight muscular enclosures called sphincter muscles. This prevents acidic juices from entering the esophagus at one end and also allows separation between the stomach and small intestine at the other end. If stomach juice is able to reflux into our esophagus it can produce a burning sensation commonly referred to as *heartburn*. This is why chronic heartburn is routinely treated with antacids, as they attempt to neutralize the acid in the stomach. Other drugs may be used that attempt to decrease acid production by the stomach.

What Happens to Food After It Leaves the Stomach?

The mixture of partially digested food drenched in acidic stomach juice is slowly sent into the small intestine. This portion of our digestive tract is the location of the majority of digestive enzyme activity and the absorption of nutrients. The wall of the small intestine presents a very sophisticated pattern of folds and projections. This design allows the small intestine to have an absorptive surface approximating the size of a tennis court. This allows for very efficient absorption.

When the food mixture is spurted into the small intestine from the stomach, it hardly resembles what we ate. Yet most of the nutrients still need further digestion to reach their absorbable state. First, bicarbonate produced by the pancreas enters the small intestine and neutralizes the acidic food mixture draining from our stomach. Then digestive enzymes that are also produced by our pancreas and bile from the gallbladder and liver make their way to the small intestine as well. These factors, along with digestive enzymes produced by the cells that line the small intestine, will complete digestion.

What Is Bile?

Bile is made up of several substances, the most outstanding being *bile acids* (bile salts). During digestion, the small intestine is a watery place to be. Along with the water entering our digestive tract in foods and beverages, water is also the basis of digestive juices. Water-insoluble substances in our diet, such as fats, cholesterol, and fat-soluble vitamins, will clump together into droplets in the small intestine. This would decrease their digestibility and absorption. This is where bile comes in. Bile acts as an emulsifier or detergent interacting with lipid droplets so that many smaller lipid droplets result instead of fewer larger ones. The advantage to creating many smaller lipid droplets is that more contact occurs between lipids and lipid-digesting enzymes. If bile were absent, as in certain disorders, lipids would stay as larger droplets in the small intestine and for the most part remain undigested and unabsorbed and end up in the feces.

Bile is produced by the liver and oozes in the direction of the small intestine 24 hours a day, 7 days a week. The liver is connected to the small intestine via a series of tubes or ducts. During periods of time in-between meals, some of the bile drains into the gallbladder, where it is stored. Then during a meal the gallbladder squeezes the bile out and it heads to the small intestine. This allows for more bile to be present in the small intestine during digestion.

What Is the Colon?

By the time the digestive mixture reaches the large intestine or *colon* most of the nutrients have been absorbed. Although some water and electrolytes will be absorbed in the colon, its primary responsibility is to form the feces that will eventually leave the digestive tract. The colon is also home to a rich bacteria colony—as many as four hundred different species of bacteria may be found. These bacteria provide some benefit to the body as they make some vitamins and fatty acids that can help nourish the body. Research is underway in an effort to better understand the relationship between the colon's bacteria and human health.

What Is the Composition of Feces?

Human feces is a combination of water, bacteria, parts of cells that line the digestive tract, and undigested food components, such as fibers. The coloring of feces is attributable to several of the substances that are removed from the body in the feces. For instance, when the body breaks down hemoglobin, coloring pigments are produced. These substances become part of bile, which empties into the digestive tract. These add color to the feces.

Hormones Are Messengers Traveling in Our Blood

What Are Hormones?

There are two ways that one region of our body can communicate with another. The first is by way of nerve impulses and the second is by way of hormones. Hormones are produced by specific organs (glands) in the body including the pituitary gland, parathyroid gland, thyroid gland, hypothalamus, pancreas, stomach, small intestine, adrenal glands, placenta, and gonads (ovaries and testicles) (Table 2.4). Hormones are released into our blood and circulate throughout our body. As they

Table 2.4 Select Hormones Related to Nutrition and Metabolism

Organ of Origin	Hormone	Primary Action
Pituitary gland	Growth hormone (GH)	Increases growth of most tissue; increases protein synthesis and fat use for energy
	Prolactin	Increases milk production in female mammary glands
	Antidiuretic hormone (ADH)	Decreases water loss by our kidneys by increasing water reabsorption by our nephrons
Thyroid gland	Thyroid hormone (T_3/T_4)	Increases rate of metabolism in our cells; normal growth
	Calcitonin	Decreases blood calcium levels by increasing kidney loss and decreasing absorption in our digestive tract
Parathyroid gland	Parathyroid hormone (PTH)	Increases blood calcium levels by decreasing urinary losses and increasing absorption in the digestive tract
Adrenal gland	Aldosterone	Increases sodium reabsorption in kidneys (decreases urinary loss of sodium)
	Cortisol	Increases glucose production in the liver and release into blood; stimulates muscle protein breakdown, promotes inflammation; increases fat release from fat cells
	Epinephrine (adrenaline)	Increases heart rate and stroke; increases glucose production in liver and release into our blood, increases fat release from fat cells
Pancreas	Insulin	Increase glucose uptake into muscle and fat tissue; increases storage of glucose as glycogen; decreases fat release from fat cells and increases fat production; increases net protein production
	Glucagon	Increases fat release from fat cells; increases glucose production in the liver and release into blood

circulate they can interact with specific cells of a specific tissue and elicit a response within those cells.

Only cells that have a specific receptor for a hormone will respond to a circulating hormone. This is an extremely accurate operation. Some hormones may have receptors on cells of only one kind of tissue in our body, while other hormones may have receptors on cells of most tissues in our body. For example, the hormone prolactin stimulates milk production in female breasts. Therefore, the cells associated with the milk-producing mammary glands will have receptors for prolactin, while most other cells in our body will not have prolactin receptors and will not be affected by prolactin. Thyroid hormone and insulin receptors, on the other hand, will be found on the cells of many kinds of tissues in our body.

Hormones are produced by specific glands and circulate in the blood to affect the operation of other parts of the body.

Are There Different Classes of Hormones?

Hormones may be grouped into one of two general categories: *amino acid-based hormones* and *steroid hormones*. The amino acid-based hormones include hormones that are proteins and those hormones that are derived from the amino acid tyrosine. Examples of protein hormones include insulin, growth hormone (GH), glucagon, and antidiuretic hormone (ADH). Examples of hormones made from the amino acid tyrosine are epinephrine (adrenaline) and thyroid hormone (T_3 and T_4). Steroid hormones are made from cholesterol and include testosterone, estrogens, cortisol, progesterone, and aldosterone.

3   The Nature of Food

All living things on this planet require nourishment to fuel and support vital operations. For instance, plants get water, minerals and nitrogen from the soil and produce their own carbohydrate, protein, and fat. Meanwhile, animals consume other forms of life, such as plants and animals or their products, in order to survive. For humans, we consume animals and their products (for example, milk, eggs) and/or plants and their products (fruits, vegetables, cereal grains). Even eating some forms of microbes (or microorganisms) such as yeast and some bacteria can help us survive and promote vitality. Humans exist at the upper end of the food chain, meaning that a large variety of life-forms are food to us, but we are not regular food for other life-forms. Plants, on the other hand, maintain a position at the other end of the food chain as they are food for many life-forms, including insects, fish, and mammals.

Nutrients Nourish Our Body

How Are Humans Nourished?

In this day and age, as food manufacturers spend millions of dollars developing new forms of food, we still must adhere to the basic rule that humans naturally nourish themselves by eating other life-forms or their products. That means that it would be impossible to nourish our bodies with completely and optimally by manufactured foods unless those foods contained the same substances and in appropriate forms, amounts and combinations that we have obtained throughout our existence by eating other life-forms on this planet.

Humans are needy from a nutritional perspective. We have an inescapable need for numerous substances, some of which we cannot make internally and others we can, which we call *nutrients*. Quite simply, a nutrient is a substance that in some way nourishes the body. It will either provide energy or promote the growth, development and maintenance of our body, or promote optimal function, health, and longevity.

What Are Essential Nutrients?

The list of nutrients includes hundreds of substances and list seems to keep getting longer. However, not all of the nutrients are deemed *essential*. Essential nutrients are those nutrients that are absolutely vital and are not made in the body either at all or in sufficient quantities to meet our needs. These essential nutrients must be in the foods we eat (or supplemented) and in sufficient quantities, otherwise signs of deficiency can develop over time. Essential nutrients can be grouped together based on general similarities, such as those that provide energy (carbohydrates, proteins, and fats), vitamins, minerals, and water. This is presented in Table 3.1

> There are more than forty essential nutrients that have to be part of our diet and at certain levels to prevent deficiency.

We can reinforce our understanding of the difference between nutrients and essential nutrients with an example. Glycine is an amino acid, which is absolutely necessary to make proteins in our cells. We have the ability to make ample glycine and therefore, theoretically, it does not need to be part of our diet. However, our body will gladly put the glycine we eat to work, so it is indeed a nutrient; it is just not considered an essential nutrient. Said another way, if glycine was lacking from our diet, it is unlikely that deficiency signs would develop because we can make plenty of it in our body.

How Much of the Essential Nutrients Do We Need?

If our diet fails to consistently provide adequate amounts of an essential nutrient, over time signs of deficiency will result. To address this notion, the first Recommended Dietary Allowances (RDAs) were developed by the United States government in the early 1940s. Other countries

Table 3.1 Essential Nutrients for Humans

Energy Nutrients	Vitamins	Minerals	Other
Protein/essential amino acids Carbohydrates Fat	Vitamins A, C, D, E, K and B_6, B_{12}, thiamin, folate, biotin, riboflavin, niacin, pantothenic acid, choline	Calcium, zinc, copper, sodium, potassium, iron, phosphorus, magnesium, chromium, chloride, molybdenum, fluoride, selenium manganese, iodide, chromium	Water

have similar recommendations. Recently, US and Canadian scientists pooled their resources to develop a more detailed set of nutrition recommendations collectively called the Dietary Reference Intakes or DRIs (Tables 3.2a–e). The DRIs include the RDAs, which speak more to preventing deficiency and promoting normal growth, development, and normal health for most people, as well as other applications such as average requirements and toxicity levels.

The DRIs are periodically scrutinized and revised based on the most current research findings. If an essential nutrient has enough research to allow for more specific recommendations to be made, then the recommendation level is called an RDA. Simply put, an RDA is the average daily level of nutrient needed to prevent deficiency and to promote general well-being for about 98 percent of a specific gender, age, and condition. On the other hand, for some nutrients such as vitamin D and calcium, an Adequate Intake (AI) level is listed instead of RDA.

Table 3.2a Recommended Dietary Allowance: Median Heights and Weights

	Age (years) or Condition	Weight		Height		Average Energy Allowance (kcal)	
		(kg)	(lb)	(cm)	(in)	(kg)	Per Day
Infants	0.0–0.5	6	13	60	24	108	650
	0.5–1.0	9	20	71	28	98	850
Children	1.0–3.0	13	29	90	35	102	1300
	4.0–6.0	20	44	112	44	90	1800
	7.0–10	28	62	132	52	70	2000
Males	11.0–14	45	99	157	62	55	2500
	15–18	66	145	176	69	45	3000
	19–24	72	160	177	70	40	2900
	25–50	79	174	176	70	37	2900
	51+	77	170	173	68	30	2300
Females	11.0–14	46	101	157	62	47	2200
	15–18	55	120	163	64	40	2200
	19–24	58	128	164	65	38	2200
	25–50	63	138	163	64	36	2200
	51+	65	143	160	63	30	1900
Pregnant	1st semester						plus 0
	2nd semester						plus 300
	3rd semester						plus 300
Lactating	1st 6 months						plus 500
	2nd 6 months						plus 500

Table 3.2b Recommended Dietary Allowance: Fat-Soluble Vitamins

	Age (years) or Condition	Vitamin A (μg)*	Vitamin D (μg)	Vitamin E (mg)	Vitamin K (μg)
Infants	0–0.5	400	5	4	2
	0.5–1.0	500	5	5	2.5
Children	1–3	300	5	6	30
	4–8	400	5	7	55
Males	9–13	600	5	11	60
	14–18	900	5	15	75
	19–30	900	5	15	120
	31–50	900	5	15	120
	50–70	900	10	15	120
	>70	900	15	15	120
Females	9–13	600	5	11	60
	14–18	700	5	15	75
	19–30	700	5	15	90
	31–50	700	5	15	90
	50–70	700	10	15	90
	>70	700	15	15	90
Pregnant	≤18	750	5	15	75
	19–30	770	5	15	90
	31–50	770	5	15	90
Lactating	≤18	1,200	10	19	75
	19–30	1,300	10	19	90
	31–50	1,300		19	90

Some of the values listed as RDA are Adequate Intake (AI) Values set by the Nutrition and Food Board. AI are similar to RDA, but lack the same knowledge base.
* Vitamin A recommendations can be expressed as Retinol Equivalents (RE) where 1 RE = μg retinal, 12 μg α-carotene, 24 μg α-carotene or α-cryptoxanthin
1 μg of vitamin D = 40 IU Vitamin D.

> An RDA is the level of an essential nutrient determined to be adequate for most people to prevent deficiency and to support well-being.

Like RDAs, AIs are also recommendations for a given nutrient, however there is not enough of a certain type of scientific information to designate a RDA quantity. Thus difference between a RDA and an AI is mostly the type and level of research studies that can be applied to the nutritional needs of a particular nutrient. An RDA is set when research allows for a more detailed understanding of how much of a particular nutrient is needed to prevent deficiency and promote general health. Meanwhile, AIs tend to be based more on studies of large populations of people and an observed level of intake of that nutrient that is associated with general health and no deficiency.

Table 3.2c Recommended Dietary Allowance: Water-Soluble Vitamins

Age (years) or Condition		Vitamin C mg/day	Thiamin mg/day	Riboflavin mg/day	Niacin mg/day*	Vitamin B₆ mg/day	Folate µg/day	Vitamin B₁₂ µg/day	Biotin µg/day	Pantothenic Acid mg/day	Choline mg/day
Infants	0–0.5	40	0.2	0.3	2	0.1	65	0.4	5	1.7	125
	0.5–1.0	50	0.3	0.4	4	0.3	80	0.5	6	1.8	150
Children	1–3	15	0.5	0.5	6	0.5	150	0.9	8	2	200
	4–8	25	0.6	0.6	8	0.6	200	1.2	12	3	250
Males	9–13	45	0.9	0.9	12	1.0	300	1.8	20	4	375
	14–18	75	1.2	1.3	16	1.3	400	2.4	25	5	550
	19–30	90	1.2	1.3	16	1.3	400	2.4	30	5	550
	31–50	90	1.2	1.3	16	1.3	400	2.4	30	5	550
	50–70	90	1.2	1.3	16	1.7	400	2.4	30	5	550
	>70	90	1.2	1.3	16	1.7	400	2.4	30	5	550
Females	9–13	45	0.9	0.9	12	1.0	300	1.8	20	4	375
	14–18	65	1.0	1.0	14	1.2	400	2.4	25	5	400
	19–30	75	1.1	1.1	14	1.3	400	2.4	30	5	425
	31–50	75	1.1	1.1	14	1.3	400	2.4	30	5	425
	50–70	75	1.1	1.1	14	1.5	400	2.4	30	5	425
	>70	75	1.1	1.1	14	1.5	400	2.4	30	5	425
Pregnant	≤18	80	1.4	1.4	18	1.9	600	2.6	30	6	450
	19–30	85	1.4	1.4	18	1.9	600	2.6	30	6	450
	31–50	85	1.4	1.4	18	1.9	600	2.6	30	6	450
	≤18	115	1.4	1.6	17	2	500	2.8	35	7	550
	19–30	120	1.4	1.6	17	2	500	2.8	35	7	550
	31–50	120	1.4	1.6	17	2	500	2.8	35	7	550

Some of the values listed as RDA are Adequate Intake (AI) Values set by the Nutrition and Food Board. AI are similar to RDA, but lack the same knowledge base.

* Niacin recommendations can be expressed as Niacin Equivalents (NE) where 1 NE = 1 mg niacin = 60 mg of tryptophan.

Table 3.2d Recommended Dietary Allowance: Minerals

	Age (years) or Condition	Calcium mg/day	Phosphorus mg/day	Magnesium mg/day	Iron mg/day	Zinc mg/day	Selenium µg/day	Copper µg/day
Infants	0–0.5	210	100	30	0.27	2	15	200
	0.5–1.0	270	275	75	11	3	20	220
Children	1–3	500	460	80	7	3	20	340
	4–8	1300	500	130	10	5	30	440
Males	9–13	1300	1250	240	8	8	40	700
	14–18	1300	1250	410	11	11	55	890
	19–30	1000	700	400	8	11	55	900
	31–50	1000	700	420	8	11	55	900
	50–70	1200	700	420	8	11	55	900
	>70	1200	700	420	8	11	55	900
Females	9–13	1300	1250	240	8	8	40	700
	14–18	1300	1250	360	15	9	55	890
	19–30	1000	1200	310	18	8	55	900
	31–50	1000	700	320	18	8	55	900
	50–70	1200	700	320	8	8	55	900
	>70	1200	700	320	8	8	55	900
Pregnant	≤18	1300	1250	400	27	12	60	1000
	19–30	1000	700	350	27	11	60	1000
	31–50	1000	700	360	27	11	60	1000
	≤18	1300	1250	360	10	13	70	1300
	19–30	1000	700	310	9	12	70	1300
	31–50	1000	700	320	9	12	70	1300

Some of the values listed as RDA are Adequate Intake (AI) Values set by the Nutrition and Food Board. AI are similar to RDA, but lack the same knowledge base.

Table 3.2e Recommended Dietary Allowance: Minerals (continued)

	Age (years) or Condition	Iodine µg/day	Chromium µg/day	Fluoride mg/day	Manganese mg/day	Molybdenum µg/day
Infants	0–0.5	110	0.2	0.01	0.003	2
	0.5–1.0	130	5.5	0.5	0.6	3
Children	1–3	90	11	0.7	1.2	17
	4–8	90	15	1	1.5	22
Males	9–13	120	25	2	1.9	34
	14–18	150	35	3	2.2	43
	19–30	150	35	4	2.3	45
	31–50	150	35	4	2.3	45
	50–70	150	30	4	2.3	45
	>70	150	30	4	2.3	45
Females	9–13	120	21	2	1.6	34
	14–18	150	24	3	1.6	43
	19–30	150	25	3	1.8	45
	31–50	150	25	3	1.8	45
	50–70	150	20	3	1.8	45
	>70	150	20	3	1.8	45
Pregnant	≤18	220	29	3	2	50
	19–30	220	30	3	2	50
	31–50	220	30	3	2	50
Lactating	≤18	290	44	3	2.6	50
	19–30	290	45	3	2.6	50
	31–50	290	45	3	2.6	50

Some of the values listed as RDA are Adequate Intake (AI) Values set by the Nutrition and Food Board. AI are similar to RDA, but lack the same knowledge base.

Currently there are RDAs and/or AI for vitamins A, D, E, K and C, thiamin (B_1), riboflavin (B_2), niacin (B_3), pyridoxine (B_6), cobalamin (B_{12}), folate, biotin, and pantothenic acid as well as calcium, phosphorus, magnesium, iron, zinc, iodine, selenium, copper, manganese, fluoride, chromium, and molybdenum. Sodium, potassium, and chloride also have AI levels. These elements are found in most foods, either naturally or after processing, and are extremely well absorbed into the body after we eat them. Therefore, a deficiency in any of these essential nutrients is unlikely, providing there are no confounding factors.

How Are the RDAs Determined?

The RDAs are determined based upon in-depth research studies, including those performed to determine "balance." Balance studies are designed to determine how much of a specific nutrient humans need to eat in order to balance that which is normally lost daily from the body and to maintain appropriate levels of that nutrient in the body. When these studies were performed, scientists observed that there was quite a bit of variability among the balances of different individuals. A hypothetical representation of a particular nutrient's balance is depicted in Figure 3.1.

Based on balance studies, researchers are able to determine estimated average requirements for specific gender and age groups for a given nutrient. Here they add up all of the individual balance levels and divide by the total number of people they assessed. The result is the Estimated Average Requirement or EAR. In this figure we see that the RDA for this nutrient is set well above the EAR. In fact the RDA is set two standard deviations (a measure of statistical variation) above the average. By doing so the RDA would be adequate to meet the needs of 97 to 98 percent of the people in the study. Knowing this, the RDAs will provide more of the nutrient than needed for balance for most individuals. From this we can certainly understand that the RDAs are not really personal recommendations but are more appropriate for making recommendations for populations. For example, the RDA for vitamin C for adult women of all ages is

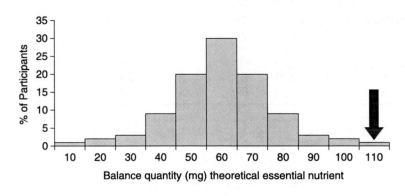

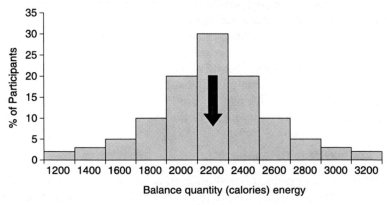

Figure 3.1 A hypothetical representation of a particular nutrient's balance.

75 milligrams, which should avoid deficiency and promote general health for about 97 to 98 percent of adult women.

It should be noted that the recommendation for energy was not set to include 97 to 98 percent of the population, but only 50 percent (see Figure 3.1). If the recommendation was set to include 98 percent of the population this might lead to weight gain for many people using the recommendation for energy as a guideline.

Beyond balance studies, other research studies involving the relationship between the essential nutrients and the body are reviewed to help determine the RDA. For example, the RDA for many nutrients during the years of rapid growth and during pregnancy must account for balance as well as an additional amount of a nutrient to allow for these periods of rapid growth. Furthermore, RDA determinations do not take into consideration acute disease, medications, or exercise training. Only recently have RDA considerations included chronic diseases such as osteoporosis and heart disease. However, at this time the RDAs and AIs are still considered to be below a level that would optimally support the prevention of several major diseases such as heart disease and cancer.

How Are Nutrition Recommendations Used on Food Labels?

By law food manufacturers must follow specific guidelines on their food labels with the purpose of informing consumers of the nutritional content of the food and to protect against misleading statements on food labels. Food labels contain the *Nutrition Facts* (Figure 3.2), which in most cases provide at least the following information:

- a listing of ingredients in descending order by weight
- serving size
- servings per container
- amount of the following per serving: total calories, total protein, calories contributed by fat, total fat, saturated fat, cholesterol, total carbohydrate, sugar, dietary fiber, vitamin A, vitamin C, calcium, iron, sodium

As many individuals try to plan their nutrient intake, the nutrition facts also include the *Daily Value* (DV). The DV uses reference nutrition standards to indicate how a single serving of a food item relates to nutrition recommendation standards and include:

- a maximum of 30 percent total calories from fat, or less than 65 grams total
- a maximum of 10 percent total calories from saturated fat, or less than 20 grams
- a minimum of 60 percent total calories from carbohydrate
- 10 percent of total calories from protein

Nutrition Facts

Serving Size 1 cup (228g)
Servings Per Container 2

Amount Per Serving

Calories 250	Calories from Fat 110

	% Daily Value*
Total Fat 12g	18%
Saturated Fat 3g	15%
Trans Fat 1.5g	
Cholesterol 30mg	10%
Sodium 470mg	20%
Total Carbohydrate 31g	10%
Dietary Fiber 0g	0%
Sugars 5g	
Protein 5g	

Vitamin A	4%
Vitamin C	2%
Calcium	20%
Iron	4%

*Percent Daily Values are based on a 2,000 calorie diet.
Your Daily Values may be higher or lower depending on
your calorie needs:

	Calories:	2,000	2,500
Total Fat	Less than	65g	80g
Sat Fat	Less than	20g	25g
Cholesterol	Less than	300mg	300mg
Sodium	Less than	2,400mg	2,400mg
Total Carbohydrate		300g	375g
Dietary Fiber		25g	30g

Figure 3.2 Example of a nutrition facts panel on a food label.

- 10 grams of fiber per 1,000 calories
- a maximum of 300 milligrams of cholesterol
- a maximum of 2,400 milligrams of sodium

> Daily Values on food labels are designed to help people make better informed nutrition choices.

Furthermore, the DV for other nutrients, such as vitamins A and C, thiamin, riboflavin, niacin, calcium, and iron, are founded upon RDA-based standards and are presented in Table 3.3. However, these standards are not as specific for gender and age as the RDAs and therefore one quantity will apply to all people.

Daily Values are expressed as a percentage and is based on a 2,000 and/or a 2,500 calorie intake, which approximates most American's recommended energy intake. Therefore a food providing 250 calories per serving will be listed as either 13 percent or 10 percent DV for a 2,000 and 2,500 calorie intake, respectively. Beyond the nutrition facts, food manufacturers must also follow federal guidelines for other statements they choose to make on a food label. Some of the statements are listed in Table 3.4.

Table 3.3 Daily Values (DV) Used for Nutrition Labeling

Nutrient	Amount	Nutrient	Amount
Biotin	300 μg	Vitamin A	5,000 IU
Calcium	1,000 mg	Vitamin B-12	6 μg
Chloride	3,400 mg	Vitamin B-6	2 mg
Chromium	120 μg	Vitamin C	60 mg
Copper	2 mg	Vitamin D	400 IU
Folic acid	400 μg	Vitamin E	30 IU
Iodine	150 μg	Vitamin K	80 μg
Iron	18 mg	Zinc	15 mg
Magnesium	400 mg	Total fat	65 g
Manganese	2 mg	Saturated fat	20 g
Molybdenum	75 μg	Cholesterol	300 mg
Niacin	20 mg	Total carbohydrate	300 g
Pantothenic acid	10 mg	Fiber	25 g
Phosphorus	1,000 mg	Sodium	2,400 mg
Riboflavin	1.7 mg	Potassium	3,500 mg
Selenium	70 μg	Protein	50 g
Thiamin	1.5 mg		

mg = Milligrams, μg = micrograms, IU = international units.

Source: Center for Food Safety and Applied Nutrition, 2002; National Academy of Sciences

What Is in My Food Besides Natural Components?

Many if not most manufactured foods contain food additives used to improve taste, texture, appearance, shelf life, safety, or nutritional value of the product. Some of the general food additive categories include: antioxidants, antimicrobials, coloring agents, emulsifiers, flavoring agents, sweeteners, pH controllers, leavening agents, texturizers, stabilizers, enzymes, and conditioners. All food additives were tested for safety and received approval by the Food and Drug Administration (FDA). This process can take years.

Nutrition Supplements—A Multibillion-Dollar Industry

What Are Nutritional Supplements?

Nutritional supplements contain ingredients that are either common or uncommon to natural foods. These substances are either extracted from a natural food or they are made in a laboratory and are provided in many forms such as pills, powders for drinks, and bars. Some examples of the early supplementation include ancient Persian physicians providing iron supplements to soldiers wounded in battle. On the other hand nutritional supplements marketed to the public began as an attempt to fill nutritional

Table 3.4 Guidelines for Food Label Claims

Fat free—must have less than 0.5 grams per serving

Saturated fat free—must contain less than 0.5 grams per serving

Cholesterol free—must contain less than 2 milligrams per serving

Sugar free—must contain less than 0.5 grams per serving

Sodium free—must contain less than 5 milligrams per serving

Calorie free—must contain less than 5 calories per serving

Low fat—must contain no more than 3 grams of fat per serving

Low sodium—must contain less than 40 milligrams per serving

Low calories—must contain less than 40 calories per serving

Low cholesterol—must contain less than 20 milligrams per serving

High or good source—one serving must contain at least 20 percent or more of the recommendation for that nutrient

Reduced, less, or fewer—must contain at least 25 percent less of a nutrient, per serving, compared with the same nutrient in a reference food

More or added—must contain at least 10 percent more of the daily value for a nutrient compared with a reference food

Light or lite—the food have at least 50 percent less fat than a similar, unmodified food which, in its unmodified form contains more than 50 percent of its calories from fat

Lean (meat, fish, poultry)—must contain less than 10 grams of fat, 4 grams of saturated fat, and 95 milligrams of cholesterol per 100 grams of the food

Extra lean—must contain less than 5 grams of fat, 2 grams of saturated fat, and 95 milligrams of cholesterol per 100 grams of the food

Fresh—food must be unprocessed, in raw state, and never frozen

---

voids in the diet. For example, a supplement may help an individual who does not eat dairy foods meet their calcium needs.

> Nutrition supplements are marketed to help ensure adequate nutrient intake to achieve a person's goal for health and/or performance.

Today, the nutrition supplements industry has evolved into a multibillion-dollar industry. Nutrition supplements are sold in supermarkets, drugstores, stores found in shopping malls, on the internet, and by direct marketing. Nutrition supplements include a broad range of individual and combinations of recognized nutrients, such as protein and amino acid preparations, essential fatty acids and fish oil, vitamins, and minerals, to more obscure substances and extracts such as co-enzyme Q10, ginseng, ginkgo biloba, hydroxy citric acid (HCA), kola nut, bilberry, grape seed extract, phytosterols, choline, lipoic acid, conjugated linoleic acid (CLA), and carnitine. As we move through the ensuing chapters we will mention different supplements as they apply to different topics of normal and applied nutrition.

Who Needs a Nutritional Supplement?

If a person's diet contains enough calories for normal weight maintenance and is well balanced, containing multiple servings of fruits, vegetables, and dairy products as well as adequate sources of protein, including fish or other seafood a couple times a week, then he or she is probably at least meeting the recommendations (RDA/AIs) for essential nutrients. Therefore, he or she would not need to supplement his or her diet to meet basic needs to prevent deficiency and to support general health.

On the other hand, if his or her diet is consistently imbalanced then that person's average daily intake for one or more essential nutrients will probably end up below recommendations. For instance, if a person doesn't eat fish or other seafood regularly, then they might not be achieving recommended levels for an essential fatty acid. Or, if a person doesn't tolerate or like milk and certain dairy foods, they might not achieve his or her AI for calcium and vitamin D on a regular basis. Therefore, unrelenting food preferences, food intolerance, and allergies, or limited availability of certain foods can certainly necessitate the consideration of a nutrition supplement. In addition, reduced calorie intakes to lose weight can often lead to inadequate intakes of one or more essential nutrients by reducing the volume of food in general or limiting the intake of certain types of foods.

Beyond achieving RDA/AI levels for essential nutrients, many people seek out supplements containing nutrition factors that are purported to optimize the fight against current conditions such as osteoarthritis and diabetes and to help prevent diseases that develop over years or decades such as osteoporosis, heart disease, and cancer. In doing so, essential nutrient levels well above the RDA/AI or other nutrients are sought out in supplementation. Often it is the case that even a well balanced diet would not provide the higher level or the unique nutrients, either at all or in adequate amounts. In this case, the diet would have to be supplemented. Excellent examples of nutrients sought out for supplementation include phytosterols and psyllium fiber for cholesterol reduction, glucosamine for joint health, lutein and zeaxanthin for eye health, and lycopene and blueberries for prostate health. Another example might be supplementation of creatine to achieve a daily level that would support the development of lean body mass for weight trainers and athletes.

What Should You Know Before You Buy a Supplement?

Before purchasing a nutritional supplement, the consumer should have an understanding of what a supplement is supposed to do and whether or not it has proven properties. The testimonial of friends and articles written in a popular magazine should not always be trusted. Freelance writers who may not have an educational background in the health sciences but can write a very believable article often author these pieces. Your most accurate source of nutritional information is people educated in nutrition/medical-related fields, preferably with a higher educational degree (PhD, MD, DO) and who study the most current nutrition research. Make sure the author of a given book or article, or an individual presenting a seminar, is well educated in that field. Ask for credentials from reputable universities and colleges that actually have campuses and accredited programs.

If you are thinking about purchasing a supplement to enhance a particular aspect of your life, such as athletic performance or disease prevention/treatment, make sure the substance has been tested under circumstances similar to those to which you want to apply the supplement. For example, just because a certain nutrient is essential for fat burning in the body does not mean that a supplemental dose of that nutrient will enhance your body's fat burning potential. Furthermore, research involving the nutrient of interest should have been published in an established scientific publication, such as the *Journal of the American Medical Association, Journal of Physiology, New England Journal of Medicine, Journal of Nutrition, Medicine and Science in Sports and Exercise*, and the *American Journal of Clinical Nutrition*. For instance, phytosterols have been shown in several research studies published in esteemed journals, such as the *Journal of the American Medical Association* to lower low density lipoprotein cholesterol, thus lowering a person's risk of heart disease.

The journals just mentioned are peer-reviewed, meaning that before a research article is published it is thoroughly evaluated by scientists who are experts in that field. Ask for this kind of information when you visit your local supplement supplier. Do not rely exclusively on the manufacturer's insert or brochure as they are trying to sell the product.

Beware of tricky marketing. Often we read articles in certain "health" magazines that convince us of the benefits of a certain substance only to find an advertisement and ordering information for that supplement five pages later. It makes you wonder if it was really a credible article or just clever advertising designed to appear as a credible article. This is especially true when the same company that published the magazine sells the supplement. Look for the word "Advertisement" written at the top of the page in tiny print.

What Are Nutraceuticals and Functional Foods?

The latter portion of the twentieth century was a time of great strides in modifying the way many nutritionists and health care practitioners viewed nutrition. For decades we made nutritional recommendations based upon what needed to be avoided or limited in our diet choices. The nutritional "bad guys" were fat, which evolved to saturated fat-rich foods, cholesterol, sodium, and arguably sugar. Today it is quite clear that the other side of the nutrition coin, or "what we should eat," is probably as significant as "what we should not eat." *Nutraceuticals* are substances found in natural foods that seem to have the potential to prevent disease or be used in the treatment of various disorders. Meanwhile, *functional foods* are the foods in which one or more nutraceuticals can be found. Nutraceutical substances include some of the more recognized nutrients such as vitamins C and E and the mineral calcium, but also include such substances as genestein, capsaicin, allium compounds, carotenoids (for example, lutein, lycopene, and zeathanxin) phytosterols, glucosamine, catechins (such as EGCG), fiber (psyllium, oat bran) (see Tables 3.5 through 3.7).

Nutraceuticals are nutrients in foods that can promote better health and/or support disease prevention.

As you may have already surmised, it is possible for a nutraceutical to be an essential nutrient. However, keep in mind that the nutraceutical

Table 3.5 Examples of Nutraceutical Substances Grouped by Natural Food source

Plants		Animal	Microbial
β-Glucan,	Allicin	Conjugated linoleic	*Saccharomyces*
Ascorbic acid	*d*-Limonene	acid (CLA)	*boulardii* (yeast)
γ-Tocotrienol	Genestein	Eicosapentaenoic	*Bifidobacterium.*
Quercetin	Lycopene	acid (EPA)	*bifidum*
Luteolin	Hemicellulose	Docosahexenoic acid	*Bifidobacterium.*
Cellulose	Lignin	(DHA)	*longum*
Lutein	Capsaicin	Spingolipids	*Bifidobacterium*
Gallic acid	Geraniol	Choline	*infantis*
Perillyl alcohol	β-Ionone	Lecithin	*Lactobacillus*
Indole-3-	α-Tocopherol	Calcium	*acidophilus*
carbonol	β-Carotene	Ubiquinone	(LC1)
Pectin	Nordihydro-	(coenzyme Q_{10})	*Lactobacillus*
Daidzein	capsaicin	Selenium	*acidophilus*
Glutathione	Selenium	Zinc	(NCFB 1748)
Potassium	Zeaxanthin		*Streptococcus*
			salvarius
			(subsp. *Thermophilus*)

Note: The substances listed on this table include those that are either accepted or purported nutraceutical substances. From: Wildman REC, *The Handbook of Nutraceuticals and Functional Foods* (Taylor and Francis, 2007).

Table 3.6 Examples Of Foods With Higher Content of Specific Nutraceutical Substances

Nutraceutical Substance/ Family	Foods of Remarkably High Content
Allyl sulfur compounds	Onions, garlic
Isoflavones	Soybeans and other legumes, apios,
Quercetin	Onion, red grapes, citrus fruits, broccoli, Italian yellow squash
Capsaicinoids	Pepper fruit
EPA and DHA	Fish Oils
Lycopene	Tomatoes and tomato products
Isothiocyanates	Cruciferous vegetables
α-Glucan	Oat bran
CLA	Beef and dairy
Resveratrol	Grapes (skin), red wine
α-Carotene	Citrus fruits, carrots, squash, pumpkin
Carnosol	Rosemary
Catechins	Teas, berries
Adenosine	Garlic, onion,
Indoles	Cabbage, broccoli, cauliflower, kale, Brussels sprouts
Curcumin	Tumeric
Ellagic acid	Grapes, strawberries, raspberries, walnuts
Anthocyanates	Red wine
3-*n*-butyl phthalide	Celery
Cellulose	Most plants (component of cell walls)

Note: The substances listed on this table include those that are either accepted or purported nutraceutical substances. From: Wildman REC, *The Handbook of Nutraceuticals and Functional Foods* (Taylor and Francis, 2007).

properties of certain essential nutrients may not be why they are essential in the first place. For instance, vitamin C is essential for making important molecules in our body such as collagen, yet its nutraceutical roles may be more related to its antioxidant activities, such as helping to prevent degenerative eye disorders—for example, cataracts and macular degeneration. We will spend more time discussing nutraceutical compounds in the later chapters. We are going to be hearing more and more about nutraceuticals for years to come.

Table 3.7 Examples of Nutraceuticals Grouped by Mechanisms of Action

Anticancer	Positive Influence on Blood Lipids	Antioxidation	Antiinflammatory	Osteogenetic or Bone Protective
Capsaicin	β-Glucan	CLA	Linolenic acid	CLA
Genestein	γ-Tocotrienol	Ascorbic acid	EPA	Soy protein
Daidzein	δ-tocotrienol	α-Carotene	DHA	Genestein
α-Tocotrienol	MUFA	Polyphenolics	Capsaicin	Daidzein
γ Tocotrienol	Quercetin	Tocopherols	Quercetin	Calcium
CLA	ω-3 PUFAs	Tocotrienols	Curcumin	
Lactobacillus acidophilus	Resveratrol	Indole-3-carbonol		
Sphingolipids	Tannins	α-Tocopherol		
Limonene	β-Sitosterol	Ellagic acid		
Diallyl sulfide	Saponins	Lycopene		
Ajoene		Lutein		
α-Tocopherol		Glutathione		
Enterolactone		Hydroxytyrosol		
Glycyrrhizin		Luteolin		
Equol		Oleuropein		
Curcumin		Catechins		
Ellagic acid		Gingerol		
Lutein		Chlorogenic acid		
Carnosol		Tannins		
Lactobacillus bulgaricus				

Note: The substances listed on this table include those that are either accepted or purported nutraceutical substances. From: Wildman REC, *The Handbook of Nutraceuticals and Functional Foods* (Taylor and Francis, 2007).

4 Carbohydrates Are Our Most Basic Fuel Source

Carbohydrates Power Our Body

The term carbohydrate was coined long ago as scientists observed a consistent pattern in the chemical formula of most carbohydrates. Not only were they composed of only carbon, hydrogen, and oxygen but also the ratio of carbon to the chemical formula of water (H_2O) is typically 1 to 1 ($C:H_2O$). Carbohydrate means "carbon with water." For example, carbohydrates glucose and galactose have the following chemical formula:

$$C_6H_{12}O_6 \text{ or } (CH_2O)_6.$$

Where Do Carbohydrates Come From?

To create energy-providing carbohydrates from the non-energy-providing molecules H_2O and CO_2 is a talent limited to plants and a handful of bacteria. In a process called *photosynthesis*, these life-forms are able to couple H_2O and CO_2 by harnessing solar energy. Along with carbohydrates, oxygen is also a product of this reaction:

$$6CO_2 + 6H_2O \rightarrow C_6H_{12}O_6 + 6O_2.$$

Humans are unable to perform photosynthesis and thus we eat plants and plant products such as fruits, vegetables, legumes, and grain products to obtain a rich supply of carbohydrates. Beyond plants and their products, milk and dairy are also good sources of carbohydrates. In fact, milk and some dairy products are the only considerable source of carbohydrate from animal foods. It should be mentioned that although humans cannot perform photosynthesis, we do possess the ability to make some carbohydrate in our body. However, in order to do so, we must start with molecules that already possess energy, as we will discuss soon enough.

> Diet carbohydrate is largely derived from plant and dairy based foods.

Are There Different Types and Classes of Carbohydrates?

As you may guess, numerous different kinds of carbohydrates are found in nature. However our discussion will be limited to those carbohydrates found in greater amounts in our diet and those important to our body. The simplest carbohydrates are the *monosaccharides*, which include glucose (dextrose), fructose, and galactose. Other examples of monosaccharides include xylose, mannose, and ribose, but these may not be as familiar to you. There are over one hundred different monosaccharides found in nature and these serve as the building blocks for larger carbohydrates, such as disaccharides, oligosaccharides, starches, and fibers (most).

What Are Monosaccharides and What Foods Have Them?

Monosaccharides are as small as carbohydrates get. Said another way, monosaccharides cannot be split into smaller carbohydrates. All other carbohydrates are made up of monosaccharides linked together. For instance, disaccharides are composed of two monosaccharides linked together. The three disaccharides found in our diet, including their monosaccharide building blocks, are listed in Table 4.1.

Glucose and fructose can be found in foods either independently or as part of larger carbohydrates. Fructose is what makes honey and many fruits sweet and is used commercially as a sweetener either as fructose or high-fructose corn syrup. On the other hand, while some galactose is found in certain foods, it is mostly found as part of larger carbohydrates.

What Are Disaccharides?

Looking at Table 4.1 we see that glucose is one-half of the disaccharides lactose and sucrose and both halves of maltose. Maltose, or malt sugar,

Table 4.1 Disaccharide Building Blocks

Disaccharide	Monosaccharide Involved
Lactose	Glucose + galactose
Sucrose	Glucose + fructose
Maltose	Glucose + glucose

may be part of our diet naturally in seeds or alcoholic beverages. Sucrose is derived from the sugar cane plant and the beet, and the sucrose-rich product is called "sugar." Lactose is the primary carbohydrate found in milk and dairy products. Nutrition scientists often refer to monosaccharides and disaccharides as "simple sugars" because of their relatively small carbohydrate size and their sweet taste. Table 4.2 presents the relative sweetness of simple sugars and compares them with sugar alcohols and artificial sweeteners.

Monosaccharides such as glucose and fructose are the smallest carbohydrate and are used to build more complex carbohydrates.

What Are Oligosaccharides and Starches?

Monosaccharides not only serve as building blocks for disaccharides but also for some larger forms of carbohydrates as well. The most recognizable larger carbohydrate is starch. Starch is found in varying degrees in plants and their products (for example, legumes, vegetables, fruits, and grains). It consists of large, straight and branching chains of the

Table 4.2 Sweetness of Sugars and Alternatives

Type of Sweetener	Sweetness (Relative to Sucrose)	Typical Sources
Simple Sugars		
Lactose	0.2	Dairy
Maltose	0.4	Germinating (sprouted) seeds
Glucose	0.7	Corn syrup
Sucrose	1.0	Table sugar
Fructose	1.7	Fruit, honey, sweetener (HFCS in soft drinks)
Sugar alcohols		
Sorbitol	0.6	Diet candies, sugarless gums
Mannitol	0.7	Diet candies, sugarless gum
Xylitol	0.9	Sugarless gum, diet candies
Artificial Sweeteners		
Aspartame (Nutrasweet®)	200	Diet soft drinks, powder sweeteners
Acesulfame-K 200	200	Sugarless gum, diet drink mixes
Saccharin	500	Diet soft drinks, powder sweeteners
Sucralose	600	Diet soft drinks, sugarless gum, cold desserts

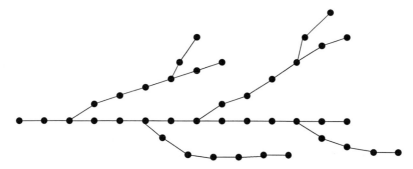

Figure 4.1 Schematic of the highly branching links of glucose that make up starch (plants) and glycogen in animals. Glycogen is more highly branched then starch.

monosaccharide glucose (Figure 4.1). Some shorter, branching chains of glucose can be found as well, and food manufacturers will also use these in the production of foods. The short, branching chains used by food manufacturers are often called maltodextrins and is typically derived from the partial digestion of corn starch.

In the human diet, we can also find a small amount of carbohydrates, called oligosaccharides, constructed from just a few monosaccharides (three to ten) linked together. Since these are found in relatively small amounts, they are not as essential to discuss. However, a few of these carbohydrates (for example, raffinose and stachyose) will require mention later on, not only for their nutritional value but for their effects within the digestive tract.

Plants make starch to store energy kind of like mammals store fat. Plant fibers, on the other hand, are not necessarily stored energy but serve more structural roles for plants. Like starch, fiber is also composed of straight and branching chains of monosaccharides, but their monosaccharides building block are not limited only to glucose. Fibers are discussed later in this chapter.

What Do Carbohydrates Do in Our Body?

Carbohydrates play quite a few roles in the human body, but perhaps none as important as being an energy source for all cells. All cells in the body will use glucose to some degree. Meanwhile, cells of the central nervous system as well as red blood cells and certain other types of cells will exclusively use glucose under normal situations. Carbohydrates also provide a limited yet readily available energy store called *glycogen*. As an energy source, carbohydrate provides 4 calories per gram.

Carbohydrates are also a modest yet vital component of cell membranes. Certain carbohydrates are also key portions of indispensable molecules. For example, molecules such as DNA and RNA contain the carbohydrate ribose. Ribose is a monosaccharide that can be made in our cells from glucose. Very complex carbohydrates called glycosaminogly-cans (GAGs) are important in connective tissue, such as in our joints. The GAGs include chondroitin sulfate and hyaluronic acid, which are popular nutrition supplements for joint inflammatory disorders. We'll spend more time discussing arthritis and nutrition in Chapter 12.

Carbohydrate serves as energy for all cells in our body and is used to make structural molecules, such as those found in joints.

Carbohydrate Is an Excellent Energy Source

How Much Carbohydrate Do We Eat?

We are eating more calories today than in the past several decades and carbohydrates are making a greater contribution to those calories. In countries such as the United States and Canada, about half of the energy adults eat comes by way of carbohydrates. About half of this carbo-hydrate is in the form of starch and the other half in the form of simple sugars. Sucrose makes up about half of the simple sugars we eat. In other areas of the world, such as Africa and Asia, sucrose consumption makes a lesser contribution while grains (for example, wheat and rice), fruits, and vegetables make a greater contribution.

The carbohydrate content of certain types of food is listed in Table 4.3. This includes easily digested carbohydrates such as sugars and starches, as well as carbohydrates that not easily digested such as oligosaccharides and fibers. Looking at this table we see that "sweets" such as candies and cakes are among those with the highest content of carbohydrate. Furthermore, nearly all of the carbohydrate in these foods comes by way of caloric sweeteners, primarily sucrose for baked sweets, which is added as a recipe ingredient.

Carbohydrates contribute half of the calories consumed in countries such as the US and Canada.

Fruits may be somewhat deceiving, according to Table 4.3, as their carbohydrate content is listed as roughly 5 to 20 percent. However, keep in mind that their water content makes up most of the remaining weight. Therefore carbohydrate is the major non-water content of fruits. Cereal grains and products such as rice, oats, pastas, and breads also have

Table 4.3 Carbohydrate Content of Select Foods

Food	Carbohydrate (% Weight)
Sugar	100
Ice cream, cake, pie	40–50
Fruits and vegetables	5–20
Nuts	<10
Peanut butter	<10
Milk	5
Cheese	1
Shellfish and other fish	<1
Meat, poultry, eggs	<1
Butter	0
Oils	0

relatively high carbohydrate content. Conversely, animal foods such as meats, fish, and poultry (and eggs) are virtually void of carbohydrate. Animal flesh (skeletal muscle) does contain a little carbohydrate, primarily as glycogen. However, the glycogen is lost during the processing of the meat. As mentioned above, milk and some dairy products (yogurt, ice cream) are the only significant animal-derived carbohydrate providers.

How Much Sugar Are We Consuming?

In 2007, the United States Department of Agriculture (USDA) estimated the consumption of caloric sweeteners (added sugars) at just under 85 pounds per adult. In a sense, sugar is the number one food additive. It turns up in some unlikely places, such as pizza, bread, hot dogs, boxed mixed rice, soup, crackers, spaghetti sauce, lunch meat, canned vegetables, fruit drinks, flavored yogurt, ketchup, salad dressing, mayonnaise, and some peanut butter. Carbonated sodas provided more than a fifth (22 percent) of the added sugars in the 2000 American food supply, compared with 16 percent in 1970.

Later in this book we will look more closely at some of the most popular diets today and yesterday including Atkins and South Beach. On these diets, the followers generally eat lower amounts of carbohydrate as well as a limited variety of carbohydrate-containing foods.

What Are the Recommendations for Carbohydrate Consumption?

The recommended range for carbohydrate intake as part of the Dietary Reference Intakes (DRIs) in the US and Canada is 45 to 65 percent of total energy. The breadth of this range allows for different people to plan their diet carbohydrate level based on their level of activity and ability to properly process food carbohydrate (see discussion of diabetes on page 83). People should focus on healthier carbohydrate sources such as whole grain products, fruits and vegetables. These foods provide vitamins, minerals, fiber and phytochemicals that promote health.

The RDA for carbohydrate energy has been set at 130 grams per day for people of all ages above 1 year of age. This would provide 520 calories of energy which is important to the central nervous system, red blood cells and other tissue dependent on glucose as their primary energy source. The RDA for carbohydrate energy would prevent ketosis, a metabolic situation that occurs when fat becomes the primary energy source for longer periods of time. Ketosis will be discussed in detail in the next chapter as well as in Chapter 8. Meanwhile, the RDA recommendation does not take into consideration exercise and additional calorie needs of working muscle.

What Are Recommendations for the Level of "Added Sugar" in the Diet?

As part of the DRIs it is recommended that the intake of "added sugar" not exceed 25 percent of calories. However, many nutritionists would like to see this recommendation lowered. That's because diets higher in added sugars are linked to excessive calorie consumption and thus obesity as well-being linked either directly or indirectly to heart disease, cancer and osteoporosis. Meanwhile the USDA recommends that an adult consuming 2,000-calorie daily, the amount that would approximate weight maintenance for an average woman not exceed 40 grams of added sugars. That level of added sugar (roughly 10 teaspoons) is the amount of sugar in a 12-ounce soft drink.

Added sugars, which could be considered the most common food additive is found in a variety of foods in the form of sucrose, corn sweeteners, honey, maple syrup, and molasses. You will find it in some unlikely places, such as pizza, bread, hot dogs, boxed mixed rice, soup, crackers, spaghetti sauce, lunch meat, canned vegetables, fruit drinks, flavored yogurt, ketchup, salad dressing, mayonnaise, and some peanut butter.

Carbohydrate Digestion and Absorption

How Are Dietary Carbohydrates Digested?

Normally, just about all non-fiber dietary carbohydrate will be absorbed across the wall of our small intestine. Monosaccharides are the absorbed form of carbohydrate, therefore disaccharides and starch must be digested into monosaccharides. Carbohydrate digestion begins in the mouth as chewing breaks up food and mixes it with saliva. Saliva contains *salivary amylase*, which is an enzyme that begins to break down starch. The activity of salivary amylase is short lived due to the rather brief period of time that food stays in the mouth. As the swallowed food/saliva mixture reaches the stomach, the acidic juice reduces the activity of salivary amylase, which halts carbohydrate digestion.

Chemical digestion of carbohydrates picks up again in the small intestine as the pancreas delivers *pancreatic amylase* along with a battery of other digestive enzymes. Pancreatic amylase resumes the assault upon starch molecules, breaking them into smaller links of glucose. The cells that line the small intestine will play the final role in carbohydrate digestion as they produce enzymes that digest the smaller carbohydrates, such as disaccharides and the remaining branch points on what was once starch. The enzymes that split sucrose, maltose, and lactose into monosaccharides are called *sucrase, maltase*, and *lactase*, respectively.

Carbohydrates are primarily absorbed as monosaccharides, thus disaccharides and starch must be digested.

Once monosaccharides are liberated they can move into the cells lining the wall of the small intestine. They can then move out the back end of these cells and then into tiny blood vessels (capillaries) in the wall of the small intestine. These capillaries drain into a larger blood vessel that leaves the intestines and travels to the liver (Figure 4.2). It should be mentioned that the absorption of glucose and galactose requires energy (ATP) but fructose does not.

What Is Lactose Intolerance?

By early childhood much of the world population, especially people of African, Asian, and Greek descent, loses the ability to produce sufficient amounts of the digestive enzyme lactase. In fact, lactase production decreases an average of 90 percent by age five, resulting in poor lactose digestion. This is believed to be the natural course for humans and a similar situation can be seen in many other mammal species after they wean from their "mother's milk." However, in some populations such as Swedes, Finns and Caucasians in United States, the incidence of lactose intolerance is low (<12 percent). It is believed that this is the result of genetic change that occurred long ago, which minimized the reduction in lactase production, resulting in this trait today.

Undigested lactose is not absorbed and continues to move through

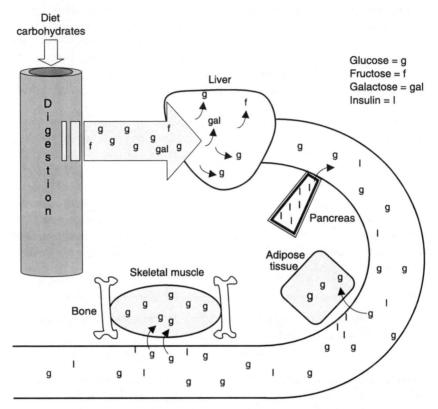

Figure 4.2 When blood glucose levels become elevated our pancreas releases insulin, which promotes the uptake of glucose in muscle and fat cells. Meanwhile, fructose and galactose are taken up by the liver.

the small intestine into the colon where it becomes available to bacteria. Bacteria easily break down lactose for energy and produce gases such as hydrogen gas (H_2) and carbon dioxide (CO_2) and other substances in the process. Lactose intolerance can be diagnosed by the Hydrogen Breath Test during which 50 grams of lactose is provided and the amount of H_2 in breath (derived from production in the intestines) is measured.

The gases produced in lactose-intolerant people can lead to bloating, cramping, and flatulence. Furthermore, as lactose moves through the digestive tract it will hold onto water, which softens feces and possibly produces diarrhea. These discomforts are collectively referred to as lactose intolerance. To deal with lactose intolerance, many people add a product called Lactaid (lactase enzyme) to their milk to predigest the lactose. Lactaid milk containing pre-digested lactose is also available. This appears to be an effective method of adapting to lactose intolerance.

Why Do Beans and Other Vegetables Produce Gas in Our Digestive Tract?

Legumes are plants that have a single row of seeds in their pods. What we commonly call legumes, such as peas, green beans, lima beans, pinto beans, black-eyed peas, garbanzo beans, lentils, and soybeans, are often the seeds of legume plants. Relatively short carbohydrate chains (oligosaccharides) such as *stachyose, raffinose,* and *verbacose* are found in legumes as well as broccoli, Brussels sprouts, cabbage, asparagus, and other vegetables, as well as whole grains. These carbohydrates are unique because they contain the disaccharide sucrose linked to one or more galactose molecules.

People (like pigs and chickens) don't produce the enzymes (for example, alpha-galactosidase) necessary to efficiently break down stachyose, raffinose, and verbacose. So, similar to lactose in lactose intolerant people, these carbohydrates remain intact in our small intestine and move into the colon. In the colon, gas-producing bacteria breakdown (ferment) these carbohydrates producing the gases methane (CH_4), CO_2 and H_2 which lead to bloating, cramping, and flatulence. A product available in stores called Beano® is an enzyme preparation (including alpha-galactosidase) that will digest these carbohydrates when it is ingested just prior to the legume-containing meal.

Carbohydrates such as stachyose, verbacose, and raffinose are responsible for the gas produced after eating beans and other vegetables.

Carbohydrate Energy Is Quickly Processed in the Body

Once Monosaccharides Are Absorbed, Where Do They Go?

As mentioned, monosaccharides (glucose, fructose, and galactose) are absorbed into the body by crossing the wall of the small intestine and entering circulation via a special blood vessel called the *portal vein.* As the portal vein carries blood from the digestive tract directly to the liver, the liver gets the first shot at the absorbed monosaccharides. The liver is able to pull most of the galactose and fructose from our blood as well as a respectable portion of the glucose (see Figure 4.2). However, much of the glucose continues past our liver and enters the general circulation where other tissue will have a shot at it. This increases the concentration of glucose in the blood from a normal or "fasting" level of 70 to 100 milligrams up to 140 milligrams of glucose per 100 milliliters of blood or higher.

How Does Our Body Respond to the Rise in Blood Glucose?

The concentration of glucose in the blood is very tightly regulated. When the level of circulating glucose climbs above the normal fasting level, the pancreas releases the hormone insulin (see Figures 4.2 and 4.3). Insulin will interact with receptors on muscle cells and fat cells and promote the movement of glucose into these cells. Because skeletal muscle and fat cells together tend to make up more than half of our total body mass, the net effect is a fairly rapid lowering of the glucose concentration. Insulin increases the movement of glucose in these cells by increasing the number of glucose transport proteins on their plasma membranes. As the level of glucose returns to the normal fasting level, the pancreas responds by releasing less insulin into circulation.

All cells in our body will continuously take glucose from our blood throughout the day to help meet their need for energy. However, after a meal, the liver, muscle, and fat cells will take a lot more glucose out of the blood than they immediately need. This allows blood glucose levels to quickly return to a normal fasting concentration.

Increased blood glucose levels causes the release of insulin to process, use, and store carbohydrate.

What Does Our Body Do with the Glucose from a Meal?

Insulin directs muscle, fat tissue, and the liver to use glucose, fructose and galactose as the primary fuel. This allows for a lot of carbohydrate entering the body from a meal to be used for energy immediately. In

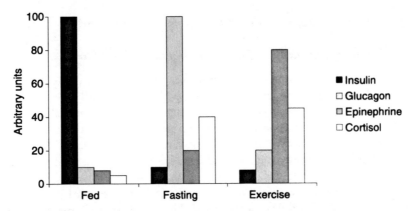

Figure 4.3 Relative levels of the major metabolic hormones during and right after a meal (fed), more than 8 to 12 hours after a meal (fasting) and during sustained moderate to higher intensity exercise. (Glucagon levels may increase during exercise if blood glucose levels decline.)

addition, insulin directs muscle and liver, and to a lesser extent other tissue, to store extra carbohydrate as glycogen. Glycogen is composed of large branching links of glucose and is very similar to plant starch. However, only so much glycogen can be made and stored, since it is meant to be a short-term not a long-term energy reserve.

How Much Glycogen Is in Our Body?

Our liver can store up to 6 to 8 percent of its weight as glycogen for about 75 to 100 grams total. Meanwhile, only about 1 percent of the weight of skeletal muscle cells is attributable to glycogen. However, since the total amount of skeletal muscle in our body far exceeds our liver, muscle will contribute much more to our total glycogen stores. Skeletal muscle can contain about 250 to 400 grams, which is about four-fifths of our total glycogen stores. Since carbohydrate provides 4 calories per gram the potential energy from glycogen is typically 1,400 to 2,000 calories, not very much. As you may expect, people with more muscle resulting from exercise training will have more body glycogen owing to increased muscle mass. In addition, their muscle will adapt to double and even triple the amount of glycogen it can store.

Interestingly, even though carbohydrates contribute approximately one-half of the energy in our diet, our body composition is not reflective. That's because only 1 percent or less of our body weight is composed of carbohydrate. This means that carbohydrate is stored with limitations, most of which is in our liver and skeletal muscle as glycogen. Other tissues, such as fat cells and the heart, contain a little glycogen as well; however, the contribution to our total body glycogen stores is very small. Since glycogen stores are relatively small there must be another means of storing the excessive energy from diet derived carbohydrate.

Can Carbohydrate from Our Diet Become Body Fat?

Since the potential to store carbohydrate as glycogen is somewhat limited, we need another means of storing excessive diet carbohydrate energy. As our liver and skeletal muscle is busy making glycogen, our liver and fat tissue will also begin to convert some of the extra glucose to fat. The fat that is made in our fat cells is stored within those cells. Meanwhile, the fat that is made in the liver is transported in the blood to fat cells and to a lesser degree other tissue such as muscle, breast tissue, etc.

> Excessive carbohydrate intake can be converted to fat and decrease daily fat use leading to increased body fat.

Interestingly, scientists have determined that our ability to convert excessive carbohydrate to fat might not be as efficient under normal conditions as we once thought. It now seems that consuming excessive carbohydrate can increase the level of body fat by decreasing our use of fat as a daily energy source. That's because our body is forced to use more carbohydrate as promoted by insulin. This situation tends to happen more when people eat too many calories and have type 2 diabetes (or prediabetes).

Can Eating a Low Carbohydrate Diet Make Us Fatter?

As will become clearer in Chapter 8, eating too much energy makes us fat, not too much of any one energy nutrient such as carbohydrate. Without question eating a high carbohydrate diet in conjunction with eating excessive energy will certainly support weight (fat) gain; so too will eating excessive fat and/or protein.

One of the reasons that carbohydrates have been bashed as of late is because of the effects of insulin upon stored fat. Insulin hinders the release of fat from adipose tissue. Therefore many dieters believe that carbohydrates, or more specifically insulin, are working against them. However, this function of insulin is very important in the normal scheme of things. By design, insulin keeps the fat tissue from breaking down and releasing fat during and for a couple of hours after a meal. At this time absorbed food energy nutrients are circulating in our blood so there would be no need to break down our fat stores. Insulin will also promote the formation of fat from excess diet energy. So, the combination of decreased fat breakdown and increased fat production may lead people to believe that insulin makes them fat!

Before we dismiss the notion that insulin is working against people in their quest to lose body fat, we should recognize that many people have elevated insulin and glucose levels during fasting. More times than not this occurs in people who have a higher level of body fat and low levels of activity. Thus eating a higher carbohydrate diet may indeed work against them to some degree. And eating a lower carbohydrate diet would allow for a higher proportion of fat to be used for energy. We discuss this more in Chapter 8.

> High carbohydrate diets can increase body fat when too many calories are consumed by decreasing the burning of stored fat and forming new fat.

Glycemic Index and Load Assess Food's Effect on Blood Glucose

What Is Glycemic Index?

As expected, the level of circulating glucose increases after eating a carbohydrate-containing meal. But to what level, and will different foods having the same amount of carbohydrate result in the same increase in blood glucose? This kind of information surely would be of interest to many people, especially those managing their blood glucose levels (such as in diabetes).

As shown in Figure 4.4, the level of glucose circulating in the blood increases after eating or drinking a carbohydrate-containing food or beverage and then is reduced back toward the normal fasting level. This response is often referred to as a *glucose tolerance curve* and it can be used to assess how well a person's body is able to take glucose out of the blood and use it for energy and to build stores.

Since different foods will produce different glucose tolerance curve patterns, scientists developed the *glycemic index*. Simply put, glycemic index is a measure of the power of carbohydrate-containing foods to raise blood glucose levels after being eaten or drunk. In addition to people managing their blood glucose levels, glycemic index has become popular for many people trying to lose weight which will be discussed this in more

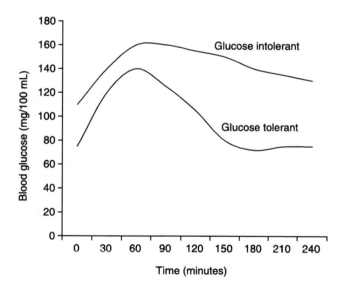

Figure 4.4 Glucose levels during an oral glucose tolerance test (OGTT). Two fasting people were provided with 75 grams of glucose and their blood glucose was measured every 30 minutes for 4 hours. Note that even after 4 hours the blood glucose level of the intolerant individual is still elevated.

detail in Chapter 11. See Table 4.4 for standard levels for glycemic index and load.

Glycemic index is a measure of a food's ability to raise the level of blood glucose.

For a long time it was assumed that because starch was more structurally complex than simpler sugars, starchy foods would be digested more slowly and therefore absorbed more slowly and evenly after a meal. On the other hand, foods containing simpler sugars (for example, soda and candy) would be digested and absorbed more rapidly, leading to a faster and greater rise in blood glucose. However, the relationship between different foods and blood glucose turned out to be more complex, which is why the determination of glycemic index for individual foods has been helpful.

Why Does Glycemic Index Vary Among Foods?

To understand why different carbohydrate-containing foods have a different glycemic index, we can start with the type of monosaccharide derived from a food. This is important because fructose and galactose do not raise blood glucose to the same extent that glucose does. For instance, the digestible carbohydrate in breads and potatoes is starch, which is made up of glucose. Meanwhile, milk and milk products contain lactose which is made up of glucose and galactose. Based on the difference in glucose content between starch and milk products, it is predictable that milk would have a lower glycemic index than bread.

Ripened fruits contain mostly fructose and glucose as well as some sucrose. For example, a medium apple contains about 8 grams of fructose and 3 grams of both glucose and sucrose. Meanwhile a medium banana contains between 5 to 6 grams of both fructose and glucose and 2 grams of sucrose. One tablespoon of honey contains 8 grams of fructose and 7 grams of glucose and less than 1 gram of sucrose, galactose, and maltose combined. So even though fruits and honey are very sweet, they will have a moderate glycemic index and load (see Table 4.4).

Glycemic load is a glycemic index adjusted for a standard serving size.

In addition to monosaccharide type, protein, fiber, and fat, as well as the processing of a food can influence its glycemic index. Fiber and

Table 4.4 Glycemic Index and Load Levels

Level	Glycemic Index	Glycemic Load	Glycemic Load/Day
Low	55 or less	10 or less	Less than 80
Medium	56 to 69	11 to 19	80 to 120
High	70 or more	20 or more	More than 120

Food	Glycemic Index	Glycemic Load	Food	Glycemic Index	Glycemic Load
All-Bran® cereal	42	8	Peanuts	14	1
Apple juice	40	11	Pears	38	4
Apples	38	6	Pineapple	59	7
Bananas	52	12	Pinto beans	39	10
Beets	64	5	Popcorn	72	8
Buckwheat	54	16	Potatoes (new)	57	12
Cantaloupe	65	4	Potatoes (russet, baked)	85	26
Carrots	47	3	rice, white	64	23
Cherrios® Cereal	74	15	rice, wild	57	18
Corn Flakes Cereal	81	21	sourdough wheat bread	54	15
Couscous	65	23	spaghetti	42	20
Fettucine	40	18	strawberries	40	1
Grapes	46	8	sucrose (table sugar)	68	7
Green peas	48	3	Shredded Wheat® cereal		
Kidney beans	28	7	Sweet corn	54	9
Life® cereal	66	16	Sweet potatoes	61	17
Linguine	52	23	Watermelon	72	4
Macaroni	47	23	Whole wheat flour bread	71	9
Navy beans	38	12	White wheat flour bread	70	10

fat seem to be able to slow the digestion process and thus can lower glycemic index. Certain types of fiber, often referred to as viscous fibers, can thicken the digestive contents in the stomach and small intestine, sort of like thickening up gravy with starch. This slows the digestion of carbohydrate and absorption of monosaccharides, which in turn reduces the rise in glucose.

Some amino acids in protein can increase the level of insulin released in response to carbohydrate and thus decrease glycemic index. Meanwhile, pasta has a lower glycemic index than what might be expected of such a high starch food. That's because starch molecules become trapped within gluten protein networks within the dough. Thus, wheat-based pastas have a relatively lower glycemic index value than expected and relatively lower than pastas made from other grains (for example, rice or corn) which don't contain gluten.

How Is Glycemic Index Determined?

Glycemic index is determined in a research lab. Fasting people are fed 50 grams of either pure glucose or enough white bread to provide 50 grams of digestible (non-fiber) carbohydrate, and blood glucose is measured over the next 2 hours. On a different day, the same people would be provided a food in an amount to allow for 50 grams of digestible carbohydrate and again blood glucose is measured over the next 2 hours. If a food raises blood glucose to 50 percent of the rise caused by glucose then the glycemic index is 50.

Because of the difference between white bread and pure glucose, glycemic indexes determined for foods using these different standards can vary. The glycemic index scale when using pure glucose is 0 to 100 and is more common because it is a little easier for the public to use. Meanwhile, when white bread is used as the standard for determining glycemic index, several foods, such as a baked potato, rice cakes, jelly beans, and Cheerios® have a value greater than 100. When this book discusses the glycemic index of foods we will use glucose as the standard as per the values of the Human Nutrition Unit at the University of Sydney (www.glycemicindex.com).

What Is Glycemic Load?

While the concept of glycemic index is pretty straight forward, it is not always easy to apply to how people eat. One issue with glycemic index is that the amount of food used to determine its glycemic index is not typically the amount of food consumed. A good example is boiled carrots which will have a glycemic index of about 90. Since one cup serving of carrots only has about 4 grams of available carbohydrate, rarely would a person eat enough carrots to achieve the level used to determine its glycemic index, which would be about 12 times that amount. That's why researchers developed a second glycemic measure more appropriate for the "real world", called *glycemic load*.

A food's glycemic load is derived by taking the glycemic index and then multiplying it by the amount of digestible carbohydrate and then dividing by one hundred. For instance, carrots have a glycemic index of 90, which multiplied by 4 (grams of digestible carbohydrate) and divided by 100 gives you a glycemic load of roughly 4. See Table 4.4 for a listing of glycemic loads of common foods relative to glycemic index.

Are Glycemic Index and Glycemic Load Important to Health?

Foods with lower glycemic responses are more desirable for people who are actively managing their blood glucose levels. This includes people with prediabetes and diabetes. The lower glycemic response could mean less medication necessary to keep blood glucose levels in check. Furthermore, lower glycemic diets are often positioned as ideal to help people lose weight. Whether or not this is true remains to be conclusively determined, however, lower glycemic foods are associated with better satiety (fullness) and hunger control, which can be helpful to people trying to shed a few pounds. Lastly, lower glycemic foods are associated with a reduced risk of heart disease. We will discuss the application of glycemic index and load to weight loss and improved fitness in Chapter 8.

Diabetes Is an Impairment of Blood Glucose Regulation

What Is Diabetes?

For many people, the fine regulation of the level of blood glucose becomes impaired. This results in chronic high blood glucose concentrations medically known as *hyperglycemia*. The impairment may be due to a decreased ability of the pancreas to produce insulin, which is the case in type 1 diabetes. The lack of insulin allows glucose levels to remain elevated even in a fasting state. Furthermore, after a meal blood glucose levels can climb exceptionally high (see Figure 4.4). For most people diagnosed with diabetes, blood glucose regulation is impaired despite their ability to produce insulin. In fact, many of these individuals produce more insulin than what seems normal, at least initially. This type of diabetes is referred to as type 2 diabetes.

In the past, type 1 diabetes has also been called insulin-dependent diabetes because medical treatment involves insulin therapy via needle injections or automated subcutaneous pumps. Insulin nasal sprays seem to be promising to simplify diabetes management. Type 1 diabetes has also been referred to as juvenile (or child-onset) diabetes because diagnosis is much more common in children. However, since type 1 diabetes can develop at any age, type 1 diabetes is the most correct terminology. Type 2 diabetes has also been called non-insulin-dependent diabetes mellitus, as medical treatment does not absolutely require insulin injections. However, because insulin injections may be prescribed from time to time this terminology is confusing. Furthermore, type 2 diabetes has been referred to as adult-onset diabetes mellitus since it is more commonly diagnosed in adults. Again, this is confusing as more children are being diagnosed with type 2 diabetes. While type 2 diabetes occurs in people of all ages and races, it is more common in US population among African Americans, Latinos, Native Americans, and Asian Americans/Pacific Islanders, as well as the aged population.

Diabetes is an impairment to the processes that regulates blood glucose.

- Type 1 is caused by a lack of insulin production.
- Type 2 is caused by a failure of insulin to effectively regulate glucose levels.

What Causes Type 2 Diabetes?

In type 2 diabetes mellitus, muscle and fat cells become less sensitive to insulin. What has become very clear to researchers, physicians, and nutritionists is that there is a strong relationship between obesity and this form of diabetes mellitus. In fact, nearly 90 percent of all individuals diagnosed with type 2 diabetes mellitus are also recognized as obese. In support of this relationship, most obese type 2 diabetics regain the ability to regulate their blood glucose as they reduce their body fat through weight loss and exercise. Although the relationship seems clear enough, the mechanism has been somewhat elusive to scientists. However, today, some evidence suggests that swollen fat cells themselves may release (and/or not release) chemicals that contribute to decreased sensitivity to insulin.

Does Sugar Cause Diabetes?

Over the years, many theories have evolved about the relationship between higher consumptions of sugar and various diseases and conditions. However, dietary sugar does not appear to promote the development of diabetes, at least not directly. As discussed above, diabetes can be largely categorized into two groups: those individuals that have a reduction in ability to make insulin (type 1 diabetes) and those individuals that appear to make insulin, but whose muscle and fat cells appear to be less sensitive to its presence (type 2 diabetes). In most cases of type 2 diabetes mellitus, one of the most significant underlying factors is an excessive body weight in the form of fat. So, if a person eats excessive amounts of sugary foods, which by simple excess of energy intake will lead to fat accumulation, obesity, and subsequent diabetes, then perhaps an argument can be made. However, sugar would then be an indirect factor, not a direct factor. On the other hand, high sugar foods such as soda, cookies, cakes, and pies can make it more difficult to manage diabetes because of their glycemic effect described above.

Blood Glucose Is Regulated Between Meals and During Exercise

How Is Blood Glucose Maintained In-Between Meals and Overnight?

The complete digestion and absorption of a meal can take several hours, depending upon its size and composition. Therefore, carbohydrate or more specifically glucose from that meal may be available for several hours as well. However, once this ends, a new blood glucose scenario begins to take shape. Cells throughout the body will continue to help themselves to glucose in the blood to help meet their energy needs. The net effect is that our blood glucose concentration will begin to decrease. When this happens the pancreas responds again. However, this time it responds by releasing the hormone *glucagon* into our blood (see Figure 4.3). In addition, *epinephrine* (adrenaline) and *cortisol* will promote efforts in different tissue that will help maintain blood glucose levels in-between meals.

How Does Glucagon Help Maintain Blood Glucose Levels In-Between Meals?

Glucagon works in a manner that is generally opposite to insulin. It will labor to increase blood glucose concentration, thereby returning it toward normal levels. To accomplish this, glucagon promotes the break-down of liver glycogen to glucose, which is released into circulation.

Glucagon will also promote another activity in our liver that will generate glucose. The process is called *gluconeogenesis*, which literally means to create new glucose if you read its root words right to left. In this process, certain amino acids, lactate (lactic acid), and glycerol from our circulation will be taken up by our liver and used to make glucose. Like the glucose generated from glycogen breakdown, this glucose can also be released into our blood to maintain blood glucose levels.

How Does Epinephrine (Adrenaline) Help Maintain Blood Glucose Levels During Fasting?

During a fasting period, a little epinephrine (adrenaline) is released into circulation from our adrenal glands (see Figure 4.3 and Table 4.5). Among epinephrine's many roles will be its influence upon the liver and skeletal muscle. It will support the effects of glucagon in the liver that were just mentioned. In skeletal muscle, the slightly elevated epinephrine will lightly promote the breakdown of glycogen to glucose. Contrary to the glucose produced from the breakdown of liver glycogen, this glucose is not released into the blood. Rather, this glucose becomes a supportive energy source for those muscle cells while fat is the major energy source. However, when this glucose is used for energy in those cells, a little bit of lactate may be produced. This lactate can enter circulation, reach the liver, and be converted to glucose. This glucose can then be released into the blood. Therefore, our skeletal muscle can modestly contribute to maintaining our blood glucose concentration during fasting.

What Does Cortisol Do to Help Maintain Blood Glucose Levels During Fasting?

Cortisol is often regarded as the "stress hormone." It is important to realize that fasting, especially prolonged fasting, is a form of stress—and stress results in the release of cortisol from the adrenal glands along with epinephrine mentioned in the previous question. Cortisol also supports the breakdown of glycogen and the conversion of amino acids, lactate,

Table 4.5 Actions Of Insulin, Glucagon, Cortisol, and Epinephrine in Carbohydrate Metabolism

Insulin	Increases the uptake of glucose by our muscle and fat cells Increases the synthesis of glycogen in our muscle and liver Increases fatty acid synthesis from excessive diet carbohydrate Decreases fat breakdown and mobilization from our fat tissue
Glucagon	Increases glycogen breakdown in our liver Increases liver glycogen-derived glucose release into our blood Increases glucose manufacturing in our liver Increases fat breakdown and mobilization from our fat tissue
Epinephrine (adrenaline)	Increases glycogen breakdown in our liver and skeletal muscle Increases liver glycogen-derived glucose release into our blood Increases fat breakdown and mobilization from our fat tissue
Cortisol (stress hormone)	Increases muscle protein breakdown to amino acids which can circulate to the liver and be used for glucose production Increases liver glycogen-derived glucose release into our blood Increases fat breakdown and mobilization from our fat tissue

and glycerol to glucose in our liver. Because cortisol also promotes the breakdown of our body protein, especially skeletal muscle protein, it ensures a supply of amino acids for conversion to glucose in our liver (Figure 4.5).

Exercise promotes the breakdown of carbohydrate stores in muscle.

What Happens to Stored Carbohydrate (Glycogen) During Exercise?

The hormone picture that develops during exercise is similar to the one discussed regarding a fasting period; however, there are relative differences. Epinephrine is released from our adrenal glands as a direct effect of exercise.

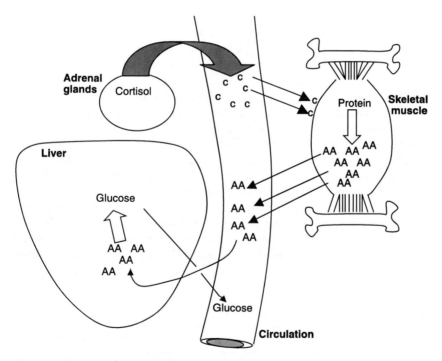

Figure 4.5 During fasting and endurance exercise (at least moderate intensity) cortisol causes the breakdown of muscle protein and some amino acids can be used to make glucose in our liver.

Quite simply, the greater the exercise intensity, the greater the epinephrine release. Epinephrine stimulates the breakdown of muscle cell glycogen (see Table 4.5 and Figure 4.3). This makes glucose available for the muscle cells hard at work. Epinephrine also promotes the breakdown of glycogen to glucose in the liver. Some of this glucose will then circulate to working muscle to provide support. Cortisol may also be released in response to moderate to intense exercise, particularly as the exercise becomes prolonged (for example, endurance cycling and running). Cortisol will also support the breakdown of glycogen as well as gluconeogenesis in our liver.

Fiber Is an Important Non-Energy Carbohydrate

What Is Fiber?

Fiber isn't a single nutrient but a family of plant-based nutrients that are generally resistant to human digestion. Since plants lack the bony skeletal design that provides much of an animal's shape and form, fibers provide much of the structural support to plant cell walls and the plant in general. Plants also use certain fiber as the foundation for their scar tissue. It is important to remember that while humans and other mammals prefer to produce proteins like collagen as the structural basis of their bodies, plants use carbohydrates.

Fiber consists of non-starch polysaccharides such as cellulose, hemicellulose, gums, mucilages, pectin, and oligosaccharides along with other plants components such as lignin. Chitin is often considered a fiber because it is a polysaccharide. Chitin is found in the exoskeletons of shellfish such as lobster, shrimp and crab as well as some insects such as beetles and ants as well as in the cell walls of some yeast and fungi. Table 4.6 lists fiber content of certain foods.

Fructooligosaccharides (FOS), which are sometimes called oligofructose or oligofructan, are short links of fructose terminating in glucose. *Inulin* is similar to FOS, however the number of fructose molecules linked together can exceed 100. Both inulin and FOS are found in many plants including Jerusalem artichoke, burdock, chicory, leeks, onions, and

Table 4.6 Fiber Content of Various Foods

Food	Fiber (% Weight)
Almonds, wheat germ	3
Lima beans, whole wheat flour, oat flakes, pears, pecans, popcorn, walnuts	2
Apples, string beans, broccoli, carrots, strawberries	1
White flour	<1

asparagus. FOS and inulin are often used as food additives as they add bulk and mild sweetness to foods while having health promoting properties.

What Is Soluble and Insoluble Fiber?

Fibers are often classified as being either soluble or insoluble; however, plants tend to contain a mixture of both. When a food is said to be a soluble or insoluble fiber it means that the majority of the fiber found within it is of that kind. For instance, prunes and plums contain both fiber types, with the skin providing more insoluble fiber and the fleshy pulp providing more soluble fiber. Psyllium fiber is referred to as a soluble fiber food source although roughly a third of its fiber is insoluble.

Dietary fiber is important for heart and gut health, immunity, and mineral absorption.

Soluble fiber sources include psyllium husk, oats, barley and legumes as well as many fruits and vegetables, particularly apples and pears. Soluble fibers used as food ingredients include inulin, FOS, guar gum, and xanthan gum.

Insoluble fiber sources include wheat bran, whole-grain cereals and breads, corn bran, flax and other seeds, as well as many fruits and vegetables, such as berries, carrots, celery, green beans, and potato skins.

As discussed in Chapter 1, solubility refers to how well a substance will interact with and dissolve in water. With regard to fiber, "soluble" refers the ability to form a gel in the digestive tract in which water is trapped. Soluble fiber supplement drinks can be used as a visual example of the gel-forming (sponge-like) properties of soluble fibers.

About How Much Fiber Do We Eat and What Are the Recommendations?

It is likely that we evolved on a high-fiber diet because of the unavailability of processing techniques. Some have estimated that our fiber consumption may have been as high as 50 grams daily when fiber-rich foods were more bountiful in our diet. Some current populations in Africa have been noted to retain high-fiber intakes. On the other hand, it is estimated the average American woman and man eats about 12 grams and 18 grams of dietary fiber daily, respectively.

The Adequate Intake (AI) recommendation for total fiber intake for adults who are 50 years of age and younger is 38 grams per day for men and 25 grams for women daily. For adults over 50 years of age, the recommendation is 30 grams per day for men and 21 grams for women. Or 14 grams per 1,000 calories consumed. Table 4.7 provides an overview of fibers commonly used in nutrition supplements and as a food additive.

What Happens to Fiber in the Digestive Tract?

Contrary to starch, fiber is not broken down well by our digestive enzymes. This is partly explained by the manner in which the monosaccharides are linked together. Whereas digestive enzymes (amylases) produced by people are very efficient in breaking the links between monosaccharides in starch, these enzymes are generally ineffective at breaking the links between monosaccharides in fiber. Plants build these bonds in a special way.

In the stomach, soluble fibers attract and bind to water and in turn form a gel-like material. This gel entraps food components such as sugars, cholesterol and fats and slowly carries them through the remaining

Table 4.7 Fiber Sources Common to Supplements and as Food Additive

Fiber Source/Type	Fiber Details	Health Benefits
Psyllium	Refers to the mucilage found in the husks of psyllium seeds from the *Plantago ovata* or blond psyllium plant. Psyllium is a good source of soluble carbohydrate.	Psyllium supplements can improve blood cholesterol levels and lower the glycemic response of food.
Fructooligosaccharides (FOS)	Contain short chains of fructose chains that end with a molecule of glucose unit.	Enhances mineral absorption in the colon
Inulin	Similar to FOS, however its chain length can be much longer	Enhances mineral absorption in the colon
Resistant starch (resistant dextrins)	Also called resistant maltodextrins, are indigestible polysaccharides formed when starch is heated and treated with enzymes. They are used as food additives.	Reduces calorie level when substituted for starches
Methylcellulose	Methylcellulose is created from the cell wall of plants. Sold as a powder, it is indigestible and does not have calories that humans can use	Relief of constipation

digestive tract. Insoluble fibers, on the other hand, tend not to contribute to the formation of gels. Because soluble fibers dissolve in water, psyllium husk, inulin, FOS and others are used in supplemental fiber drinks as discussed below and in Chapter 13.

As fiber reaches the colon, bacteria begin to breakdown (ferment) some of the fibers for energy and in the process produce gases such as carbon dioxide, methane gas, and hydrogen gas. These gases often lead to uncomfortable bloating and flatulence associated with higher fiber intakes. Soluble fibers are more fermentable than insoluble ones. In addition other molecules, such as short-chain fatty acids, are produced by bacteria, which can be absorbed into the body. These fatty acids yield a small amount of energy and health benefits. Therefore, foods or supplements providing psyllium, beta-glucan (oats or barley), inulin, FOS, cellulose, guar gum, xanthan gum, and oligosaccharides will be fermented and you can expect gas production.

What Is Diverticulosis and Can Fiber Help?

Diverticulosis is a situation in which there is an out-pouching of the inner wall of the colon. This disorder is believed to be the result of increased pressure within the colon. In turn, this increased pressure is most likely the result of the highly refined diet that people choose to eat in the United States. A refined diet results in less fiber or "roughage" and thus less digestive leftovers or "residue" making its way into the colon. Less content in the colon results in a smaller diameter and greater pressure exerted upon its walls from within. It is a matter of physics, as there is an inverse relationship between the radius (r) of a collapsible tube and pressure (P) as follows:

$$P = 1/r^4$$

So you see, if the radius of the colon increases due to increased content then the internal pressure decreases, and vice versa. Researchers have clearly shown that those populations in the world that eat more fiber have a lower incidence of diverticulosis. Diverticulosis can lead to a medical concern called *diverticulitis*. Here the out-pouchings become impacted with bacteria and debris, leading to irritation, inflammation, pain, and sometimes bleeding.

Insoluble fibers like cellulose and hemicellulose appear to have a beneficial effect upon the formation of feces and their evacuation. Bran is an excellent source of these insoluble fibers and explains the popularity of bran breakfast cereals, muffins, and other products among individuals experiencing constipation and *diverticulosis*. Soluble fibers can contribute to mass and moistness of feces but not to the same extent as insoluble fiber. However, it is important to recognize that both types of fibers are beneficial and should be sought out for general digestive health.

Can Fiber Promote General Gut Health?

Beyond diverticulosis, fiber supports general gut health. Certain fibers, particularly soluble fibers, are probiotic. Probiotic nutrients support the health of beneficial bacteria in the digestive tract. These bacteria include bifidobacteria and lactobacilli, which are major types of bacteria found in the digestive tract. These bacteria improve the health of the digestive tract and can decrease the likelihood of gut-related issues such as irritable bowel disorders and certain tumors.

Are Certain Types of Fiber Good for Lowering Blood Cholesterol Levels?

Soluble fibers include beta-glucans, mucilages, pectins, gums, and some hemicelluloses and are purported to reduce blood cholesterol. Soluble fibers may bind to cholesterol in the digestive tract rendering them unavailable for absorption. Psyllium, oat, and barley fiber are among the most advantageous providers of soluble fiber and the Food and Drug Administration (FDA) allows claims on food packages linking the consumption of these fibers to a reduction in cholesterol. Look for the following health claim on a food containing psyllium fiber: "The soluble fiber from psyllium seed husk in this product, as part of a diet low in saturated fat and cholesterol, may reduce the risk of heart disease."

A product must contain at least 1.7 grams of soluble fiber from psyllium seed husk per serving in order to have the health claim on its label.

Additionally, there is evidence to suggest that the short-chain fatty acids (acetic, butyric, propionic, and valeric acids) and lactate produced in the colon by bacterial breakdown of soluble dietary fibers may reduce cholesterol formation in the liver. Thus, soluble fibers can inhibit cholesterol absorption from the digestive tract as well as cholesterol production in the liver. These two factors may lead to reductions in the level of cholesterol in blood; this will be explored more thoroughly in Chapter 13.

Is Fiber Good for Diabetics?

Fiber is important to people who have diabetes for two reasons. First, fiber lowers the glycemic index and load of a food by adding bulk. In addition, soluble fibers promote the formation of gels in the stomach which slows the digestion and absorption of carbohydrates. These effects lower the glycemic response of a food and contribute to better blood glucose management. Fiber consumption, particularly whole grains, seems to increase insulin sensitivity. This means that the level of circulating insulin will be lower throughout the day, which can lower the risk of heart disease (see Chapter 13). Lastly, fiber promotes satiety and can reduce total food consumption at a meal leading to less carbohydrate and fewer calories consumed. In turn, reducing the number of calories consumed can promote weight loss in overweight people with diabetes, which is important as most are overweight, primarily those with type 2.

Can Fibers Enhance Mineral Absorption?

Soluble fibers such as inulin and FOS enhance the absorption of some minerals in the colon, namely calcium and magnesium. While researchers are trying to better understand how this occurs, it would seem that there are a couple of possibilities. First, minerals such as calcium and magnesium can bind to fibers further up in the digestive tract. Then when soluble fibers are broken down in the colon they are released and available for absorption. The creation of acids (short-chain fatty acids and lactate) when soluble fiber is broken down by bacteria decreases the pH of the colon, which in turn enhances the absorption of calcium and magnesium.

Can Fiber Support Immune Function?

In addition to supporting heart and gut health as well as enhancing the absorption of key minerals, dietary fiber can also enhance the immune system. When soluble fibers are broken down by bacteria in the colon the by-products seem to increase the production of T helper cells and antibodies, as well enhance key immune system operations that provide immune protection.

Are There Other Dietary Considerations When Eating a High-Fiber Diet?

Perhaps the most obvious consideration is the production of gases, which may lead to bloating and cramping and the possibility of diarrhea. These symptoms seem to be most common when people who are not fiber consumers increase their fiber intake dramatically. It is recommended that people who are sensitive to fiber and these effects ramp up their intake slowly. Because fiber binds water, which is used to soften stool, there might be an additional need for water. This is easily solved by consuming fiber foods and supplements with water or other fluid.

FAQ Highlight

What Are Noncalorie and Low Calorie Sweeteners and Are They Safe?

Monosaccharides and disaccharides make foods like fruits and honey sweet. They can be used by food manufacturers to make recipe foods sweet and are referred to as natural sweeteners. However, since natural sweeteners come with an energy value, food manufacturers and people often try to substitute an alternative sweetener that does not carry the same energy content. This in turn lowers the calorie level of a food, thereby making it more attractive for weight loss and management. And because simple sugars in food can adhere to our teeth and promote the formation of dental caries, many candies and gums are manufactured with alternative sweeteners to reduce their potential to promote tooth decay. As a food additive, these substances must be approved for use by the Food and Drug Administration (FDA), who determines the safety.

Saccharin—Discovered in 1879, saccharin is three hundred times sweeter than sucrose. Saccharin has long been a controversial sweetener and the FDA proposed a ban in 1977. The reasoning behind this action was studies conducted in the 1970s that linked saccharin consumption to bladder cancer in rats. However, the media brought question to the methods used in these studies and concerns regarding the applicability to people. For instance, the rats used in studies were fed very large doses of saccharin, equivalent to several hundred diet sodas daily. Saccharin, which at this time was the only artificial sweetener on the market, was allowed continued use by food manufacturers. A follow-up population study by the FDA and the National Cancer Institute found that in general people who used saccharin were not at greater risk than people who didn't. However, the findings of the study suggested that heavy use of saccharin (more than six servings daily) might increase cancer risk. Thus the cancer-promoting potential of saccharin in people is still debated and products containing saccharin carry a warning on their labels. Saccharin is sold under the trade name Sweet'N Low®.

Aspartame—Aspartame is a dipeptide (two amino acids) and typically, amino acids alone or together are not known for their sweetening abilities. However, when these two amino acids (phenylalanine and aspartic acid) are linked together along with methanol, the result is a very potent sweetener. Since aspartame consists of amino acids, the building blocks of proteins, it has an energy value. However, because aspartame is about two hundred times sweeter than sucrose, a little bit goes a very long way as a sweetener. Thus its energy value is nominal and certainly not a concern for those who count their calories.

You will find aspartame in food substances that are served chilled, not heated. Examples include diet drinks, gelatins, and diet gums. Aspartame is subject to breakdown when heated and therefore it is not ideal for use in baked sweets. Concern has been expressed regarding consumption of aspartame and the development of neurological abnormalities such as headaches, dizziness, nausea, and other side effects. Many individuals have filed complaints with the FDA about aspartame. Some scientists think that these people may be more sensitive to one of the components of aspartame or to the small amount of formaldehyde and formate produced. Both formaldehyde and formate are considered toxic at higher intake levels, however the FDA believes the risk to be extremely low under typical circumstances. It is important to point out that since aspartame contains phenylalanine, people with a genetic condition called phenylketonuria (PKU) should avoid aspartame. Aspartame is sold under the trade name NutraSweet® and Equal®.

Sucralose—Sucralose was discovered in 1976 and the FDA approved it for use in food and beverages in 1998. Sucralose is six hundred times sweeter than sugar and unlike aspartame it is appropriate for most home cooking and baking recipes because it won't breakdown when heated. Sucralose is made by exchanging three chlorine atoms for hydroxyl (OH) groups on the sucrose molecule. Sucralose is not digested and therefore doesn't provide calories. However some of it is absorbed into the body. By and large sucralose is urinated out of the body within a few days. Some concern has been expressed by the public regarding the safety of sucralose. Despite several research studies suggesting that sucralose is safe for general use, some argue that not enough is known about long-term consumption of sucralose and whether or not some of the chlorine can be released and be problematic like other chlorine-based molecules.

Acesulfame K—Approved for use by the FDA in 1988 and has an intensity of sweetness about two hundred and fifty times that of sucrose. Acesulfame is used as a sweetener in many countries other than the United States and it appears to be usable with cold and hot food preparation. It is considered safe sweetener and is marketed under the name Sunette®.

Stevia—Stevia is not an artificial sweetener as it is derived from a South and Central American shrub. Stevia is approximately three hundred times as sweet as sucrose. Recently Stevia has been approved for use in foods and beverages in Australia and New Zealand, and there is growing pressure for the FDA to approve its use in the US. At this time, Stevia is only available in the US as a dietary supplement.

Sugar Alcohols—Since these substances can be found in plants, sugar alcohols such as sorbitol, xylitol, lactitol, mannitol, and maltitol are recognized as artificial sweeteners. Sugar alcohols are used mainly to sweeten sugar-free candies, cookies, and chewing gums as they do not promote the formation of cavities in the same way as sugars.

5   Fats and Cholesterol Are Not All Bad

Over the past couple of decades fat and cholesterol have taken a beating in the press, being labeled as the nutritional "bad boys." Often we are told to avoid them as much as possible. However, today we are told that we do indeed need fat, especially certain types of fat that might support cardiovascular and joint health as well as help support the maintenance of memory and cognition later in life. Cholesterol from food, on the other hand, might not be as potent a blood-cholesterol raiser as we once thought. So which types of fat are better for you and which are more expendable from the diet? Furthermore, how much cholesterol is okay and are some sources healthier than others? In this chapter we will answer basic questions related to fat and cholesterol, and continue to set up later chapters related to metabolism, weight loss, joint health, heart disease, and more.

The Basics of Fats and Cholesterol

What Are Lipids?

Fats and cholesterol belong to a special group of molecules called *lipids*. The members of this club have something pretty significant in common: they are relatively insoluble in water. This might not seem like a big deal, but keep in mind that most of our planet's surface is water and, more important to our topic, most of our body is water as well. Because of their inability to dissolve into water, we must make special concessions to accommodate lipids both during digestion and also inside of the body.

> Fat and cholesterol are lipids, which are a group of molecules that don't dissolve well into water.

During digestion, an emulsifying substance called *bile* is called to action to facilitate lipid digestion and absorption. As for fat and cholesterol inside of the body, they require special transport shuttles to circulate. Fat also has its own cell type specifically designed for storage. These cells are called *adipocytes*, or more commonly "fat cells," and large collections of adipocytes are called *adipose tissue*. Adipose tissue is found under the skin (subcutaneous fat) and in deeper deposits (visceral fat) such as in the abdomen, around vital organs, and throughout skeletal muscle.

What Is the Difference Between Fat, Oils, and Triglycerides?

Fats and oils are terms commonly used to refer to food sources of *triglycerides*. Often fat and oil are considered to be different based on appearance: fat is solid at room temperature and oil is liquid. However, they are really two of the same thing, generally speaking. They are both collections of triglycerides. For simplicity, we will use "fat" to include all sources of triglycerides.

A triglyceride molecule is a combination of three *fatty acids* linked to a *glycerol* molecule backbone (Figure 5.1). Although a triglyceride molecule will always have this general design, there can be great variability in the type and combinations of fatty acids that link to glycerol. Only one glycerol molecule exists, but like monosaccharides there are numerous different types of fatty acids in nature. Furthermore, if a triglyceride involves three fatty acids then monoglycerides and diglycerides will have one and two fatty acids attached to glycerol, respectively. Technically, they can be considered fat as well.

What Is Cholesterol and Can We Make It in Our Body?

Cholesterol has received its share of negative press over the years, however it is important to realize that cholesterol is absolutely vital to our

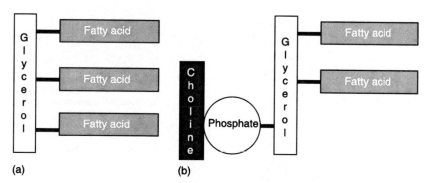

Figure 5.1 (a) Triglyceride (fat) has a glycerol "backbone" with three fatty acids attached. Thus a monoglyceride and a diglyceride would only contain one and two fatty acids, respectively. (b) Phospholipids are diglycerides with phosphate and something else attached in place of the third fatty acid. This molecule is lecithin (phosphotidylcholine).

existence. Cholesterol can be made in many cells, and under normal situations we seem to make all that we need. In fact, we will make about 1 gram of cholesterol each day depending on how much cholesterol is in the diet. The liver is by far the most productive organ when it comes to making cholesterol and one of its jobs is to share with the rest of the body. Cholesterol is a necessary component of cell membranes and many vital substances in the body are made from cholesterol (Figure 5.2). These substances include bile components, vitamin D, testosterone, estrogens, aldosterone, progesterone, and cortisol.

> Cholesterol is needed for cell membranes and to make certain hormones, digestive factors, and vitamin D.

Fatty Acids: A Closer Look

Can Fatty Acids Vary in Length?

For the most part, the length of fatty acids can vary by as much as twenty carbon atoms or so. If a fatty acid has four carbon atoms or fewer, it is referred to as a short-chain fatty acid. On the other hand, if a fatty acid chain has six to twelve or greater than twelve carbon atoms, it would be referred to as a medium-chain fatty acid or a long-chain fatty acid, respectively. Often, fatty acids with twenty or more carbon atoms are referred to as very-long-chain fatty acids. Most fatty acids in nature have

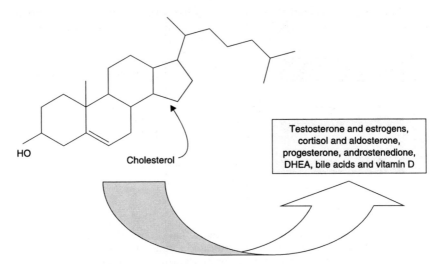

HO

Cholesterol

Testosterone and estrogens,
cortisol and aldosterone,
progesterone, androstenedione,
DHEA, bile acids and vitamin D

Figure 5.2 The cholesterol molecule and its derivatives (steroid hormones and other cholesterol-derived molecules.

an even number of carbons, yet some fatty acids do indeed have an odd number of carbons.

What Are Saturated and Unsaturated Fatty Acids?

Fatty acids can differ in their degree of saturation. Saturation refers to whether all of the carbon atoms between the end carbons are linked to two atoms of hydrogen. If this is the case, then the carbons are saturated with hydrogen and that particular fatty acid would be called a *saturated fatty acid* (SFA) (Figure 5.3). However, if, at one or more points, adjacent carbon atoms are bonded to only a single hydrogen atom each, the fatty acid would then be an *unsaturated fatty acid* (see Figure 5.3).

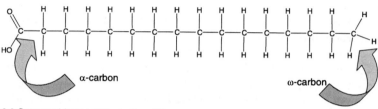

(a)   16:0 Saturated fatty acid (palmitic acid)

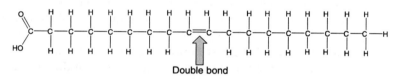

(b)   18:1 ω-9 Monounsaturated fatty acid (oleic acid)

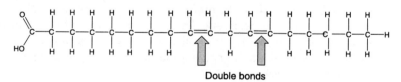

(c)   18:2 ω-6 Polyunsaturated fatty acid (linoleic acid)

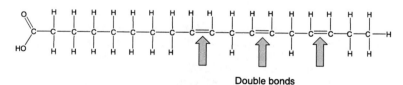

(d)   18:3 ω-3 Polyunsaturated fatty acid (linolenic acid)

Figure 5.3 (a) Saturated fatty acid showing the alpha (α) and omega (ω) carbons. (b) The monounsaturated and (c,d) polyunsaturated fatty acids have their unsaturation points indicated.

By nature, when two adjacent carbon atoms in a fatty acid are linked to only one hydrogen atom each, the carbon atoms must bond to each other twice. Chemists call this a *double bond* and if a fatty acid has only one double bond, it is referred to as a *monounsaturated* fatty acid (MUFA). Meanwhile, if there is more than one double bond, then it is a *polyunsaturated* fatty acid (PUFA).

What Does "Omega" Mean with Regards to Fatty Acids?

Because fatty acids can vary greatly, scientists will indicate the number of carbons and double bonds in a fatty acid. For instance a 18:3 fatty acid will be 18 carbons long and have three double bonds. Scientists also use *omega* system to indicate where double bonds are in a fatty acid. It works like this. If a fatty acid is linked to glycerol, the second carbon closest to the link is referred to as the *alpha* (α) carbon (see Figure 5.3). Meanwhile, the carbon furthest from the linkage with glycerol is called the omega (ω) carbon.

The omega system is based on the Greek alphabet. Alpha is the first letter of the alphabet and omega is the last. No matter how many carbons are in your fatty acid chain, these carbon atoms will always be addressed in this manner. Looking at a fatty acid not linked to glycerol, the alpha carbon would be the first carbon atom adjacent to the carbon bonded to two atoms of oxygen. Table 5.1 lists common fatty acids and their abbreviations.

To indicate position of the first double bond we count the number of carbons to the first carbon of the first double bond from the omega end. For instance, if the first double bond starts at the third carbon atom in, it is an omega-3 (ω-3) fatty acid (see Figure 5.3). Likewise, if the first double bond appears at the sixth or the ninth carbon atom in, these would be ω-6 and ω-9 fatty acids, respectively. For the most part, when addressing polyunsaturated fatty acids, we indicate only the position of the first double bond because subsequent double bonds seem to occur in series after one saturated carbon atom.

Table 5.1 Common Fatty Acids

Acetic acid (2:0)	Myristic acid (14:0)	Arachidic acid (20:0)
Butyric acid (4:0)	Palmitic acid (16:0)	Arachidonic acid (20:4 ω-6)
Caproic acid (6:0)	Palmitoleic acid (16:1 ω-9)	Eicosapentaenoic acid (EPA)
Caprylic acid (8:0)	Stearic acid (18:0)	(20:5 ω-3)
Capric acid (10:0)	Oleic acid (18:1 ω-9)	Docosahexaenoic acid
Lauric acid (12:0)	Linoleic acid (18:2 ω-6)	(DHA) (22:6 ω-3)
	Linolenic acid (18:3 ω-3)	

What Are "Trans" Fatty Acids?

Taking a closer look at double bonds in Figure 5.4, we see that there can be some variation in the position of the hydrogen atoms. If the hydrogen atoms attached to the carbon atoms of a double bond are positioned on the same side of the double bond, it is a *cis* bond that is the predominant way they are found in nature. If the hydrogen atoms bonded to the carbon atoms are on opposite sides of the double bond, it is referred to as a *trans fatty acid*.

Interest has been growing regarding the presence of *trans* fatty acids in our diet and their potential impact upon health. Although *cis* versus *trans* may seem like a very minor point in regard to fatty acid design, these contrasting forms can impart different properties to a fatty acid. *Cis* double bonds cause a kinking or bending of the fatty acid, while *trans* double bonds do not. This makes unsaturated fatty acids with *trans* double bonds similar to saturated fatty acids in that they do not bend or kink. We will discuss *trans* fatty acids in more detail below as well as in Chapter 13.

Trans fats are like saturated fats in that they don't bend, and increase the risk of cardiovascular disease.

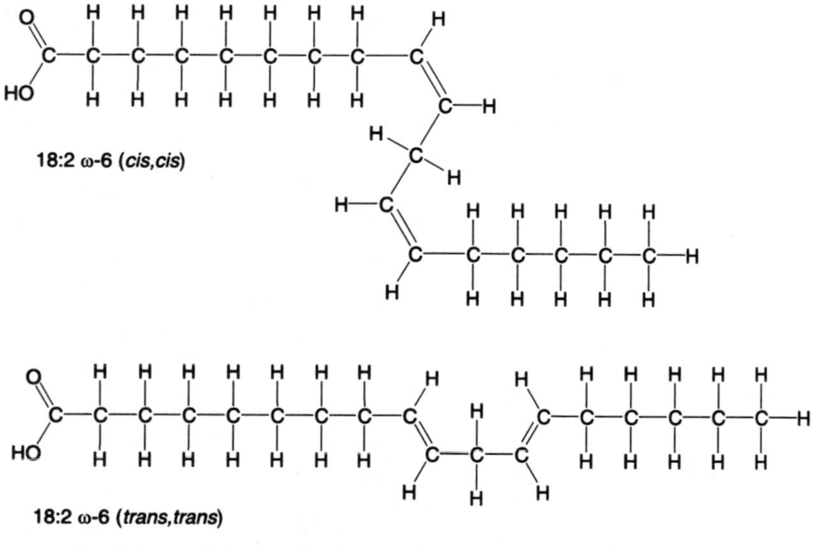

18:2 ω-6 (*cis,cis*)

18:2 ω-6 (*trans,trans*)

Figure 5.4 The top fatty acid is the same as in Figure 5.3c and it demonstrates its true three-dimensional design. The bottom fatty acid is the same as the top fatty acid, except that the double bonds are *trans* instead of *cis*. The *trans* double bonds fail to effectively kink the fatty acid chain.

What Do We Mean by Saturated and Unsaturated Fats?

Regardless of the origin of a triglyceride source (plant or animal), the triglycerides will contain a mixture of fatty acids. When we say that a fat source is *saturated*, we are indicating that the majority of the fatty acids within the source are saturated. For instance, we often refer to butter and beef fat as saturated fats. This is because the majority of their fatty acids are saturated. Table 5.2 lists the approximate percentages of fatty acids for each food source.

Why Are Oils Liquid at Room Temperature While Fats Are Solid?

In general, if the majority of fatty acids in a triglyceride source are saturated, then it most likely will be solid at room temperature. Contrarily, if a triglyceride source contains a greater percentage of unsaturated fatty acids, especially PUFA, then this source will most likely be liquid at room temperature. Saturated fatty acids are straighter than unsaturated fatty acid. This allows them to pack closer together and to be more solid. Take a look at Table 5.2 and notice how the oils have a higher percentage of unsaturated fatty acids while the more solid fats (lard, tallow, etc.) have a high percentage of saturated fatty acids. Despite their names, palm oil and palm kernel oil are more solid at room temperature.

Table 5.2 Approximate Fatty Acid Composition of Common Triglyceride Sources

Type of Fat	SFA (%)	MUFA (%)	PUFA (%)
Butter fat	66	30	4
Beef fat	52	44	4
Lard	41	47	12
Coconut oil	87	6	2
Palm kernel oil	81	11	2
Palm oil	49	37	9
Vegetable shortening	28	44	28
Peanut oil	18	49	33
Margarine	17	49	34
Soybean oil	15	24	61
Olive oil	14	77	9
Corn oil	13	25	62
Sunflower oil	11	20	69
Safflower oil	10	13	77
Canola oil	6	62	32

SFA = saturated fatty acid; monounsaturated fatty acid (MUFA); polyunsaturated fatty acid (PUFA).

Can Different Kinds of Fatty Acids Be Part of the Same Triglyceride Molecule?

There are probably no definite rules as to the selection of fatty acids that make up a triglyceride molecule. One triglyceride molecule may be composed of one saturated, one monounsaturated, and one polyunsaturated fatty acid, all of the same or varying lengths. However, the types of fatty acids found within triglyceride molecules will depend on the plant or the animal source. For instance, the triglycerides in olive oil largely contain the MUFA oleic acid (18:1 ω-9) (about 82 percent), while about two-thirds of the fatty acids in butter are SFAs of varying length.

The presence of certain types of fatty acids in either a plant or an animal largely depends upon the nature of the plant or animal and the purpose of the fat for that life-form. For instance, fish that live in deeper water tend to be better sources of ω-3 PUFA because these fatty acids are found in the cell membranes of these fish and play a protective role against the increased pressure and decreased temperatures at greater depths as well as help regulate their buoyancy. Land animals create storage fat that is largely composed of saturated fatty acid. Since these fat molecules can pack tightly in fat cells it minimizes the necessary space.

Fat and Cholesterol Requirements and Food Sources

What Foods Provide Us with Triglycerides and Cholesterol?

As displayed in Table 5.3, fats and oils, and thus triglycerides, are present in both animals and plants. Oil is a natural component of many plant tissues including leaves, stem, roots, kernels, nuts, and seeds. Common edible oils include sunflower, safflower, corn, olive, coconut, canola, and palm oil. Contrarily, butter is made from the fat in milk, while lard is hog fat, and tallow is the fat of cattle or sheep. Other animal flesh will contain fat, including poultry and their eggs.

Cholesterol is not a necessary substance for plants; therefore they do not need to make it. Contrarily, mammals will make cholesterol to help meet their body needs. As a result, cholesterol intake in the diet is attributed only to consumption of animal foods or foods that have animal products in their recipe. It should be mentioned though that plants do create molecules that are similar to cholesterol called *phytosterols* which we will discuss in Chapters 12 and 13.

How Are Vegetable Oils Produced?

Vegetable oils are the edible oils extracted from seeds, nuts, kernels and other plant tissue. Edible vegetable oils are extracted from plants using solvents such a hexane and/or through mechanical processes such as cold pressing and expelling. Mechanical processing does not involve solvents

Table 5.3 Approximate Fat and Cholesterol Content of Various Foods (by Weight)

	Fat (%)	Cholesterol (%)
Animal foods		
Beef	32	<1
Bologna	29	1
Butter	82	2
chicken, white meat	4	<1
Cheese, cheddar	32	1
Cheese, cottage (4%)	4	1
Codfish	<1	Trace
Egg, whole	12	4
Egg, white	<1	Trace
Halibut	3	Trace
Hamburger	13	<1
Lamb chops	36	1
Mackerel	6	Trace
Margarine	82	0
Milk (whole)	3	<1
Milk (skim)	Trace	Trace
Pork chops	21	1
Pork sausage	46	1
Salmon	4	Trace
Plant foods		
Avocados	13	0
Bread (white)	4	<1
Cereals and grains	1–2	0
Crackers	1	0
Fruits	<1	0
Leafy vegetables	<1	0
Legumes	<1	0
Margarine	82	0
Root vegetables	<1	0

Percentage of a food's mass that is attributable to fat. To determine grams of fat in a food simply multiply the percentage by the weight (grams) of the food.

and the major difference is the temperature of the extraction processes. Cold pressing involves a hydraulic press between two plates and the temperature tends to stay below 120°F. Meanwhile, expelling involves a screwing mechanism which results in more frictional heat allowing the temperature to reach as high as 185°F.

How Much Fat Do We Need in Our Diet?

At this time there is not a Recommended Dietary Allowance (RDA) (or Adequate Intake (AI)) for total fat. Meanwhile an Acceptable

Macronutrient Distribution Range (AMDR) has been declared as 20 to 35 percent of energy, which would be practical for most people based on today's food supply. It is important to realize that the AMDR is not a requirement level and many nutrition scientists believe that the absolute lowest requirement for fat in our diet could be as little as 5 percent of calories (for weight maintenance) as long as it is derived from healthier sources including seeds, plant oils, as well as fish and other marine life.

Some fat is needed in the diet to provide essential fatty acids, which are important regulatory factors.

Are There Essential Fatty Acids?

The need for dietary fat is not necessarily for energy purposes. Fat is needed in our diet as a means of providing two essential fatty acids, *linoleic acid*, an ω-6 PUFA, and α-*linolenic acid*, an ω-3 PUFA. Since the amount of these fatty acids in fat storage (adipose tissue) is limited, this suggests that their role in our body isn't really to provide calories, although they will be used for energy. Linoleic and α-linolenic acid are used to make longer, more complex fatty acids that have special functions.

Linoleic acid is used to make a longer ω-6 fatty acid called arachidonic acid (ARA) while α-linolenic acid is used to produce longer ω-3 fatty acids, namely eicosapentaenoic acid (EPA) and docosahexaenoic acid (DHA). Both ARA and DHA are found in higher concentration in the brain and are vital for the development of the central nervous system and eyes. Meanwhile, EPA and ARA can be used to make factors called eicosanoids (for example, prostaglandins, thromboxanes, and leukotrienes) that help regulate many bodily functions as discussed below and in later chapters.

What Foods Are Good Sources of Essential Fatty Acids?

Good sources of linoleic acid are safflower oil, sunflower seeds (oil roasted), pine nuts, sunflower oil, corn oil, soybean oil, pecans (oil roasted), Brazil nuts, cottonseed oil, and sesame seed oil. Dietary surveys in the United States suggest that the intake of linoleic acid is about 12 to 17 grams for men and 9 to 11 grams for women.

Good plant sources of α-linolenic acid are flaxseed and walnuts—their oils are among the best sources of α-linolenic acid—as are soybean, canola, and linseed oil as well as some leafy vegetables. Diet surveys in the United States suggest that typical intakes of α-linolenic acid are about 1.2 to 1.6 grams daily for men and 0.9 to 1.1 grams daily for women.

Therefore the ratio of linoleic acid to α-linolenic acid is about 10 to 1, a point that will become more important later in this chapter and in Chapters 12 and 13.

Marine mammals (for example, whale, seal, and walrus) and the oil derived from cold-water fish (cod liver, herring, menhaden, and salmon oils) provide *eicosapentaenoic acid* (EPA) and *docosahexaenoic acid* (DHA). EPA and DHA are fatty acids that are made from linolenic acid in marine animals. A lot of interest in the ω-3 PUFA was created when researchers reported that there is a lower incidence of heart disease in some populations, such as Greenlanders. Diet patterns showed high fish consumption in these people, which leads to greater ω-3 PUFA intake and a reduced incidence of heart disease. In addition, there are links between the consumption of fish and cognitive development as well as reducing age-related losses in memory and cognition.

> Fish and fish oil supplements are good sources of the omega-3 fatty acids DHA and EPA.

What Foods Contain Trans Fatty Acids?

Trans fatty acids can be found in many fat sources although its prevalence is very low. Bovine (cows, steer, oxen, etc) food sources are probably the greatest natural contributors of *trans* fatty acids to the human diet. For instance, beef, butter, and milk triglycerides may contain 2 to 8 percent of their fatty acids as *trans* fatty acids. Interestingly, cattle are not solely responsible for generating this *trans* fatty acid content. It is actually the bacteria in their unique stomachs that produce the *trans* fatty acid. These fatty acids are then absorbed by the cow and make their way into the tissues and milk of these animals.

In addition, *trans* fatty acids can be created during the processing of oils (that is, margarine and other hydrogenated oils), which will be described later, and when cooking oils are re-used over long periods, such as in fast-food restaurants and diners. In more recent decades, more than half of the *trans* fatty acids in the human diet were derived from processed oils either consumed plain or used in recipes (for example, fried foods, baked snack foods). Cookies, crackers, and other snack foods that utilize hydrogenated vegetable oil may contain up to 9 to 10 percent of their fatty acids as *trans* fatty acids.

Because the consumption of higher amounts of *trans* fatty acids is linked to increased risk of heart disease and stroke, the American Heart Association, and the most recent Dietary Reference Intakes (DRIs) in the United States and Canada, recommend limiting the *trans* fat level of the diet. In addition, food manufacturers in many countries, including the

United States and Canada, are required to list the *trans* fat levels in the Nutrition Facts on food labels. Because of this, snack-food manufacturers are choosing hydrogenated oils with lower *trans* fat content to produce snack foods. Furthermore, in 2006 New York City placed a ban on *trans* fat in restaurants, a public health initiative that is being followed by other cities.

What Is Margarine?

Margarine was first developed in the nineteenth century as an alternative for butter. Early on it was a popular butter substitute for people who could not afford butter or to whom butter was not available. Margarine can be made from animal fats and/or vegetable oils; however, the bulk of margarine containing products today use vegetable oil based margarines. This is partly attributable to the relationship between a diet high in saturated fat in animal fat and the risk of heart disease. Plant oils tend to have fewer saturated fatty acids and do not contain cholesterol. More specifically, plant oils have much lower amounts of three types of saturated fatty acids (that is 16:0, 14:0, and 12:0), which are the SFAs that seem to be most associated with raised blood cholesterol levels.

Today, margarine from plant oils is made by adding hydrogen to unsaturated fatty acids in plant oils. Scientists called this process *hydrogenation*, during which some PUFAs are converted to MUFAs and some of the MUFAs are converted to SFAs (Table 5.4). This converts the liquid oil to semisolid or to solid fat. Hydrogenation occurs when the oils are heated up in a container and hydrogen gas is applied. The degree of change depends upon how much hydrogenation is allowed to take place. For instance, margarines that come in stick form are typically more hydrogenated than softer tub margarine.

> Margarine is typically made by solidifying plant oils in a process called hydrogenation.

Table 5.4 Margarine Made by Hydrogenating Corn Oil

Fat Source	SFA (%)	MUFA (%)	PUFA (%)
Corn oil	13	25	62
Margarine (from corn oil)	17	49	34

SFA = saturated fatty acid; monounsaturated fatty acid (MUFA); polyunsaturated fatty acid (PUFA).
During hydrogenation some of the PUFA become MUFA and some of the MUFA became SFA.

The most popular plant oil used for hydrogenation is soybean oil. Because of their relatively high content of MUFA and PUFA, margarines made from soybean, sunflower, safflower, olive, and cottonseed oils are perceived to be healthier than butter. However, when energy (heat) is applied to plant oils during hydrogenation, a small number of the *cis* double bonds can be converted to *trans* double bonds, which helps solidify the oil. In fact, conventional margarines have a higher *trans* fatty acid content than butter and typically the harder the margarine the higher the *trans* fatty acid level. Food companies have been working successfully over the past decade to alter their process for forming margarine to lower and eliminate the *trans* fat content, which is reflected on the food labels.

Digestion and Absorption of Fat and Cholesterol

How Are Lipids Digested in the Watery Digestive Tract?

Digestion is a watery affair and has been loosely compared to whitewater rafting. In addition to the water-based fluids we drink, liters of water-based fluid enter the digestive tract daily as part of saliva and other digestive juices. Dissolved in those fluids that our body provides are digestive enzymes. This means that our digestive enzymes are water soluble, while their task is to interact with and break down water-insoluble lipids for absorption. This presents an interesting yet readily solved problem.

When lipids are present in the small intestine the natural course would be for these substances to clump together. This is analogous to oil clumping together in the kitchen sink when we wash dishes, or to the separation of oil from the watery portion of traditional salad dressings. If lipids remain clumped together in the small intestine, surely the efficient digestion of these substances would be hindered? To solve this potential problem, *bile* is delivered to the small intestine and serves as an emulsifier or detergent during lipid digestion. Here, components of bile coat smaller droplets of lipid, rendering them water soluble, as depicted in Figure 5.5. Bile activity keeps larger lipid droplets from reforming. So instead of having a few very large droplets of lipids, the result is many tiny droplets. When lipids are present as tiny droplets, digestive enzymes have no problem attacking them and efficiently doing their job.

Which Enzymes Digest Fat and Cholesterol?

Although a triglyceride-digesting enzyme called *lingual lipase* is present in saliva, the job of digesting triglycerides is mostly handled by another lipase enzyme delivered by the pancreas. Pancreatic lipase detaches two fatty acids from glycerol, which results in a monoglyceride and two fatty

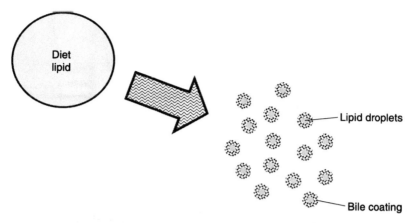

Figure 5.5 Small lipid droplets are created because of the mixing actions of our
stomach and small intestine. Bile components coat the little lipid droplets making them water-soluble and rendering fats, cholesterol, and
other lipids easier to digest and absorb.

acids (Figure 5.6). In turn, the remaining fatty acid may be detached by
yet another enzyme from some of the monoglycerides. This would then
produce glycerol and a fatty acid. Thus, the products of triglyceride digestion are fatty acids, monoglycerides, and glycerol, which are now small
enough to move into the cells lining the small intestine. Meanwhile, some
of the cholesterol in our diet is actually linked to other molecules, with
the most prevalent attachments being fatty acids. These are often referred
to as *cholesterol esters*. Other digestive enzymes *(cholesterol esterase)* will
liberate cholesterol so that it can be absorbed.

> The digestion of fat and cholesterol requires bile and lipase enzymes
> and the assistance of the lymphatic circulation.

How Efficient Is Fat Digestion and Can We Decrease Fat Absorption?

The efficiency of the digestion and absorption of the fat and cholesterol
we eat is greater than 90 percent. Certain drugs and dietary supplements
have been marketed to reduce the absorption of fat from the diet. For
instance, the supplement chitosan is fiber-like substance derived from
chitin. Chitin is a polysaccharide-like structure made up of amino sugars
(sugars with nitrogen) which helps harden the shells of shellfish (shrimp,
lobster, crab), insects (beetles), and is also found in some other animals
and the cell walls of some fungi. Chitosan is a processed form of chitin

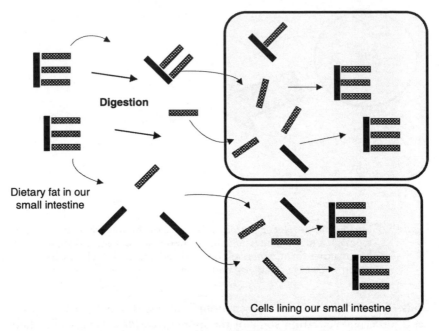

Figure 5.6 Triglyceride are digested to fatty acids, monoglycerides and some glycerol, all of which move into the cells lining our small intestine. Triglycerides are put back together inside these cells and put into chylomicrons to enter circulation (lymphatic).

and it is used in the food and drug industry and in supplements. Chitosan is more water soluble than chitin and is often marketed as a fat binder in the digestive tract.

In addition the drug xenical (Orlistat) hinders the actions of pancreatic lipase, the principal fat-digesting enzyme. This results in less absorption of diet-derived fat and more fat in the feces. Orlistat has been shown in research studies to be an effective therapy for weight loss and is recommended in conjunction with a healthy, reduced calorie and fat diet and exercise program. Because Orlistat can increase the amount of fat in the lower digestive tract there is the potential for side effects such as loose, oily stools and flatulence. Furthermore, because there is the possibility of reduced absorption of fat-soluble vitamins, manufacturers recommend the use of a supplement at least 2 hours before the use of Orlistat.

Will Gall Bladder Removal Stop Fat Digestion?

Bile is made in the liver and stored in the gallbladder in-between meals. Disorders involving the liver or gallbladder can lead to reduced bile production and/or delivery to the small intestine. When fat-containing food particles arrive in the small intestine, bile is squeezed out of the gallbladder and travels to the small intestine through a duct. Some people have their gallbladder removed for medical reasons. Since bile is made in the liver and the gallbladder merely functions as a temporary storage depot for bile, this is not a serious concern. In many cases, the liver sends adequate amounts of bile directly to the small intestine to support adequate digestion of a reasonably sized meal. However, if fat is not efficiently digested and absorbed, a lower-fat diet might be prescribed by a physician. The presence of increased amounts of fat in feces can be used to gauge the efficiency of fat digestion and absorption. Feces will become more pale and greasy in appearance when proper absorption does not occur. In addition, bacterial metabolism of some of the fat may result in some discomforting symptoms as well.

How Are Triglycerides and Cholesterol Absorbed?

Absorbing lipids into the body requires special consideration. Since the blood is water-based, how can these water-insoluble substances circulate? Cells lining the wall of the small intestine reassemble triglycerides and package them up along with cholesterol into shuttles called chylomicrons. Chylomicrons can leave these cells and enter the lymphatic circulation before enter the blood. Chylomicrons are very large and are unable to squeeze through the entry holes to the blood stream. Instead they drain into the larger openings to the lymphatic circulation. Within minutes, chylomicrons will circulate to a duct in the chest that gives them access to the blood (Figure 5.7). Once in the blood, a chylomicron will circulate for about a half hour, delivering its lipid bounty to tissue throughout the body.

Fat Storage, Mobilization, and Use

What Happens to Dietary Fat in Our Body?

When we eat a meal containing fat, it is absorbed and circulates within chylomicrons. As it circulates, fat is slowly transferred from chylomicrons to fat cells as well as skeletal muscle, heart, and other organs (breast tissue, for example) (see Figure 5.7). In order to transfer diet-derived fat to our tissue, an enzyme must be present in that tissue. The enzyme is called *lipoprotein lipase* (LPL) and just like lingual lipase and pancreatic lipase, LPL also removes fatty acids from glycerol. The fatty acids liberated by LPL move out of the chylomicrons and enter the nearby cells. Scientists have studied LPL for years and it now seems that differing levels of LPL activity in different locations of adipose tissue may partly explain why people seem to accumulate more fat stores in some regions of their bodies and not as much in other areas.

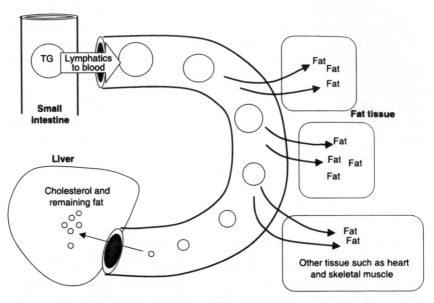

Figure 5.7 Chylomicrons are made in the cells that line the wall of our small intestine and they carry a lot of fat and a lesser amount of cholesterol from the diet. They enter the lymphatic circulation and then the blood and then deposit nearly all of their fat before being removed by our liver.

While a little bit of dietary fat can be used for energy very early during a meal as the body shifts from a fasting to a fed state, by and large dietary fat is destined for storage or put to use in other ways. By design, fat cells will store loads of fat and insulin promotes this activity. On the contrary, skeletal muscle cells and the heart have a limited ability to store fat. However, the amount of fat that skeletal muscle can store can be increased by aerobic training (such as running and biking). The importance of this fat is related to performance, as during exercise this fat is readily available to the muscle cells in which it is stored. In addition, aerobic exercise training also promotes adaptations in muscle cells, making them better fat burners during and after exercise. More on the relationship between exercise and fat burning and storage will be discussed in later chapters.

Body fat is primarily derived from food fat and secondarily from fat production in fat tissue and the liver.

Can We Make Fat?

While diet-derived fat is being deposited in tissue throughout the body, if a lot of carbohydrate and/or protein were consumed, some can be converted to fat. This takes place in the liver and fat cells, with the latter only able to use glucose to make fat. Insulin promotes this activity, which makes sense since diet-derived carbohydrate and some amino acids raise insulin levels. The principle fatty acid products are palmitic acid (16:0) and oleic acid (18:1 ω-9) and palmoleic acid (16:1 ω-9). The fat made in fat cells is stored within those cells, while the fat made in the liver is packaged up and relocated mostly to fat cells for storage.

Contrary to popular belief the ability of the body to make fat from excessive dietary carbohydrate and protein is not as strong as once thought. However it does occur and for some people and situations, such as long-term excessive calorie intake, the involved processes are stronger. On the other hand, deriving more fat from polyunsaturated fat sources such as plant and fish oils can reduce these processes.

While fat manufacturing from diet-derived energy building blocks such as carbohydrates (glucose and fructose) and protein (some amino acids) does occur, it only explains a portion of the accumulated body fat during weight gain. The majority of the fat accumulated is from the diet. Since fat is mostly consumed with carbohydrate and protein, both of which raise insulin levels, more dietary fat is directed to storage. Since too many total calories are being consumed more fat will be directed into storage than broken down for use as fuel. Thus there is a net gain of body fat which in turn increases body weight.

How and When Do We Remove Fat from Our Fat Cells?

The fat stored in fat cells is available to us when food energy is not being absorbed (fasting) and when we exercise. Just as the hormone insulin promoted the storage of fat when energy was coming into our body, the process of mobilizing fat from fat cells is promoted by the hormones released into our blood when we are fasting and/or exercising (Figure 5.8). These hormones are glucagon, epinephrine, and cortisol, and all promote the release of fat from fat stores.

In order for fat to be released from fat cells, fat is first broken down to fatty acids and glycerol, which then enter our blood and circulate. However, because of their general water insolubility, the fatty acids will hitch a ride aboard a protein in the blood called *albumin*. On the contrary, glycerol is fairly water soluble and can dissolve into blood. In fact, researchers will measure the level of glycerol in the blood to estimate how much fat is being broken down.

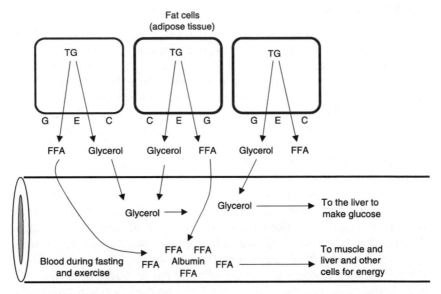

Figure 5.8 Circulating glucagon (G), epinephrine (E) and cortisol (C) tell our fat cells to breakdown their triglyceride (TG) to free fatty acids (FFA) and glycerol.

> Body fat is broken down to serve as energy in-between meals and during exercise.

Circulating fatty acids are removed by cells, especially skeletal muscle and our heart, liver, and other organs and then used by those tissues primarily for energy. However, keep in mind that cells of the brain and red blood cells (RBC) cannot use fatty acids for energy and will continue to use glucose. Conveniently the glycerol released from fat tissue can be used to make glucose in the liver and released into circulation to help maintain a desirable level of circulating glucose during prolonged exercise and fasting.

Fat and Cholesterol Need Special Help to Get Around in Our Body

How Are Lipids Shuttled Around in Our Blood?

Not only will our liver make a fair amount of cholesterol and fat on a daily basis, but it will also receive these nutrients from diet-derived chylomicrons. Like fat, most cholesterol is housed in the liver for only a short period of time as it is destined for other tissues throughout the body. Once cholesterol reaches other tissues, it can be used to make some of the substances listed previously or to become part of cell membranes. Some of the cholesterol in our liver is also used to make bile salts, a key component of bile.

Whether they are coming from the digestive tract or the liver special transportation vehicles or *lipoproteins* are needed to circulate lipids. Generally speaking, lipoproteins are a protein-containing shell encasing the lipid substances in need of transportation (Figure 5.9). Lipoproteins can be divided into four general classes based upon their densities (see Figure 5.9). In order of increasing density lipoproteins are chylomicrons, *very low density lipoproteins* (VLDLs), *low density lipoproteins* (LDLs), and *high density lipoproteins* (HDLs). Looking at the composition of these lipoproteins in Figure 5.9, we see that the greater the lipid to protein ratio, the lower the density. This makes perfect sense because lipids are less dense than proteins.

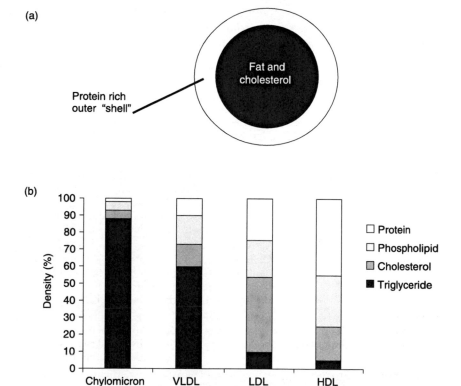

Figure 5.9 (a) Lipoproteins are lipids encased in a water-soluble protein shell. (b) Our blood contains several types of lipoproteins, which can be separated based upon their density (lipid to protein ratio). Chylomicrons are the biggest and have the highest ratio, opposite to HDL.

The proteins that help make up the lipoprotein shell are called *apoproteins*. Not only do they make the lipoprotein more soluble in water, but they will also function in helping the lipoprotein be recognized by specific tissues throughout our body. This allows a lipoprotein either to unload some of its lipid cargo or to be removed from the blood and broken down. For instance, the receptor for LDLs is located in the liver tissue and also in other tissue throughout the body. When a specific apoprotein on an LDL docks on the LDL receptor, this allows the LDL to be removed from the blood.

What Is the General Activity of Chylomicrons?

As summarized in Table 5.5, chylomicrons are made by the cells lining our small intestine and transport diet-derived lipids throughout the body. Chylomicron composition reflects our dietary lipid intake; therefore, they contain mostly fat. As chylomicrons circulate they unload most of their fat in fat tissue and other tissues such as muscle, as described previously. Once most of the fat has been removed the chylomicron is much smaller and is recognized and removed from the blood by the liver where it is broken down. Any cholesterol and leftover fat becomes the property of the liver.

Table 5.5 The Most Abundant Lipoproteins

Lipoprotein Class	Site of Production	General Activity	Fate
Chylomicrons	Small intestine	Transport dietary fat and cholesterol from digestive tract. Much of the fat is deposited in fat and muscle tissue	Chylomicron remnants containing cholesterol and remaining fat are removed from the blood by the liver
Very low density lipoproteins (VLDLs)	Liver	Delivery of fat and cholesterol from the liver to tissue throughout the body	As they circulate they deposit fat in fat tissue and other tissue and become LDLs
Low density lipoproteins (LDLs)	Derived from VLDL in circulation	Deposit cholesterol in tissue throughout our body	Eventually removed from the blood by the liver and to a lesser degree other tissue
High density lipoproteins (HDLs)	Produced by the liver and small intestine	Circulate and pick up cholesterol from tissue throughout the body	Eventually removed from circulation primarily by the liver

What Are Low Density Lipoproteins and How Do They Function?

As mentioned earlier, not only will the liver receive cholesterol and some fat from chylomicrons, but it is also a primary cholesterol- and triglyceride-producing organ in the body. Fat and cholesterol in excess of the liver's needs are packaged up into VLDLs and released into our circulation. As VLDLs circulate throughout our body, they unload a lot of their fat, mostly in fat cells. As a result their lipid to protein ratio decreases, which renders them denser, and they become LDLs (Figure 5.10). Therefore, LDL is derived from circulating VLDL.

LDL has two fates. One fate is to continue to circulate throughout the body and deposit cholesterol in various tissues. The second fate is to be recognized by tissue, removed from the blood, and broken down. Many tissues throughout our body can do this, but the liver handles more than half of the task. The longer LDLs circulate, the more opportunity there is for cholesterol to be deposited throughout our body.

> LDLs contain mostly cholesterol and serve to deliver it throughout the body.

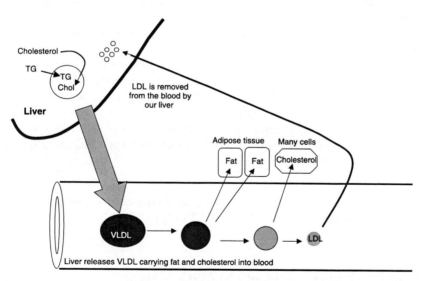

Figure 5.10 Very low density lipoproteins (VLDLs) release their fat to tissue (mostly adipose tissue) yielding low density lipoproteins (LDLs), which continue to circulate and to deliver cholesterol to tissue. LDLs are then removed from blood mostly by the liver.

Where Do High Density Lipoproteins Come From and What Do They Do?

The last type of lipoprotein is HDL. HDL is made in our liver and to a lesser extent in our intestines. It is HDL's job to circulate and pick up excess cholesterol from tissues throughout our body and return it to the liver. The whole process is very interesting because in order for circulating HDL to return the cholesterol to our liver, some of the cholesterol is first passed to circulating LDLs. The LDL is then subject to removal from our circulation by the liver and broken down. HDL delivers the rest of its cholesterol directly to the liver. In regard to heart disease, if LDL wears the villain's black hat, as higher levels are linked to increased risk of a heart attack and stroke, then HDL wears the hero's white hat, as higher levels are linked to lower risk. We will spend more time talking about blood lipids and cardiovascular disease in Chapter 13.

What Information Can We Derive from a Blood Cholesterol Test?

When a health professional refers to our blood cholesterol level it is usually total cholesterol. Total cholesterol is the sum of the cholesterol in all of the lipoproteins circulating in our blood at the time of the blood draw. Since chylomicrons will circulate only for a couple of hours after a meal, they should be absent from blood drawn after an overnight fast. If there are chylomicrons in a fasting blood sample it could indicate a medical condition whereby chylomicrons are not rapidly and efficiently processed.

The fractions of total cholesterol are the amount of cholesterol found in each type or class of lipoproteins. Thus LDL-cholesterol is the cholesterol only found in LDL. And likewise HDL-cholesterol is the cholesterol found only in HDL. With regard to heart attacks and strokes, having a total cholesterol level greater than 200 milligrams per 100 milliliters of blood and elevated LDL- and low HDL-cholesterol levels increase the risk (Table 5.6 has a sample lipid profile).

> A total cholesterol level is the sum of all the cholesterol in lipoproteins primarily LDLs, HDLs and VLDLs.

Body Fat: Energy Source and So Much More

Where Is Body Fat Stored?

Fat (triglyceride) is an energy source for many of our cells (in particular muscle and liver) and is our primary means of storing the excessive energy

Table 5.6 Lipid Profile Example

Blood Lipid or Ratio	Measurement (milligrams/100 milliliter)	Normal Range (milligrams/100 milliliter)
Triglyceride	137	0–200
Cholesterol (total)	163	50–200
HDL-cholesterol	42	30–90
VLDL-cholesterol	27	5–40
LDL-cholesterol	94	50–130
Cholesterol:HDL	3.9 (ratio)	3.7–6.7
LDL-cholesterol:HDL-cholesterol	2.2 (ratio)	

HDL = high density lipoprotein; VLDL = very low density lipoprotein; LDL = low density lipoprotein.

from the foods we eat. Although some fat can be found in several cell types in our body (such as skeletal and cardiac muscle cells), by and large most of the fat stored in our body is housed in fat cells. Collections of fat cells or *adipocytes* are commonly referred to as fat tissue or *adipose tissue*. Because a larger percentage of the fatty acids stored in adipose tissue are monounsaturated and saturated, the fat tissue is more semisolid than liquid. This can contribute to the dimpling appearance in the layer of fat found beneath our skin (subcutaneous fat) that is often referred to as *cellulite*.

Are There Advantages to Storing Energy as Fat?

Storing excess energy as fat rather than as protein or carbohydrate has great advantages. First, we are able to store more than twice the amount of energy in 1 gram of fat (9 calories) as we can in 1 gram of carbohydrate or protein (4 calories). Second, stored fat will have a lot less water associated with it than would be stored in carbohydrate and protein. The net effect of storing excess diet energy as fat versus carbohydrate or protein is that our body weight and volume are minimized. Said differently, it allows the human body to be lighter and smaller despite significant energy stores.

> Storing energy as fat, versus carbohydrate or protein, allows our body to remain smaller and lighter.

Are We Born with All of the Fat Cells We Will Ever Have?

We are not born with a full complement of fat cells as some scientists once thought. The number of fat cells in the body increases at various stages throughout growth, but by the time adulthood is reached the total number of these cells can become fixed. This means that if our body fat mass does not change, we probably would not produce new fat cells as adults. However, if we consume excessive calories, the number of fat cells can increase. In adipose tissue there is a small number of so-called *pre-adipocytes* or fat *stem cells*. When these cells are signaled, they will produce new fat cells. As you may have guessed, the signals are chemicals, many of which are released by existing fat cells when they become swollen with an increased bounty of stored fat.

Do Fat Cells Do More Than Store Energy?

For a long time fat tissue and their cells were viewed as somewhat inert containers of energy storage. However, today we know that adipose tissue functions as a gland with the capability to release a variety of factors relative to its size and endowed energy. As mentioned previously, some of these factors may promote the formation of more fat cells. Perhaps some of the most interesting released factors are those that circulate to the brain and provide insight to our energy storage status. One of the most important factors seems to be the hormone *leptin*. Fat cells release more and more leptin into our circulation when fat cells accumulate more fat. Leptin then signals the brain to reduce appetite. In addition, as fat cells swell due to excessive calorie consumption, some of the chemicals they release can promote the development and worsening of diabetes, high blood pressure and other medical conditions.

Can Fat Help Protect the Body?

Fat tissue provides some protection to various tissues in the body. For instance, fat tissue around our internal organs provides some cushioning. This helps protect the organs against external trauma. Furthermore, the subcutaneous layer of fat storage also provides some cushioning, which protects muscle. Subcutaneous fat is not well vasculated, meaning that there aren't a lot of blood vessels in that tissue relative to other tissue. Meanwhile, skeletal muscle is heavily endowed with blood vessels which provide oxygen and energy nutrients during activity and exercise. In the absence of subcutaneous fat it would be easier to rupture smaller blood vessels in skeletal muscle, which then would be evident in bruises. As an example, prior to competition, bodybuilders will be very cautious not to bang into things or play contact sports (rugby, football, roller hockey, etc.). As they attempt to "lean out" for the competition, they reduce their subcutaneous fat to nadir levels, which would allow them to bruise more easily. This then would impact their aesthetic presentation during the bodybuilding competition.

Does Body Fat Help Our Body Conserve Body Heat?

Subcutaneous fat not only helps protect skeletal muscle from trauma but it also helps conserve our body heat. This is because fat tissue is a relatively good insulating tissue. Maintaining our body temperature allows cell operations to function optimally. Interestingly, too little subcutaneous body fat might allow for greater heat losses daily. This might partly explain why a leaner person may have a higher energy expenditure than another person having the same body weight but who is less lean. Following this line of thinking it would be easier for a leaner person to maintain their body weight than a heavier person. We'll take a closer look at this in Chapter 7.

> Body fat is important to maintain body temperature and to protect organs and muscle.

What Is Brown Adipose Tissue?

While most of the fat tissue in an adult's body is somewhat pale (white adipose tissue), infants tend to have a fair amount of *brown adipose tissue* (BAT). This type of fat tissue is a little different from white adipose tissue as it contains a lot more blood vessels. This is one reason why it appears darker in color. BAT is especially important for infants to help them maintain their body temperature. When infants are born, they are fairly lean and it is easy for heat to leave their bodies. BAT has the ability to increase some of its metabolic events, which results in the generation of extra heat. BAT is able to uncouple the process of ATP formation via the breakdown of energy nutrients. Although this may seem somewhat "futile" when it comes to making ATP, the molecule that cells use to power most operations, it does allow for the generation of heat which will help maintain the body temperature of the baby. For adults, this may seem like a great way of burning unwanted fat, but this isn't to be, because as babies become children and then teens, the amount of BAT is reduced and becomes almost nonexistent by adulthood.

Does Fat Play a Structural Role in Our Body?

Our cell membranes contain molecules, called *phospholipids*, that seem to have structural similarities to triglycerides (see Figure 5.1). Like triglycerides, phospholipids contain a glycerol backbone to which fatty acids are attached. However, phospholipids contain only two fatty acids, not three as in triglycerides. The third fatty acid is replaced by phosphate combined with another molecule, such as choline, serine or inostiol. This helps make the phospholipids special and appropriate to be part of the membrane.

Phospholipids provide the basis for the water-insoluble properties of our cell membranes. In turn, then, the barrier-like properties of membranes allow each cell to regulate the movement of water-soluble substances into and out of cells and their internal organelles. In addition, the attached fatty acids can be removed and used to make other molecules that help regulate bodily function.

Does Fat Play a Role in Regulating Body Function?

Phospholipids in the plasma membrane of cells may contain special fatty acids which can be detached and modified when the need arises. These special fatty acids include EPA and ALA discussed above and modified versions of these fatty acids (eicosanoids) will help regulate processes such as blood pressure, inflammation and the actions of platelets (blood clotting factors). These eicosanoids include *thromboxanes, leukotrienes* and *prostaglandins*.

In general, the eicosanoids that result from either EPA or ARA have opposite effects. For instance, eicosanoids from ARA promote vaso-constriction, inflammation, and blood clotting, while those from EPA have an opposite effect. Interestingly, EPA and ARA compete for the same processes (enzymes) that convert them to eicosanoids (Figure 5.11). That means the relative availability of ARA and EPA will be a principal factor in determining the eicosanoids produced and thus the action. We will discuss eicosanoids in more detail in Chapters 12 and 13.

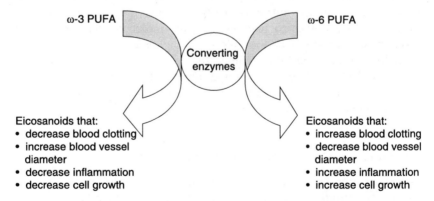

Figure 5.11 Essential fatty acids are used to make eicosanoid molecules. Those eicosanoids that are made from omega-6 PUFA are associated with events related to heart disease, cancer, and arthritis, while those derived from omega-3 PUFA are associated with reducing the risk and incidence of heart disease, cancer, and arthritis.

FAQ Highlight

What Are Fat Substitutes?

Fat tends to impart a smooth texture and tastier quality to many foods. For example, most of ice cream's taste and mouth-feel are the result of its rich fat content. However, along with the positive attributes associated with fat in foods, there are some potential negative attributes as well. Fat enhances the energy content of a food. Furthermore, a diet rich in fatty foods contradicts nutritional recommendations. Therefore, food manufacturers have long searched for fat substitutes that would provide the desirable mouth-feel and taste of fat but not the energy content of fat itself.

Earlier substitutes were fairly successful but unable to completely capture the true characteristics of fat. These include plant gums, cellulose, Caprenin, Paselli SA2, N-Oil, Sta-Slim 143, and Maltrin. Researchers have developed several newer fat substitutes, some of which are used in food production today, while others are still awaiting FDA approval. Olestra and Simplesse are two substitutes that offer much promise.

Olestra—Approved for use in savory snack foods, such as chips, in 1996, Olean is the commercial name for Olestra which consists of several fatty acids attached to a molecule of sucrose. The fatty acids provide many of the desirable qualities of fat to be experienced by the mouth. However, since olestra is not digested and absorbed, it comes without an appreciable energy expense. Some scientists have raised concerns associated with the large-scale use of olestra in foods. One concern is that olestra might bind to vitamin E and other fat-soluble vitamins in the digestive tract and decrease their absorption. Furthermore, some nutritionists have expressed concern that olestra can cause digestive discomforts, such as cramping or diarrhea. To accommodate these concerns, fat-soluble vitamins were added to olestra-containing products and a warning statement was mandated by the FDA for a couple years. Although excessive intakes of olestra may have this effect, lower and more typical consumption of olestra-containing products probably does not cause any more digestive problems than regular snacks.

Simplesse—Simplesse is the product of milk and egg proteins, mixed and heat-treated until fine, mist-like protein globules are formed. These protein globules seem to taste and provide a mouth-feel similar to fat. On the contrary, however, this substitute yields much less energy than fat. Simplesse's application is limited to cool or cold items, such as cheese, cold desserts, mayonnaise, yogurt, and salad dressings. Heat will break down the fine protein globules, therefore Simplesse is inappropriate for baked or fried items.

6   Proteins Are the Basis of Our Structure and Function

The name protein is derived from the Greek term *proteos*, which means "primary" or "to take place first." Protein was first identified in a laboratory about a century ago at which time scientists described it as a nitrogen-containing part of food that is essential to human life. While protein has long been the darling of the weight lifting and sport community, over the past few years there has been more attention focused on the importance of protein during weight loss and general health.

Proteins Are Combinations of Amino Acids

What Are Amino Acids?

We now know that all proteins are collections of amino acids. Said another way, amino acids are the "building blocks" of proteins. Although the final functional form of some proteins may contain minerals or other nonprotein components, the basis for these proteins is still amino acids.

All amino acids have the same basic design, as shown in Figure 6.1. There is both a nitrogen-containing amino portion and carboxylic acid portion attached to a central carbon atom. The presence of both an amino and an acid portion on each molecule led to the name *amino acid*

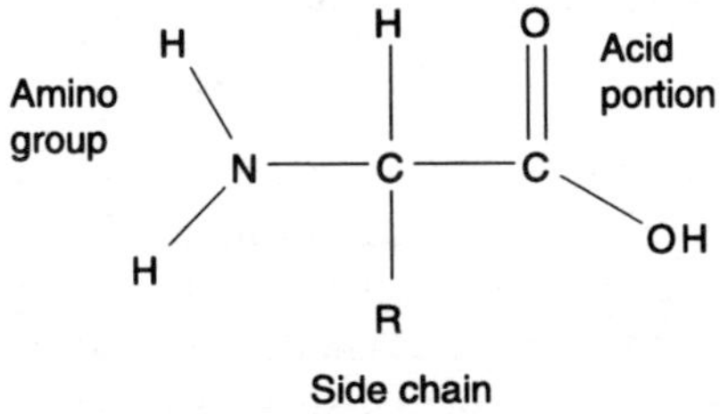

Figure 6.1 Basic components of amino acids. An amino acid contains a central carbon atom (C) with the following attachments: amino group, carboxyl (carboxylic acid) group, hydrogen (H), and a side chain (R group).

for this family of molecules. There is also a hydrogen atom attached to the central carbon, as well as a mysterious "R" group.

> Twenty amino acids serve as the building blocks of protein; ten of them are dietary essential.

The R group denotes the portion of an amino acid that will be different from one amino acid to the next. The R portion of an amino acid may be as simple as a hydrogen atom, as in glycine, or much more complex to include carbon chains and rings, acid or base groups, and even sulfur (S). The structure of the twenty amino acids used to make protein is shown in Figure 6.2.

How Many Amino Acids Are in Proteins?

There are probably hundreds of different amino acids found in nature, but only twenty are incorporated into the proteins found in living things (Table 6.1). This means that these twenty amino acids are the basis of protein found in birds, lizards, plants, bacteria, fungi, yeast, and so on. This is a very profound and also convenient situation. First, it allows us to further appreciate that, despite the obvious structural and functional differences between the different life-forms on this planet, there is common ground and more than likely common ancestry. Second, it somewhat simplifies human nutrition as we are able to obtain all of the amino acids we need to make our body proteins by eating the proteins of other life-forms.

Table 6.1 The Twenty Amino Acids Used to Make Proteins

Essential Amino Acids	Nonessential Amino Acids
Tryptophan	Alanine
Valine	Proline
Threonine	Tyrosine
Isoleucine	Cysteine
Leucine	Serine
Lysine	Glutamine
Phenylalanine	Glutamic acid
Methionine	Glycine
Arginine*	Asparagine
Histidine*	Aspartic acid

* Essential during growth.

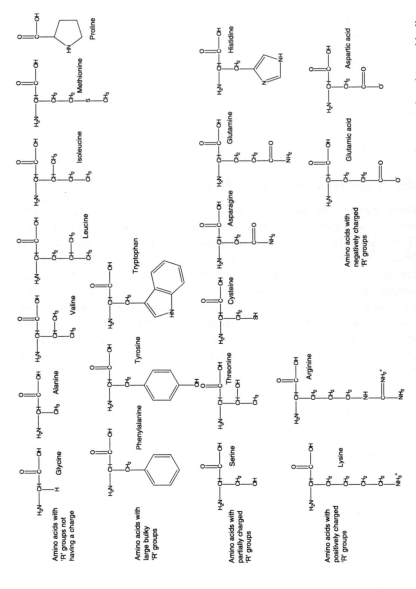

Figure 6.2 The twenty amino acids used to make the proteins of life. The "R" or side groups can be neutral, or big and bulky, or charged. The sequence of amino acids in a protein will then determine the final shape.

Some proteins contain just a few amino acids linked together, while others contain hundreds of amino acids. Scientists often refer to the links of amino acids in the following manner.

- Peptides are 2 to 10 amino acids including dipeptides, tripeptides, etc.
- Polypeptides are 11 to 100 amino acids.
- Proteins are over 100 amino acids.

Other scientists will describe protein size based on the weight of the protein molecule (molecular weight) and sometimes use the term daltons as a unit of weight. When we discuss proteins in this book we will refer to protein size and design only if its helps us understand a protein's unique function.

What Do Proteins Look Like?

As mentioned above, peptides and proteins are composed of links of amino acids. Some smaller proteins will exist as a somewhat straight chain of amino acids; however, most proteins will exist in a complex three-dimensional design (Figure 6.3). Links of amino acids will contort themselves based upon the specific sequencing of the amino acids.

How links of amino acids contort depends on the interaction between the side groups (R groups) on the different amino acids. For instance, some amino acids are attracted to other amino acids in the chain while others are repulsed. This is due to either opposing or similar charges. An analogy would be children holding hands to form a chain. As you can imagine, within a short period of time the chain would bend in a manner specific to the children. Some children would want to be closer (or further away) from others. As amino acid chain bends, twists, and warps about three dimensionally, some amino acids will form bonds with other amino acids. This helps stabilize the three-dimensional design.

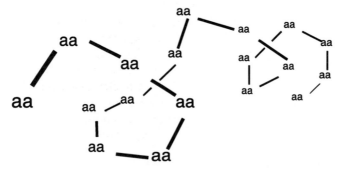

Figure 6.3 The specific sequence of amino acids will determine the final three-dimensional structure of the protein. For instance, this one is starting to look a little like a spiral staircase.

> Most proteins have a complex, three-dimensional design that enables each protein's unique function.

It will be the final structure that determines the functional properties of a protein. It is interesting that many proteins are actually all globbed up, somewhat like crumpled paper or loosely packed yarn. In fact, the names of some proteins, such as hemoglobin and immunoglobin, reflect their globbed (globular) nature. On the contrary, many proteins have more of a filament design, meaning that they are much longer than they are wide. Many of these proteins are like stretched-out coils. This is the case with collagen. In fact, numerous collagen proteins come together, side by side, to form a ropelike fibrous super-protein. Further still, it is possible for a protein to demonstrate both globular and filament attributes as is the case with muscle proteins actin and myosin.

What Role Do Proteins Play in the Human Body?

Much of the structure and function of our body is based on proteins. Thus, protein and individual amino acids must function in our body in a number of ways. For instance, proteins can function as:

- enzymes (regulate chemical reactions)
- structural proteins (yield form to cells and tissue)
- contractile proteins (provide basis for muscle contraction)
- antibodies (help protect us from foreign entities)
- transport proteins (help transport substances in our blood)
- protein hormones (insulin, glucagon, and growth hormone)
- clotting factors (allow our blood to clot to stop a hemorrhage)
- receptors on cells (allow hormones and neurotransmitters to function)

Individual amino acids can be used to make certain hormones and neurotransmitters such as epinephrine, serotonin, norepinephrine, and thyroid hormone (Table 6.2). In fact, most neurotransmitters are derived from amino acids. Amino acids are also used to make other important substances such as creatine, choline, carnitine, nucleic acids, and the vitamin niacin. Last, amino acids can be used by some tissue as an energy source or can be converted to glucose or fat depending upon our current nutritional/metabolic state (that is, fasting, fed, exercise).

Table 6.2 Select Substances Made from Amino Acids

Amino Acid	Substances Made From the Amino Acid(s)
Tryptophan	Serotonin
Lysine and methionine	Carnitine
Methionine, glycine and arginine	Creatine
Aspartic acid and glutamine	Pyrimidines
Aspartic acid, glutamine and glycine	Purines
Tyrosine or phenylalanine	Epinephrine, norepinephrine, thyroid hormone, dopamine

Food Protein Nourishes Our Body as Amino Acids and Peptides

What Foods Contain Protein?

Because protein is vital to life, all life-forms will contain protein; however, the protein content will vary. In general, foods of animal origin will have greater protein content than plants and plant-derived foods (Table 6.3). Among the foods that have the highest protein content (percent of calories) are water-packed tuna and egg whites. Being an animal, tuna (and other fish) contain skeletal muscle for locomotion. Thus, eating finned or shellfish provides protein sources that are fairly similar to human skeletal muscle proteins. Meanwhile, the predominant protein in egg whites is

Table 6.3 Approximate Protein Content of Various Foods

Food	Amount	Protein (g)
Beef	3 ounces	22
Pork	3 ounces	21
Cod, poached	32 ounces	21
Oysters	32 ounces	14
Milk	1 cup	8
Cheddar cheese	1 ounces	7
Egg	1 large	6
Peanut butter	1 tablespoon	5
Potato	1	3
Bread	1 slice	2
Banana	1 medium	1
Carrots, sliced	2 cups	1
Apple	1	2
Sugar, oil		0

albumin (for example, ovalbumin and conalbumin) and ovomucoid, globulins, and lysozymes. Another popular protein source with this group, because of its protein density, is milk. The principal proteins in milk are caseins and whey, which are actually families of related proteins.

Cereal grains produce a vast array of proteins (including albumins); however, the most interesting proteins may be gliadin and glutenin. When these proteins are mixed with water, such as when we make dough, gluten is formed. Gluten provides the structural basis for the network that traps gases produced by yeast when dough rises. Soy lacks these proteins, and ingredients need to be added to soy flour to make it rise to a light bread. Gluten continues to be a topic of interest as many people either experience an allergy or intolerances to foods that contain it. We will discuss gluten intolerance in the FAQ Highlight at the end of this chapter.

What Are Some Foods with the Highest Protein Content?

Egg whites, fish, leaner meats, and low-fat milk are popular with people seeking concentrated protein sources such as athletes, body-builders and other weight trainers. For instance, water-packed tuna such as Albacore can have 80 percent of its calories from protein or 20 grams per 3 ounce serving. One 3-ounce steak of yellowfin tuna also has about 20 grams of protein, which is about 87 percent of the calories. Meanwhile, egg whites and many egg-white products such as Egg Beaters® are largely protein as well. Protein supplements also provide a concentrated protein source and are extremely popular with athletes and fitness enthusiasts. Protein supplements provide isolated protein sources or blends of sources. By and large these sources are whey protein isolate and concentrate, casein isolates, milk protein isolates, soy protein isolate, and egg white isolate (for example, egg albumin). Protein supplements for muscle mass and strength development will be discussed in Chapter 11.

> Fish, egg white, and low-fat dairy and protein supplements are concentrated sources of protein.

How Are Proteins Digested?

The goal of protein digestion is to disassemble proteins to their constituent amino acids and smaller peptides that can be absorbed. Protein digestion begins in our stomach, as swallowed food is bathed in the acidic juice. In fact, the presence of protein/amino acids along with distension of the stomach causes stomach juice to ooze from glands in the wall of the stomach. The acid serves to straighten out the complex three-dimensional design characteristic of many proteins. Scientists refer to this as denaturing the protein or changing its natural three-dimensional design. This will make it easier for protein-digesting enzymes in the stomach and small intestine to do their job. This is analogous to straightening out a ball of yawn so that you can cut small lengths.

An enzyme called *pepsin* is found in stomach juice and begins to break the bonds between amino acids. The impact of pepsin is significant yet incomplete, as most of the bulk of protein digestion takes place further along in the small intestine. As partially digested proteins make their way into the small intestine, a battery of protein-digesting enzymes attack and break down protein into very small amino acid links and individual amino acids. Most of these enzymes come from the pancreas and include *trypsin, chymotrypsin, carboxypeptidase A and B, elastase,* and *collagenase*. These enzymes are made, packaged, and released by our pancreas in an inactive form. It is not till they reach the small intestine that these enzymes are activated by another enzyme produced by the small intestinal called *enterokinase (enteropeptidase)*. The reason for this complex system is to protect the pancreas and the duct that connect to the stomach from the protein-digesting activity of these enzymes.

How Are Amino Acids Absorbed?

Amino acids are taken up by the cells that line the small intestine, then move out of the backside of those cells and enter the bloodstream. Meanwhile, small peptides, consisting of just a couple or a few amino acids linked together can also be brought into these cells where final digestion to amino acids can take place. Therefore, as a general rule, the absorbed form of protein will be individual amino acids. Fragments of proteins and some peptides can also be absorbed and are important in developing the immune system during infancy, and are linked to many food allergies reactions. Food allergies will be addressed in Chapter 12.

Amino acids and some peptides are absorbed into circulation, more specifically the portal vein, which delivers the amino acids to our liver. The liver removes a lot of amino acids from circulation. In fact it is typical for only about one-fourth of the absorbed amino acids to circulate beyond the liver, much of which will be the branched-chain amino acids, namely leucine, isoleucine, and valine. This is probably because these essential amino acids are needed by our skeletal muscle to replace what was used for energy during fasting or exercise. Additionally these amino acids play a role in maintaining and developing muscle mass, which is important for weight lifters as well as for people losing weight.

> A lot of the amino acids absorbed into circulation go to the liver while the branched-chain amino acids go to skeletal muscle.

How Are Amino Acids from the Diet Processed in the Body?

The amino acids that enter our blood from our digestive tract evoke a release of insulin from our pancreas. However, the ability of elevated blood amino acid concentrations to cause the release of insulin is nowhere near as potent as elevated glucose. Regardless, the increased presence of circulating insulin will promote the uptake of amino acids in certain tissue, primarily muscle, as well as support the building of new protein in muscle and tissue throughout our body. And, as mentioned in the previous chapter, the increase in insulin will also lower glucose levels. Thus, amino acids can have a glycemic lowering effect.

The increase in the level of circulating amino acids after a meal can slightly increase the level of glucagon as well. Considering this, aren't the actions of insulin and glucagon opposite, thus making this scenario counterproductive? Consider the following scenario. What if our sole source of food was wild game for a period of time? Having the effects of insulin and glucagon would allow the conversion of some amino acids to glucose in the liver while insulin would promote the formation of glycogen and muscle protein as well as promote the production and storage of some fat if enough protein is consumed. All of these efforts would leave that person in better shape for enduring an extended period of time before they ate again. This certainly may have been the case for our distant ancestors when enduring winters or prolonged dry seasons when vegetation might not have been available.

What Happens to Excess Amino Acids Absorbed from the Diet?

Amino acids from diet protein in excess of the needs of cells are not stored as protein. So, unlike fat, we do not store excessive diet protein as body protein. Instead our liver breaks down amino acids in excess of our needs and several of these amino acids can be used to make fat. Insulin promotes this process of making fatty acids from excessive amino acids. However, the conversion of excessive amino acids (like carbohydrate) to fat is not as efficient as was once thought and it turns out that more of the excessive amino acids will be used for immediate energy.

> Excessive diet protein is largely used for energy and to a minimal degree for fat production.

Protein and Amino Acids Are Essential Components of Our Diet

How Much Protein Should We Eat Daily?

The RDA for protein for adults is set at 0.8 grams of protein per kilogram of body weight. This works out to about 54 to 60 grams for most men and about 44 to 50 grams for most women. You can estimate basic protein needs based on percent of total calories, where by 12–15 percent will give you approximately the same level. This level of protein merely compensates for normal daily body protein loss; however it is not an optimal level of protein in various situations such as weight loss, exercise, and illness. In these situations a protein level of 25 percent of calories is more appropriate. Higher protein needs in these situations are discussed more in Chapters 8 and 11.

Are High-Protein Diets Dangerous?

At one time there was a belief that higher intakes of protein can be problematic to health. Today we know that for most people this isn't the case. In fact, diets with a higher level of protein then the RDA are encouraged for athletes as well as people during weight loss. Two areas of health have been the target for concern regarding higher protein intakes. The first is kidney health. It was long believed that since higher intakes of protein leads to the formation of more nitrogen-based compounds such as urea, this work become detrimental to the kidneys. However we now know that this isn't the case unless a person has a special situation related to the kidneys and receiving guidance from his or her physician.

The second area is in relation to bone. Some research efforts have determined that when diet protein levels increase, so too does the level of calcium in the urine. This lead to the conclusion that high-protein diets cause a loss of calcium from bones, rendering a person more prone to osteoporosis. However, follow up research has shown that the higher protein intake also increases calcium absorption, thus leading to a corresponding increase in calcium in the urine. So, like kidney dysfunction, the notion that a high protein intake, such as 25 percent of calories for weight loss or maintenance, leads to osteoporosis has not been shown to be true.

What Are Essential Amino Acids?

From a nutritional standpoint, only ten of the twenty amino acids found in protein are *essential* to the diet. These amino acids present us with the same situation as do the other essential nutrients. We simply cannot make them or at least not in the amounts necessary to promote growth, development, and health throughout the lifespan. As a result, these amino acids must be provided by our diet. As listed in Table 6.1, arginine and histidine are noted as essential during periods of growth and maybe at an advanced age but not at other times.

The easiest way to remember the essential amino acids is by the acronyms TV-TILL-PM-AH. These are the first letters of the essential amino acids tryptophan, valine, threonine, isoleucine, leucine, lysine, phenylalanine, methionine, and the two semi-essential amino acids arginine and histidine. Other acronyms include PVT TIM HALL or VP MATT HILL where PVT is the abbreviation for the military rank of private.

What Are Nonessential Amino Acids?

The remaining amino acids used to make protein in our body are called *nonessential*. That's because they can be made in our body by using essential amino acids and/or other molecules. It should be understood that dietary essentiality or nonessentiality by no means is meant to imply biological essentiality or nonessentiality. All twenty amino acids must be present in cells to make proteins which support the health of those cells and our body in general. Further, if a problem exists in making a nonessential amino acid, as is the case in some genetic anomalies, then that amino acid would also become a dietary essential for that person as well. This is the case with some individuals who lack the ability to produce the appropriate enzyme to convert phenylalanine (essential amino acid) to tyrosine (nonessential amino acid). In these cases (that is, people with phenylketonuria [PKU]), tyrosine becomes an essential amino acid.

What Are "Complete" Proteins?

The goal of protein nutrition is fairly simple—to provide our body with food protein that closely resembles our own protein and in adequate amounts. Furthermore, since the nonessential amino acids can be made in our body, it is desirable for food protein to provide the essential amino acids, in proportion to human protein. Food sources with levels of essential amino acid content similar to our essential amino acid requirements are considered more "complete" and sometimes referred to as higher biological value. Those that don't measure up to the standard are considered incomplete.

Complete Protein Sources: Animal based protein sources from such as beef, pork, fish, poultry, eggs, milk, and milk products are among the more complete protein sources. In addition, soy, quinoa, amaranth, buckwheat, and spirulina are complete or nearly complete plant based protein sources.

Incomplete Protein Sources: Plant-based foods such as wheat, corn, fruits, and vegetables are considered incomplete or lower biological value as the levels of essential amino acid within their protein does not match our essential amino acid needs as closely.

Complete proteins contain all essential amino acids in proportion with human protein.

How Can Incomplete Protein Foods Be Combined to Form a Complete Protein?

When we compare the essential amino acid composition of an incomplete food, we find that one or more of these amino acids is in a limited quantity relative to our protein (Figure 6.4). These amino acids are referred to as "limiting amino acids" because our cells' ability to make new protein will be limited to the level in that protein. This is analogous to building a brick wall with alternating rows of red, white and blue bricks. If there are only enough red bricks to build the wall 4 feet tall, that is as tall as the wall could be built even if there are abundances of blue and white bricks.

What Does It Mean to "Complement Protein"?

Because the limiting amino acids within plant foods varies, strategic combinations of different plant foods will provide adequate quantities of all the essential amino acids. This practice is called "complementing" proteins (Table 6.4). For example, we could combine cereals (oats, wheat, rice, rye) or nuts and seeds (walnuts, cashews, almonds, pecans, and sunflower, pumpkin, and sesame seeds) which are low in lysine but a good source of methionine, with legumes (beans, peas, lentils, garbanzos (chick peas)) which are low in methionine but a good source of lysine. While considered a complete protein source, soy is limited in lysine as well and often used in a complementing scheme. The practice of complementing proteins may be best served within the same or adjacent meals for strict vegetarians with lower daily protein intakes (for example, below RDA); however, for less restrictive vegetarians, complementing within the same day is fine.

How Important Is Complementing Protein to Vegetarians?

Vegetarians either partially or totally restrict animal based foods and those containing animal based ingredients from their diet. Vegetarians

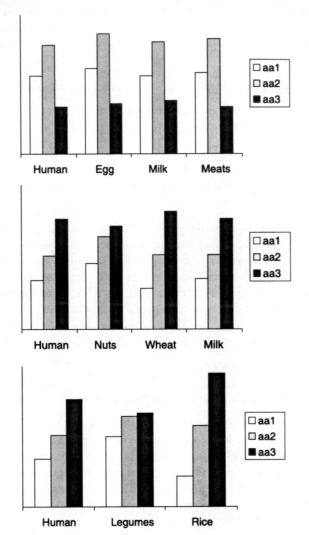

Figure 6.4 Example content of three essential amino acid (aa) in human protein and three high biological value protein sources (top). Comparison of two lower biological value protein sources (nuts and wheat) to human protein and milk (middle). Eating two lower biological value foods allows them to complement each other to make a higher biological value meal (bottom). Here, the limitations of legumes to provide aa3 is compensated for by the abundance of aa3 in rice. The opposite is true for rice and aa1. (Note: the three amino acids are not necessarily the same in the different graphics)

Table 6.4 Simple Solutions for Complementing Proteins

Combination	Examples
Legumes and grains	Rice and black beans (or kidney beans, lentils, or black-eyed peas)
	Tortillas and beans
	Barley and bean soup
	Peanut butter sandwich with whole grain bread
Legumes and nuts or seeds	Hummus
	Bean soup with sesame seeds or nuts
	Combine beans, chickpeas, and various nuts in a salad.
Eggs and dairy products with any vegetable source	Oatmeal with milk
	Cheese sandwich
	Cheese pizza with vegetable toppings
	French toast, pancakes, waffles
	Dry cereal and milk
	Quiche
	Meatless lasagna
	Fried rice with egg
	Macaroni and cheese

with more restrictive practices will have to be more conscious of complementing protein, especially since their overall protein intake tends to be lower than non-vegetarians.

Fruitarians—Levels of fruitarianism vary. Diet tends to include what certain plants bear (that is, fruits, nuts, some or all vegetables) but not the plant sources that would be harvested, such as grains. Strict fruitarianism is meant to simulate the diet in the Garden of Eden, therefore cooked vegetables will not be included. Complementing protein sources is very important and can be challenging depending on diet criteria.

Vegans—Vegans tend to restrict their dietary choices to what plants bear as well as food produced from harvested plants (for example, cereal grain products, sprouts). A vegan diet tends to include cooked foods such as oatmeal, breads, and some vegetables to enhance their palatability (for example, corn, potatoes, beans). Vegans have numerous options for complementing proteins and soy-based foods also provide a complete protein source.

Lactovegetarians—Include milk and dairy products to a vegan diet. Since milk is a good source of complete protein, there is less concern for complementing proteins, especially if milk-based products are consumed at different meals or if soy foods are part of the daily intake.

Ovovegetarians—Include eggs and foods containing eggs to a vegetarian diet. Like the vegan, there are multiple options for complementing proteins and there is less concern for complementing proteins, especially if eggs are consumed throughout the day or the diet includes ample soy foods.

Lactoovovegetarians—Include dairy, eggs, and recipe foods that include eggs and dairy products as ingredients. Minimal concern exists for complementing protein if these foods are found in meals and snacks throughout the day or ample soy is part of the diet.

Body Protein Is Turned over Daily

Are Body Proteins Broken Down Daily?

During a single day, roughly ¼ to 1 pound of our body protein is broken down to amino acids. The lower end of the range would apply more to a smaller woman while the higher end of the range would be more applicable to a larger, more muscular man. Much of the breakdown occurs in the liver and muscle and during the same day an equivalent amount of protein is made (synthesis). Protein breakdown and production considered together is called "protein turnover" and even though there is this significant quantity of protein turnover we are mostly the same from one day to the next.

Protein is either broken down or manufactured to allow us to adapt to the most current metabolic situation within cells, and also in our body. This process also allows us to maintain the integrity of proteins subjected to daily wear and tear. These activities allow cells to make or break down enzymes, which are either involved or not involved in different metabolic states such as fasting, feeding, and exercise. These processes also allow us to remodel tissue such as muscle and bone and to make and break down hormones and neurotransmitters. It is important to remember that our cells are constantly active. This allows us to grow, heal, remodel, and internally defend ourselves on a continual basis.

> Protein turnover refers to the constant break down and production of protein throughout our body.

How Long Do Body Proteins Last?

All proteins in our body have a certain life expectancy. For instance, when insulin and glucagon are released into our blood an individual molecule of either will circulate for about 5 to 10 minutes before they are removed and broken down. Meanwhile, some enzymes within cells may exist only for a few minutes or so before they are replaced or not remade. This can allow cells to shift metabolic gears, so to speak, when going from a fasting to a fed state, resting to exercise state, and so on.

Contractile proteins in muscle (for example, myosin and actin) may last only a couple of days, while connective tissue proteins, such as collagen, may last weeks to months before they are broken down and replaced. The rate of turnover or remodeling of skeletal muscle contractile proteins and connective tissue proteins helps us understand why the human body seems to get bigger and stronger in just a couple of weeks or so when lifting weights regularly. Meanwhile, it seems to take months and years for scar tissue, which is largely connective tissue, to change.

Are There "Free" Amino Acids in the Body?

Free amino acids are found in the body as a result of digestion of food protein and the absorption of amino acids as well as a product of protein breakdown in cells. Free amino acids account for about 1 percent of the amino acids in our body, the rest of course would be part of peptides and proteins. Most cells in the body have a small assortment of free amino acids, meaning they are independent and not linked to other amino acids as part of peptides and proteins. In addition there is a small amount of amino acids circulating in the blood, although this increases after a protein containing meal. Circulation provides a delivery system for diet derived amino acids to get to all tissue as well as a means for amino acids to be exchanged between tissue such as during fasting and exercise. Free amino acids in cells and in the blood are collectively referred to as the "amino acid pool" and these amino acids are available to make new body protein or amino acid-derived substances (for example, neurotransmitters, hormones, metabolic factors).

Body Protein Can Be Used For Energy

Are Amino Acids Used for Energy?

In addition to the amino acids used to make important body chemicals, such as certain hormones and neurotransmitters, as well as key metabolic factors (for example, carnitine, creatine), amino acids are used for energy. Typically 20 to 40 grams of body protein, in the form of free amino acids, is utilized to make each day as energy. If our diet failed to include protein we would lose a significant amount of body protein over time. The RDA level for protein factors this in and has provides some padding as well. Some situations can increase the reliance on amino acids as a fuel source such is the case of weight loss and higher levels of exercise as discussed soon.

> Amino acids can be used for energy during fasting and endurance exercise.

What Happens If We Do Not Eat Enough Protein?

Our diet needs to at least replace a quantity of protein equivalent to what is lost to energy pathways and processes that produce amino acid-derived molecules such as neurotransmitters, nucleic acids, some hormones, niacin, etc. If one or more amino acids are in limited quantity in our cells, then protein synthesis is limited to that level as discussed above. If this continues over time, there will be a decrease in total body protein content. This would be visually obvious as skeletal muscle mass is reduced. If the deficiency continues, the level of various proteins in blood would decrease and our immune system could become compromised, leaving us more prone to infections.

What Happens to Body Protein When We Don't Eat Enough Calories?

Situations can occur that increase the use of body protein for energy. Eating too few calories or fasting increases the reliance on body protein as an energy source. In these situations the level of circulating glucagon and cortisol increase. Cortisol, the stress hormone, will promote the breakdown of our body proteins to amino acids. Meanwhile, both of these hormones promote the conversion of amino acids to glucose in our liver which is released to serve as fuel. The amount of amino acids used to make glucose is related to the length and degree of caloric restriction and the intensity and duration of exercise. Simply stated, as glycogen stores in the liver and muscle become depleted, as in prolonged fasting and aerobic exercise, the reliance upon amino acids to make glucose increases.

During a longer period of fasting (for example, more than a week) the reliance on amino acids lessens as our brain adapts to utilize more ketone bodies. This is one way that our body attempts to slow the loss of protein, however the use of amino acids for energy is still greater than during more normal times. If the loss of body protein continues for months, a person can reach a critical level of body protein whereby normal function is compromised and illness can occur and over more protracted periods, death is possible. Even if the cause of death is due to an infection, the true cause is probably a failure to maintain an optimal immune defense because of poor protein status.

What Happens to Body Protein When We Exercise?

During prolonged aerobic (cardiovascular) exercise, muscle protein is broken down and amino acids, mostly alanine and glutamine are released into the blood. Alanine is one of the principal amino acids used to make glucose in the liver and the new glucose can help maintain blood glucose levels and fuel muscle during long aerobic exercise bouts. This process is driven by primarily by cortisol as well as epinephrine, both of which are elevated in circulation during exercise. Cortisol promotes muscle protein breakdown during the exercise while epinephrine promotes the conversion of amino acids to glucose in the liver. Since cortisol is a stress-related hormone, the degree to which this happen depends on how hard you exercising and for how long. Thus for shorter, less intense exercise sessions (for example, walking and casual bicycling) this isn't a consideration; however for recreational and competitive endurance athletes and heavy-weight trainers it is. We will explore this further in Chapter 11.

What Happens to the Nitrogen When Amino Acids Are Used for Energy Purposes?

Amino acids are different from carbohydrate and fat because they contain nitrogen (N). This creates an additional consideration for the body if it wishes to use amino acids for energy or to make fat (in an overfed state) or glucose (in a fasting or exercise state). Thus an important step in using amino acids for any of these purposes is to remove the nitrogen-containing portion of the molecule. Once removed the nitrogen portion of amino acids becomes ammonia (NH_4^+), which is potentially toxic to the brain. Thus it must be removed from the body before it builds up in the blood.

The most prevalent way to rid the body of the nitrogen removed from amino acids is as *urea* (Figure 6.5). Urea is made by the liver and released into the blood, circulates to the kidneys and is subsequently lost from the body in urine. Each molecule of urea allows for the efficient removal of two nitrogen atoms from our body.

> The nitrogen from amino acids used for energy is mostly removed from the body as urea.

Special Applications of Amino Acids and Protein

How Important Is Protein During Weight Loss?

Although this will be discussed in more detail in Chapter 8, certain beneficial roles of protein pertaining to weight management should be introduced here. Protein can be advantageous to weight loss for a couple of reasons. First, current research suggests that when a meal derives more of its calories from protein, versus saturated fat and simpler carbohydrates the meals can promote greater satiety (fullness) and possibly reduce hunger a couple of hours later. Furthermore, amino acids require special

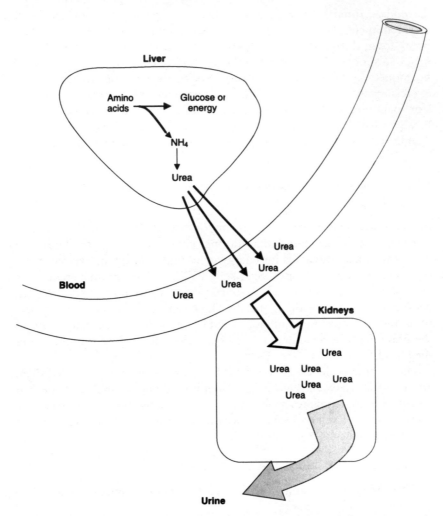

Figure 6.5 The nitrogen that is removed from amino acids is used to make urea in our liver. Urea then circulates to our kidneys and is removed from our body in urine.

(energy requiring) processing if they are to be used for energy. That means that more calories are burned to use protein for energy during weight loss than many carbohydrates and saturated fat. This could promote greater weight loss over time. Furthermore, eating more protein during weight loss may help a person maintain more muscle mass during the weight loss process, which in turn can be more beneficial to his or her metabolism (the number of calories burned).

Can Amino Acids Affect Our Mood and Sleep?

Because certain neurotransmitters in the brain are made from amino acids, amino acids from the diet or supplements are often touted to be able to influence mood, memory, and emotions. For instance, tryptophan and tyrosine are used by brain cells to make serotonin and the catecholamines, namely norepinephrine and dopamine, respectively. Furthermore, choline, which can be made from the amino acid serine, is a building block for the neurotransmitter acetylcholine.

Serotonin is a neurotransmitter mostly associated with a calming and sleepy feeling. In order for serotonin to be produced, tryptophan must exit the blood and enter our brain cells. The movement of tryptophan out of the blood requires a special transport system. However, tryptophan must compete with several other amino acids, namely valine, leucine, tyrosine, and phenylalanine, to do so.

One of the most commonly associated foods with calmness and sleepiness is milk, particularly warm milk. Some of this notion is derived from watching what happens to babies after they drink warm milk (either from the breast or milked-based formula). While some of calming effect is related to the suckling action itself, some the remaining effect might be related to protein fragments created during the digestion of milk. So, the old belief that warm milk can produce tiredness, which lacks scientific confirmation to date, might have some merit and future research should add greater clarity to this issue.

FAQ Highlight

Is Gluten a Problem for Some People?

Many people experience an adverse reaction to gluten, the principal protein in many cereal grains. The symptoms have long been associated with the digestive tract; however, other parts of the body can be affected and are currently being used in the diagnosis of gluten sensitivity. Celiac disease is the diagnosis made as a physician brings together many of the hallmark and perhaps more obscure symptoms.

Celiac disease can occur at any time in a person's life and often the onset is triggered after surgery, viral infection, emotional stress, pregnancy or child birth. The impact of celiac disease can affect several areas and systems of the body often making the diagnosis challenging. In fact the symptoms associated with the digestive tract can mimic other digestive disorders. Symptoms often include:

- abdominal cramping, bloating, gas
- diarrhea and constipation

- vomiting
- fatty (pale) stools
- anemia
- weight loss
- failure to grow properly (infants and children)
- behavioral changes (infants and children)
- dental enamel defects
- osteopenia or osteoporosis
- fatigue, weakness.

For some people, gluten sensitivity can led to very frustrating skin condition called *dermatitis herpetiformis* or DH. This condition, typically involving blistering and itching is more common on the hands, face, buttocks, and knees and involves. Small packets of immune factors (IgA) and an enzyme called *transglutaminase* can be found in the skin layers and used to make the diagnosis. Additionally, people experiencing DH might have damage to the lining of the small intestine, but without symptoms, making diagnosis of gluten sensitivity more difficult.

Gluten is the dominant protein class in cereal grains and most of it is *gliadin* and *glutenin*. Gluten is responsible for the elastic and structural properties of dough used in baking as it allows products to rise. As gases are produced by yeast in dough, they get trapped in the gluten-based network causing the dough to rise. People diagnosed with celiac disease need to avoid all foods containing gluten and thus must be attentive recipe/ingredient readers.

Gluten is most notably found in wheat, rye, barley, and grains grown in regions with more extreme weather conditions (for example, Canada and northern parts of the United States) tend to have more gluten. Gluten is not found in oats, rice, millets, buckwheat, sorghum, quinoa and amaranth. However it should be mentioned that many of the gluten-free grains can acquire some gluten if they are milled in the same facility as wheat, barley and rye or even grown next to these crops. It should also be mentioned that some people who are gluten sensitive will also react with a protein in oats called *avenin*. Lastly, soy is not a grain and does not contain gluten and it is tolerated well by most gluten sensitive people.

7   Water is the Basis of Our Body

We bath in it, swim in it, and seek out vacation destinations based on its presence. Water is one of the most important aspects of our everyday life. We thirst for water to maintain good hydration status for optimal health. In fact it is easy to argue that water is our most important nutrient. Each day we must match water intake with losses in order to risk dehydration. In this chapter we will discuss the importance of water to our body as well as its source and how much we need.

Body Water Basics

How Much of Our Body Is Water?

Water makes up about 60 percent of our total body weight, typically a little more for men and a little less for women. For instance, a 175-pound man might attribute more than 100 pounds of his weight to water. Roughly two-thirds of our body water is found within our cells as intracellular fluid, while the remaining one-third is extracellular fluid found bathing our cells. As mentioned earlier, extracellular fluid includes both the fluid between our cells and also the plasma portion of our blood.

When looking at certain body tissue, skeletal muscle is a little more than 70 percent water (by weight), while fat tissue is less than 10 percent water (Figure 7.1). By and large, it is the ratio of skeletal muscle to fat tissue that has the greatest impact on the amount of water in the body. Because men tend to have a higher percentage of muscle and a lower percentage of fat compared with women, they tend to have a higher percentage of body water. However, regardless of gender, a lean muscular person will have a higher percentage of body water while a non-muscular, overweight person will have a lower percentage of body water.

> The percentage of body water is largely determined by the relative amount of muscle to body fat.

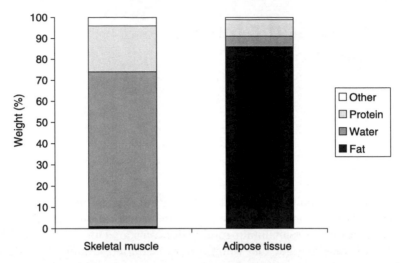

Figure 7.1 Difference in composition between skeletal muscle and adipose (fat) tissue. Skeletal muscle is largely water and then protein while adipose tissue is mostly fat and very little water, protein, and other material.

Why Do We Have So Much Water in Our Body?

Water is the most abundant substance in the body because it provides the medium or environment for the body. That means that all other substances within the body are either dissolved, suspended, and/or bathed within water. In general, substances such as carbohydrates, protein, and electrolytes dissolve well into body water. Meanwhile, lipids do not and the transport of lipid materials in our blood requires water-soluble transporters such as proteins or lipoproteins. For instance, fat-soluble vitamin D hitches a ride upon a vitamin D binding protein (DBP), while sex hormones (estrogen, testosterone) can latch onto sex hormone binding protein (SHBP). In the meantime, fats and cholesterol are transported in lipoproteins, which are in essence "submarines" carrying lipid cargo.

How Does Water Help Us Regulate Our Body Temperature?

Water has the capability to absorb heat to keep us from overheating (hyperthermia) as well as help keep us from overcooling (hypothermia). In comparison with other materials, water can absorb a lot of heat before its own temperature changes. This allows body water to absorb the heat generated during normal metabolism and during times of extra heat production such as exercise. Water then facilitates the removal of extra heat from our body by sweating (discussed below). On the other hand water can give up heat to help keep tissue warm when we are in cooler environments.

What Other Roles Does Water Play?

Water also provides the basis for the lubricating substances found in our joints. This helps cushion the joint and reduce the physical stress and friction between the bones in the joint. Water is the basis of amniotic fluid that cushions and protects a fetus during pregnancy. In addition, of our urine, bile, saliva, mucus, lacrimal fluid (tears), and digestive secretions, all are water based.

Daily Body Water Losses

How Much Water Do We Lose Daily?

Our body loses water constantly and through more than one route (Figure 7.2 and 7.3). In fact, no other essential nutrient is lost from the body by as many routes and at the same levels as water. Water is lost as urine and through breath as well as from skin surfaces as sweat. For an average

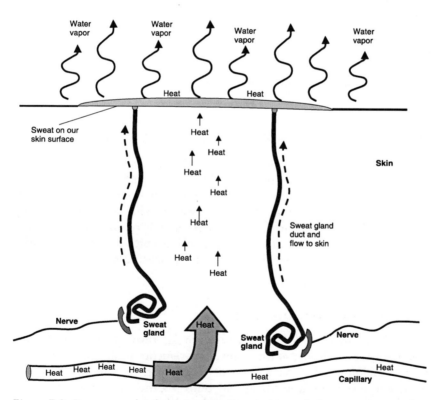

Figure 7.2 Our sweat glands begin deep in our skin and they ooze sweat when they are stimulated by our brain when our body temperature rises and by circulating epinephrine during exercise.

adult it is typical to lose as much as 2 to 3 liters (quarts) daily. As one milliliter of water is the same as one gram of water, this equals 2 to 3 kilograms or 0.9 to 1.4 pounds. This means we need to replace water at the same level as what is lost in order to prevent dehydration. This requirement is higher than all other essential nutrient requirements combined.

How Much Water Is Lost Daily as Urine?

Every day our kidneys process about 180 liters (47.5 gallons) of blood-derived fluid to regulate blood composition. Of the 180 liters, more than 99 percent is returned to our blood, while the remaining 1 percent becomes urine. Dissolved in our urine will be waste products of our metabolism (such as urea) and other substances in excess of our needs (excessive sodium, for example). About 1 to 2 liters (about 4 to 8 cups) of our body water is lost daily as urine. This quantity will change relative to our water consumption. For instance, people who drink a lot of fluids will produce more urine daily, and that urine will probably seem clearer (more dilute).

We lose about 2 to 3 liters of water from our body daily, which is largely recovered in foods and beverages.

How Do We Know If We Are Not Getting Enough Water?

People who aren't getting enough water will void less urine which is more concentrated with waste products and excess substances. For these reasons people sometimes look at the color of their urine to gauge their body water or "hydration" status. However, while this can certainly provide insight, food factors, such as the vitamin riboflavin, can darken the color of urine and/or alter its odor, such as with coffee. Researchers use more objective measures such as urine specific gravity to suggest hydration status.

How Much Water Is Lost in Feces?

Water helps moisten feces for easier transit through and out of the colon. Typically, during normal bowel movements adults lose about 100 to 200 milliliters of water as part of feces daily. As you might expect, we would lose more water from our body via the feces during bouts of diarrhea. This also means that we need to drink more fluids as tolerated during, as well as after, these unpleasant episodes.

Do We Lose Body Water When We Breathe?

Water is also lost from our body through breathing. When we inhale, air moving through our air passageways (that is, the trachea and bronchi) becomes humidified. This means that we are adding moisture to it. Subsequently, when we exhale, much of the humidified air is lost to the outside environment. This is noticeable on a cold day as humidified exhaled air condenses to form little clouds. The amount of body water lost in this process is about 300 to 500 milliliters, depending on the humidity level of the air. For instance, in a dry environment, such as a desert climate or at higher altitudes, a little more of our body water is used to humidify the air we inhale. This in turn means that a little more water would be lost during exhalation. Conversely, breathing more humid air decreases the amount of water lost through our lungs.

Do We Lose Body Water in Sweat?

We sweat throughout the day to help remove extra body heat produced by normal cell operations, but most of time we do not even notice it because it is so minimal. For an adult this can add up to about ½ liter or 2 cups (see Figure 7.2). However, when we exercise or find ourselves in a hot environment, sweating certainly becomes more obvious. This is especially true if it is humid. Increased moisture in the air can hinder the evaporation process, allowing sweat to accumulate on our skin.

Sweating and Water Loss

What Is Sweat?

Sweat is mostly water with a varying amount of dissolved substances, such as sodium and chloride. In addition, a little potassium, calcium, iron, and other minerals are found in sweat, but the levels of these substances is much lower than sodium and chloride. Sweating is a principal means of getting rid of body heat and keeping the body from overheating. Each liter of sweat can remove 580 calories of heat from the body. Other methods of removing heat from our body include convection, conduction, and radiation (Table 7.1).

Why Do We Sweat?

When "core" body temperature, which is the temperature in and around our vital organs increases, our brain prompts sweating. Sweating is also stimulated by circulating epinephrine, which is released into the blood by our adrenal glands during exercise. This helps us understand why we sweat more when we exercise and why we sweat even more while

Table 7.1 How We Lose Heat from Our Body

Method	Mechanism	Factors
Evaporation	Transfer of our body heat to sweat water. This warms the water to its vapor point. Heat leaves body in evaporated water.	Sweating is increased relative to the intensity of exercise and/or as temperature increases.
Convection	Transfer of our body heat into the surrounding air or water (such as swimming in a pool).	Convection increases as air or water temperature decreases, and vice versa.
Conduction	Transfer of our body heat to a object or surface. This could be a chair, bed, bare feet on the floor, etc.)	The warmer the objects the less heat that is transferred, and vice versa.
Radiation	Transfer of our body heat to other entities by radiating energy waves. This is similar to the energy waves from the sun warming our body on a sunny day.	The warmer the objects the less heat that is transferred, and vice versa.

exercising in warmer climates. Excessive body heat warms the sweat reaching our skin until the water reaches its vapor point. Sweat water changes from a liquid to a vapor which then lifts off into the air, thus taking heat with it.

> Sweating is our principal mean of releasing heat in warmer environments and during exercise.

How Much Sweat Do We Produce?

Typically sweating occurs all the time, at least to some degree, even if you are not moving and the temperature seems comfortable. For instance, if you are sitting in your living room, the sweating process is still lightly stimulated by the brain to rid excessive heat. At this low level, sweating might only yield two cups in an entire day (500 ml) Therefore, as that produced sweat moves slowly through the tubes, practically all of the sodium and chloride are brought back into our body along with some water. This results in only tiny amounts of water reaching our skin. In fact, you probably do not even realize that you are sweating, but you are. Oppositely, in a warmer environment and/or during exercise, when sweating is more strongly stimulated, it becomes very noticeable.

Can Sweat Composition Change?

Not only can sweat vary in how much is produced but it can also vary in composition. By and large the final concentration of sweat depends on how rapidly it is produced. As shown in Figure 7.2, our sweat glands are based pretty deep in our skin. When we sweat, the initial fluid oozing into the tubes leading to our skin surface is concentrated with sodium and chloride and similar to the concentration in our blood (plasma). As that sweat flows through the tube, sodium and chloride can be absorbed back into our body along with some of the water. What is most important in determining the final amount and composition of the sweat reaching our skin surface is how rapid the sweat flows through the tubes, which itself is related to the strength of stimulation. When the flow of sweat through the tubes is faster, more sweat reaches the skin and less and less sodium, chloride, and other factors are reabsorbed. As the sweat evaporates it leaves the once-dissolved substances on our skin, which can cake on a drier day.

Is It Possible to Increase the Amount We Sweat?

Because sweating is such an important means of removing heat, distance runners and other endurance athletes become "better sweaters." This

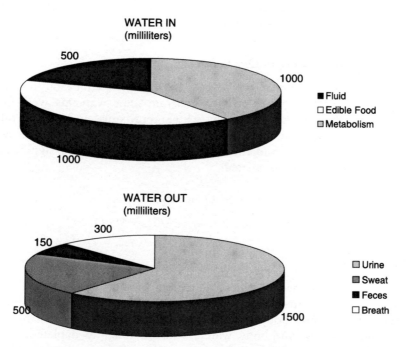

Figure 7.3 Typical volumes of water intake and loss on a daily basis for a man who does not exercise and is not exposed to a hot environment.

means that their sweat glands and tubes have adapted during the athlete's training to produce larger volumes of sweat but containing less sodium and chloride. This helps keep them from overheating but at the same time it keeps them from losing excessive amounts of the key electrolytes in sweat. A well trained endurance athlete may sweat 2 to 3 liters per hour of exercise. That's more than 8 to 12 cups.

Water Is an Essential Nutrient

What Foods and Beverages Provide Water?

If we combine the routes of water loss from our body, it totals about 2 to 3 liters (2 to 3 quarts or 8 to 12 cups) per day. If the amount of water lost from the body is not at least matched by the amount of water provided to the body, then dehydration can occur. However, this does not necessarily mean that we need to drink 8 to 12 cups of pure water every day because there is water in most of the foods we eat, including water-based fluids such as milk, coffee, tea, juices, and drinks such as soda, Kool-Aid®, sport drinks, etc. On the average we drink about 1 liter of water daily in the form of water or other fluids such as soft drinks. Furthermore, we receive about 1 liter of water in the foods we eat. Foods such as fruits and vegetables will have a relatively high water content compared with meats, breads, and fats (Table 7.2).

Can We Produce Water in Our Body?

In addition to the water we ingest, we can also count on normal metabolic reactions in our cells to generate some water as well. On average an adult will generate about ½ liter (approximately 2 cups) in our normal metabolic reactions. When our cells completely break down (combust) the glucose and the fatty acid, two of our most significant energy nutrients, water is created:

glucose: $C_6H_{12}O_6 + 6O_2 \rightarrow 6CO_2 + 6H_2O$

palmitic acid: $C_{16}H_{32}O_2 + 23O_2 \rightarrow 16CO_2 + 16H_2O.$

What is Thirst?

When our body needs water, a region of our brain called the hypothalamus initiates thirst. Thirst is a symptom of dehydration and is a signal to replenish body water. However, this also means that by the time thirst occurs, our body water is already slightly depleted. This probably is not that big a deal for most of us; however, to an athlete engaged in competition, this can result in decreased performance and the

Table 7.2 Water Content of Common Foods

Food	% Water
Collards, lettuce (iceberg)	96
Radishes, celery, cabbage (raw)	93–95
Watermelon, broccoli, beets	90–92
Snapbeans, milk, carrots, orange	87–90
Apples, cereals (cooked)	83–85
Potatoes (boiled), banana, egg (raw), fish (baked flounder)	74–78
Corn, prunes	70
Chicken (roast)	67
Beef (lean sirloin)	59
Cheese (Swiss)	42
Bread (white)	37
Cake (devil's food)	24
Butter	16
Almonds, soda crackers (e.g. saltines)	4
Sugar (white), oils	0–5

difference between victory and defeat. Most athletes who compete in endurance sports will drink prior to and during an event. A common rule among endurance athletes is that they need to "drink before they are thirsty."

Can Dehydration Affect Sport Performance?

By the time we have lost about 2 percent of our body weight as water we will become thirsty and may experience a slight reduction in strength. By the time we are dehydrated by 4 percent of our body weight, muscular strength and endurance are significantly hindered, while a 10 percent reduction of our body weight as water is associated with heat intolerance and general weakness. If dehydration continues, life itself becomes threatened. If dehydration continues to a 20 percent loss in our body weight, we become susceptible to coma and death. We will discuss the need for proper hydration in the Chapter 11.

FAQ Highlight

Is Water Our Most Essential Nutrient?

Many people regard water as our most important essential nutrient. This is because of three principal concepts. First, when we do the math, our dietary need for water far exceeds any other essential nutrient. For instance, 1 milliliter of water weighs exactly 1 gram, therefore daily need for water for an adult would be approximately 2,000 to 3,000 grams

(2 to 3 kilograms). This is about 30 to 60 times greater than our need for protein and millions of times greater than our need for different vitamins and minerals.

Second, signs and symptoms of water deficiency begin to show much more rapidly than any other essential nutrient. If we abstain from all food and drink, we would develop signs of water deprivation by the end of the first day or two. Furthermore, we may die from severe dehydration by the week's end.

Third, as water is the basis of the human body, water imbalance (dehydration or toxicity) could not occur without influencing the metabolism of all other nutrients in some way.

8 Energy Metabolism, Body Weight and Composition, and Weight

The old saying goes that little girls were made of "sugar and spice and everything nice" and little boys were made of "snakes and snails and puppy-dog tails." That definition might have sufficed when we were young, but as adults we know that what we are made of is a lot more complex. Furthermore, changing what we are made of through weight loss and improved fitness all too often proves very challenging. In this chapter we will explore the basis of body weight and composition and what it takes to lose weight and keep it off. We will also take a close look at the two biggest contributors to our body weight, namely muscle and fat, and how they impact our health.

What Is the Composition of Our Body?

What Kind of Stuff Are We Made of?

When we step on a scale, it registers the total weight or mass of our body. However, this is just a general measurement and does not really provide us with an accurate assessment of the individual contributions made by the different types of substances to our weight. Said another way, the scale is not sensitive to body composition. In the first chapter we recognized that the elements carbon, hydrogen, oxygen, and nitrogen make up greater than 90 percent of our body weight. We also acknowledged that these elements are components of the major types of molecules in our body. These molecules are by and large water, protein, fat (triglycerides), and carbohydrate, as well as variations and combinations of the latter three molecule types. Meanwhile, minerals make up most of our remaining body weight. Table 8.1 presents examples of body compositions of what are deemed to be average adults.

If we were able to remove the water from our body, we would find that our body is mostly made up of energy molecules such as protein, fat, and carbohydrate. In fact, greater than 80 percent of what would be left over is energy-providing substances in one form or another. So we can be viewed as a container of energy similar to the foods we eat. This is

Table 8.1 Theoretical Contributors to Body Weight for a Lean Man and Woman

Component (Substance)	Lean Man (%)	Lean Woman (%)
Water	62	59
Fat	16	22
Protein	16	14
Minerals	5–6	4–5
Carbohydrate	<1	<1

important, for when we are not satisfying our energy needs with external sources (food), we are able to power bodily functions by tearing down internal energy sources. Keep in mind that our cells are tireless in their operational efforts and must be fed 24 hours a day.

> Skeletal muscle and fat (adipose tissue) make up more than half of our body.

How Do the Different Tissues Contribute to Our Weight?

While it is interesting to know how much water, protein, fat, carbohydrate, and minerals are found in the body, it is often more helpful to take it up a level and look at the contributing tissue. In fact, the contribution of various tissues explains the relative contributions made by the different molecules and minerals.

Muscle and fat (adipose tissue) are typically the greatest contributors to body weight. For instance, a generally lean man will be about 40 to 45 percent muscle and 14 to 18 percent body fat. That means that muscle and fat make up half to about two-thirds of his body mass. For this man, bone might contribute about 8 percent and the skin 2 percent. The rest of body weight is composed of organs and tissue such as the heart, lungs, liver, kidneys, intestines, pancreas, brain, spinal cord, and our circulations (blood, lymphatic). The American Council on Exercise has classified body fat levels as shown in Table 8.2.

Why Do We Store Excessive Energy as Fat?

As discussed in Chapter 5, fat is how we store most of the excessive energy we consume. It is a matter of efficiency as more than double the amount of energy can be stored in a gram of fat than in carbohydrate and protein (9 calories versus 4 calories per gram). Furthermore,

Table 8.2 Body Fat Classifications

Description	Women (%)	Men (%)
Essential fat	10–12	2–5
Athletes	13–20	6–13
Fitness	21–24	14–7
Acceptable	25–31	18–25
Obese	32+	25+

Source: American Council on Exercise (ACE).

carbohydrate and protein attract water, thus storing excessive energy exclusively as glycogen or protein would increase body water tremendously. For instance, each gram of glycogen attracts about 3 grams of water. Thus storing energy primarily as carbohydrate or protein would make us much heavier, larger, and somewhat waterlogged. This would be a huge disadvantage, as body weight would probably triple!

The Basis of Body Weight Change

How Does Body Weight Change?

Body weight changes as components of body composition change. That means that a loss of body fat would decrease weight and a gain of body fat would increase it. However it is important to realize that gains in body fat are often accompanied by minor changes in supportive tissue such as muscle, skin, and bone. The same can be said of muscle. Changes in muscle mass can result in minor changes in bone, skin, and blood mass as well.

For most people body weight will change largely due to alterations in either or both body fat and muscle. Increases in muscle mass result from resistance exercise as discussed below and in Chapter 11. For regular exercisers and athletes, muscle mass becomes a significant consideration in understanding why they weigh what they weigh. Meanwhile, for most people though, the scale goes up as body fat is accumulated. In either case, changes in body weight will depend on their energy (calorie) balance. In addition, reduced physical activity, which often happens during adulthood, can reduce muscle mass and theoretically lower body weight. However, what's more typical is that losses in muscle are paralleled by gains in fat tissue which counterbalances the weight loss or can lead to weight gain if the accumulation of fat exceeds loss of muscle.

> For most people body weight changes are due to calorie imbalances and changes in physical activity.

What Is the Basis of Weight Loss or Gain?

For most people the basis for weight loss and weight gain is energy or calorie balance (Figure 8.1). To an economist, it would be a simple model of supply and demand; for us, it allows us to use those algebra skills we developed in high school. If the calories contained in the food we eat (supply or positive) exceeds the calories expended ("burned") by our body (demand or negative), then we will store the surplus.

Quantifying the energy content of foods is easy. We can simply read the food label or look at a calorie chart. A food's energy content is the sum total of the energy contributions of its protein, carbohydrate, fat, and alcohol. However, quantifying the energy that we expend over the course of a single day and assessing how our energy expenditure may fluctuate over time with respect to different situations is a bit more complicated.

How Do We Know How Much Energy Is in Food?

When scientists want to know the energy content of a food, they can place the food in an insulated chamber, called a *bomb calorimeter*, and "combust" it. Combustion requires oxygen and the products of combusting foods in a bomb calorimeter include carbon dioxide, water, and heat. In addition, if the food contains protein or amino acids, some nitrogen-containing gases will also be produced.

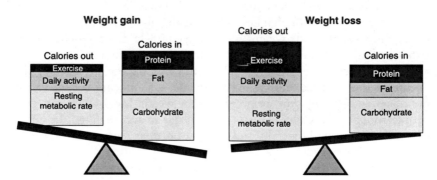

Figure 8.1 Weight gain is caused by an energy imbalance, whereby the calories expended by the body are fewer than those coming into the body in food. Weight loss is caused by an energy imbalance, whereby the calories expended by the body (metabolism) exceeds the calories brought into the body in food. Note: the mild resting metabolism and low level of daily activity and exercise in the weight gain imbalance and the increase in exercise and physical activity driving a higher "calories out" in the weight loss.

Since heat energy is typically measured in calories* it is applied to food energy and the energy used in our body. In separate experiments, scientists can also determine the individual amounts of carbohydrate, protein, fat, and alcohol in a given food. The approximate energy equivalent of 1 gram of these substances is as follows:

- 1 gram of carbohydrate = 4 calories
- 1 gram of protein = 4 calories
- 1 gram of alcohol = 7 calories
- 1 gram of fat = 9 calories

If we were to add up the energy contribution of the individual energy nutrients in a food, it should approximate the total calories of heat measured by the bomb calorimeter.

Do We Generate the Same Amount of Energy When Using Energy Nutrients in Our Body as Generated in a Bomb Calorimeter?

We combust energy nutrients in our cells and in the process generate the same amount of energy as in the bomb calorimeter. In fact, the reason we bring oxygen into our body is so that it can be used in the combustion of energy nutrients within our cells. Furthermore, carbon dioxide is produced during the combustion of these energy nutrients in our cells and we must breathe it out.

Despite several similarities between the combustion of energy nutrients in a bomb calorimeter and in our cells, there are a couple of fundamental differences. First, when amino acids and proteins are combusted in a bomb calorimeter, nitrogen-containing gases are produced. Contrarily, when amino acids are used for energy in our cells, most of the nitrogen is ultimately used to make urea. Second, the combustion of energy nutrients in a bomb calorimeter is for the most part an instantaneous process, while the combustion of energy nutrients occurring within our cells happens over a series of many chemical reactions (energy pathways). Last, unlike a bomb calorimeter, when we combust energy nutrients in our cells, we capture roughly 40 percent of the energy released in the formation of ATP and to a lesser degree guanosine triphosphate (GTP) (see Chapter 1). Meanwhile, the remainder of the energy released in the breakdown of energy nutrients is converted to heat.

---

* It is common to use calories (lower case "c") to express energy in relation to the body. To comply with common use, this book uses calorie generally to imply kilocalorie. However it is recognized that a calorie is a thousandth of a kilocalorie or Calorie (capital "C"). Food labels correctly use Calories.

How Are Energy Nutrients Used by Our Cells?

Carbohydrates, amino acids, fat, and alcohol can all be used by our cells to make ATP. Although the energy pathways involved in the metabolism of these substances are unique, they are indeed interconnected at various points. This allows us to convert glucose and certain amino acids to fatty acids and also to convert amino acids, glycerol, and lactate to glucose. However, only certain tissue will engage in these conversion activities.

> Carbohydrate use for fuel begins with an anaerobic pathway and becomes aerobic like fat and amino acids.

What Is Anaerobic Energy Metabolism?

Energy pathways in our cells occur in either the mitochondria or the intracellular fluid (cytoplasm). In the latter, monosaccharides such as glucose become engaged in an energy pathway called *glycolysis*. All cells can use glucose for energy; meanwhile fructose and galactose are used by the liver mainly. Glycolysis converts glucose to two molecules of *pyruvate*. In this process, two ATP molecules and heat energy will be generated (Figure 8.2). Since these ATP will be generated without the need for oxygen, glycolysis is often referred to as *anaerobic* energy metabolism.

Pyruvate has several options, depending on the type of cell and what is going on inside of that cell (Figure 8.3). If the cell lacks mitochondria, such as in RBCs, pyruvate is converted to *lactic acid* (lactate). This lactate enters the blood and can serve as fuel for certain other organs such as the kidneys. Meanwhile, *astrocytes* that create the blood-brain barrier produce lactate which neurons in our brain can use. The blood-brain barrier is a special molecular fence that separates the cerebral spinal fluid, which nourishes the brain and spine, from the general circulation. Perhaps the most famous source of lactic acid is muscle during intense exercise such as weight lifting or sprinting.

What Is Aerobic Energy Metabolism?

In order for pyruvate and lactate from glycolysis or fatty acids and amino acids to be used for energy in cells there need to be two things—mitochondria and ample oxygen. Because of the need for oxygen, energy generation in mitochondria is called *aerobic*. In most cells the pyruvate generated by glycolysis enters mitochondria for combustion. In addition, cells in certain tissue such as kidneys, liver, brain, and muscle will convert circulating lactate to pyruvate which can enter the mitochondria.

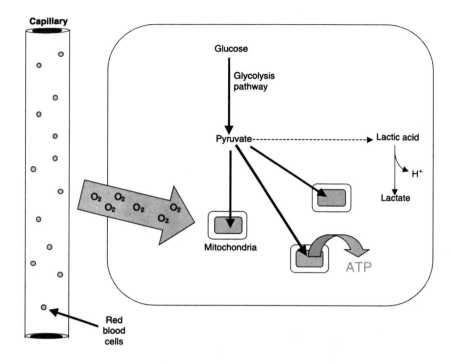

Figure 8.2 In our cells pyruvate can enter mitochondria where it is broken down further to produce energy (ATP). Because oxygen is needed for our mitochondria to produce ATP the processes are called "aerobic." If oxygen is not abundant in that cell or if the cell does not have mitochondria—a red blood cell, for example—then pyruvate is converted to lactic acid.

Meanwhile some amino acids are converted to pyruvate as well or enter mitochondria directly like fatty acids.

Aerobic energy metabolism takes place in mitochondria and requires oxygen, and produces water and carbon dioxide.

Once inside the mitochondria, pyruvate can be converted to another molecule called *acetyl CoA*. Acetyl CoA can then enter another energy pathway called the *Krebs' cycle* (Figure 8.4).

During several of the chemical reactions that take place in our mitochondria, electrons are removed by carrier molecules and transported to special links of proteins embedded in the inner membrane of mitochondria. These special links of protein are called the *electron-transport chain* (Figure 8.5). The electrons are passed from the carrier molecules to

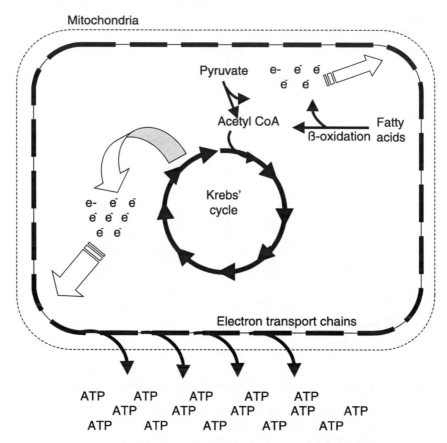

Figure 8.3 In the mitochondria of our cells, pyruvate and fatty acids are broken down to acetyl CoA which then is broken down in a series of chemical reactions called the Krebs' cycle. During the breakdown of fatty acids, pyruvate and acetyl CoA, electrons are removed and carried to the electron transport chains that are stitched into the inner membrane. The electrons then become important in the making of ATP, which can be used by that cell to power an operation! It should also be mentioned that these processes also produce carbon dioxide and water.

the electron-transport chain and then, like a bucket brigade, are passed along its length. As electrons are passed along the electron-transport chain, energy is released which drives the formation of ATP. Each of our mitochondria contains thousands of electron-transport chains.

What Are the By-Products of Energy Metabolism?

When energy nutrients are combusted by aerobic processes, the end products will be carbon dioxide, water, ATP, and heat. The carbon dioxide is actually a product of several reactions in our mitochondria.

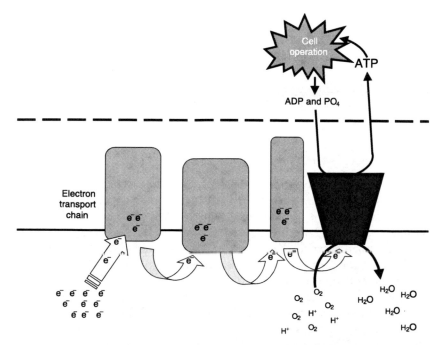

Figure 8.4 Electrons are moved down the electron transport chain allowing the production of energy (ATP). The electrons reaching the end of the chain are used to make water from available oxygen and hydrogen ions.

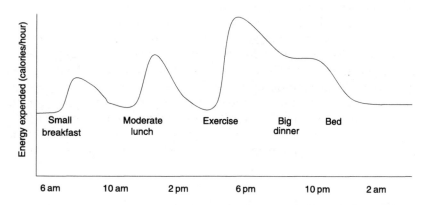

Figure 8.5 Example fluctuations in energy expenditure over a 24-hour period. This would include periods of sleep (12 am), eating (7 pm) and physical activity (4 pm). As shown in Figure 8.4, oxygen is needed to receive the electrons reaching the end of the electron-transport chain. Subsequently, the oxygen and electrons are coupled with hydrogen to make H₂O. This serves to generate water in our body on a daily basis.

Since the need for carbon dioxide is somewhat limited in our body, it is considered a waste product and must be removed by our lungs. If oxygen is absent from a cell, the electron-transport chain will become jammed up with electrons and stop functioning. At this point that cell will have to rely more heavily upon anaerobic ATP generation. This is perhaps most obvious in skeletal muscle during heavy exercise. The increased reliance on anaerobic energy metabolism in skeletal muscle leads to the production of more and more lactic acid.

What Processes Use Fat for Energy?

When we use fat (triglyceride) for energy, both the fatty acid and glycerol can be used in energy pathways. Fatty acids enter an energy pathway called *beta-oxidation* (β-oxidation), which takes place within the mitochondria. Beta-oxidation produces several molecules of acetyl CoA, which can then enter the Krebs' cycle. Also during β-oxidation electrons are removed and transported to the electron-transport chain by the special carriers mentioned previously and discussed in more detail in Chapter 9. Therefore, fatty acids require mitochondria and oxygen in order to be used for energy; they are completely aerobic. Meanwhile, glycerol's importance, from an energy standpoint, lies mainly in its ability to be converted to glucose in the liver during fasting or exercise.

How Are Amino Acids Broken Down?

Amino acids can be used for ATP production in several ways. By consuming a lot of protein, excessive amino acids will be broken down in the liver mainly. Once the nitrogen is removed from the amino acids, the remaining molecule can be converted to molecules in the energy pathways such as pyruvate, acetyl CoA, or those that are part of the Krebs' cycle. This makes the generation of energy from amino acids aerobic. Meanwhile, during fasting and endurance exercise some amino acids can be converted to glucose in the liver. And, some amino acids can be used during fasting to produce ketone bodies. Both the glucose and ketone bodies produced via amino acids will be used by other tissue such as the brain and muscle.

Metabolism Equals Energy Expenditure

What Is Metabolic Rate?

The chemical reactions that take place in our cells release energy, and this energy is ultimately derived from the breakdown of energy nutrients namely carbohydrate, protein, fat and alcohol. Over the course of the day almost all of the energy released will be converted to heat and lost from the body. Metabolism refers to the sum of the energy (calories) generated in our body and lost as heat. To go a little further, metabolic rate is the amount of heat we produce within a specified period of time, such as over an hour or a day.

If energy expenditure is measured over an hour's time, it only estimates the expenditure during that hour and cannot be confidently extrapolated to longer periods of time. For instance, if energy expenditure is measured for 1 hour after lunch or during a morning exercise session, surely it would be greater than when you are sleeping. On the contrary, if energy expenditure is expressed over a period of a day, it will not indicate periods within the day when the metabolic rate was higher, such as in more active times of the day, or lower, as in less active times of the day or when sleeping (see Figure 8.5).

> Metabolism is the sum of all chemical reactions in the body and is assessed as heat release or oxygen use.

How Do We Measure Metabolic Rate?

Our body works very hard to maintain its temperature at around 37°C (98.6°F). This means that excess heat generated by chemical reactions in cells must be dissipated. Because this dissipated heat is a direct indicator of our metabolism, we can use an insulated chamber sensitive to temperature change to determine how much heat we produce (energy expenditure). This method of estimating metabolic rate is often referred to as *direct calorimetry*. Calorimetry literally means "heat measurement." However, since the operational expense for this scientific tool is overwhelming, facilities designed to perform direct calorimetry may be found at only a handful of universities and research institutions.

One alternative method can be employed to assess metabolic rate called *indirect calorimetry*. Because ATP is generated from the combustion of energy molecules which requires oxygen and produces carbon dioxide, it is possible to estimate energy expenditure based upon these gauges. Representative chemical reactions for the combustion of carbohydrates, protein, and fat are shown below. You see that oxygen is used as a reactant for each reaction while carbon dioxide is a product. Utilizing mathematic equations we can estimate the amount of heat produced in a given period of time based upon the amount of oxygen inhaled or the amount of carbon dioxide expired. As it turns out, indirect calorimetry is not only a very accurate indicator of metabolism, but it also gives us an idea of the mixture of energy substances our body is using during that time.

Carbohydrate:

$$C_6H_{12}O_6 + 6O_2 \rightarrow 6CO_2 + 6H_2O$$

Triglyceride (fat):

$$2C_{57}H_{110}O_6 + 163O_2 \rightarrow 114CO_2 + 110H_2O$$

Protein:

$$C_{72}H_{112}N_2O_{22}S + 77O_2 \rightarrow 63CO_2 + 38H_2O + SO_3 + 9CO(NH_2)_2.$$

Based on the amount of oxygen used during a period of time, researchers can estimate the amount of energy used or more commonly calories burned. For instance, we can use 4.8 calories burned per liter of oxygen used to estimate calorie needs. If a man uses 20 liters of oxygen an hour (360 liters/day) this would translate to around 96 calories/hour or 2,300 calories daily.

How Can We Know What Our Body Is Using for Energy?

Based on the chemical reactions shown above, we can calculate what researchers call the respiratory exchange ratio (RER) (or respiratory quotient (RQ)) for a given time period. RER is equal to the amount of carbon dioxide exhaled divided by the amount of oxygen inhaled.

$$RER = CO_2/O_2$$

- RER of glucose $6CO_2/6O_2 = 1.0$
- RER for the triglyceride $114CO_2/163O_2 = 0.70$
- RER for the protein $63CO_2/77O_2 = 0.82$

If we measure a person's gases during a period of time we can calculate a few things. For example, say that during 1 hour a person consumed 15 liters of oxygen and expired 12 liters of carbon dioxide; we can first calculate their RQ for that hour:

$$RER = 12/15 = 0.80$$

We can find the RER of 0.80 on Table 8.3 and follow it over to the calorie source columns. At an RER of 0.80 this individual would be using approximately 33 percent carbohydrates and 66 percent fat to fuel his or her metabolism. We will assume that the contribution from amino acids toward energy production during that time is minimal. This is a fair assumption for a healthy person not engaged in prolonged fasting or endurance exercise during this time. Furthermore, we can estimate metabolic rate by multiplying the amount of oxygen consumed (15 liters) by the caloric value for 1 liter of oxygen for an RER = 0.80. Their metabolic rate would be:

$$15 \times 4.801 = 72 \text{ calories/hour}$$

Table 8.3 Thermal Equivalent of O_2 and CO_2 for Nonprotein Respiratory Quotient

Nonprotein RQ	Caloric Value 1 Liter O_2	Caloric Value 1 Liter CO_2	Carbohydrate (%)	Fat (%)
0.707	4.686	6.629	0	100.0
0.71	4.690	6.606	1.1	98.9
0.72	4.702	6.531	4.76	95.2
0.73	4.714	6.458	8.4	91.6
0.74	4.727	6.388	12.0	88.0
0.75	4.739	6.319	15.6	84.4
0.76	4.751	6.253	19.2	80.8
0.77	4.640	6.187	22.8	77.2
0.78	4.776	6.123	26.3	73.7
0.79	4.788	6.062	29.9	70.1
0.80	4.801	6.001	33.4	66.6
0.81	4.813	5.942	36.9	63.1
0.82	4.825	5.884	40.3	59.7
0.83	4.838	5.829	43.8	56.2
0.84	4.850	5.774	47.2	52.8
0.85	4.862	5.721	50.7	49.3
0.86	4.875	5.669	54.1	45.9
0.87	4.887	5.617	57.5	42.5
0.88	4.899	5.568	60.8	39.2
0.89	4.911	5.519	64.2	35.8
0.90	4.924	5.471	67.5	32.5
0.91	4.936	5.424	70.8	29.2
0.92	4.948	5.378	74.1	25.9
0.93	4.961	5.333	77.4	22.6
0.94	4.973	5.290	80.7	19.3
0.95	4.985	5.247	84.0	16.0
0.96	4.998	5.205	87.2	12.8
0.97	5.010	5.165	90.4	9.58
0.98	5.022	5.124	93.6	6.37
0.99	5.035	5.085	96.8	3.18
100	5.047	5.047	100	0

What Are the Major Factors That Contribute to Our Metabolism or Energy Expenditure?

Since all bodily operations and activities burn calories we can categorize them to determine the number of calories we expend daily. Classically, researchers defined the following four principal factors that contributed to our total calories burned daily.

- *Basal metabolism*—Calories burned by basic bodily operations and measured in a laboratory setting while laying down after a good night's sleep and fasted for at least 12 hours.

- *Physical activity*—Calories burned performing all physical movement.
- *Thermal effect of food*—Calories burned to digest food and process nutrients internally.
- *Active thermogenesis*—Changes in calories burned due to changes in environmental temperature.

Total energy expenditure (calories burned) = basal metabolic rate + physical activity + thermal effect of food + active thermogenesis.

A simpler and more common way to estimate the total number of calories we burn daily is to use Resting Metabolic Rate (RMR), which includes the thermal effect of food, and to ignore adaptive thermogenesis, since for most people it really isn't a factor. By doing so you focus on the number of calories your body burned in a resting (not moving) state and the number of additional calories you burn when you are moving (physical activity).

Total energy expenditure = RMR × physical activity factor (daily activities + exercise)

What Is "Resting" Metabolic Rate?

Resting metabolic rate is the number of calories your body burns while not moving (rest) to function normal and to keep you alive and well. This includes the beating of the heart, breathing, making urine, thinking, and making new molecules and cells. For instance, every second our body generates two million new red blood cells. RMR tends to account for 50 to 75 percent of total calories burned daily. That means that physical activity contributes between 25 to 50 percent depending on how active someone is throughout the day and the amount and type of exercise they do.

How Do We Estimate RMR?

RMR can be estimated using equations. One of the most common ways to assess RMR is the Mifflin–St Jeor equation. The Mifflin–St Jeor equation for RMR is:

for men

$$(10 \times \text{Wt}) + (6.25 \times \text{Ht}) - (5 \times \text{Age}) + 5$$

for women

$$(10 \times \text{Wt}) + (6.25 \times \text{Ht}) - (5 \times \text{Age}) - 161$$

Note: Wt = weight in kilograms, where 1 pound = 0.454 kilograms and Ht = height in centimeters, where 1 inch = 2.54 centimeters.

Here is an example RMR for a 35 year old man who weighs 180 pounds (82 kilograms) and is 5 ft and 11 inches tall (180 cm) using the Mifflin–St Jeor equation:

RMR = (10 × 82) + (6.25 × 180) – 5 × 35) + 5

RMR = 1,775 calories.

How Much Does Different Tissue Contribute to RMR?

Looking specifically at basal metabolism occurring within different tissues in the body we find that the most metabolically active tissue (calories expended/gram tissue) are the vital organs, namely the heart, kidneys, lungs, pancreas, brain, and liver. While only making up roughly 10 percent of our body weight, these organs accounts for as much as 50 to 60 percent of our RMR. Interestingly, the retina of the eye is the most metabolically active tissue (per gram of tissue). Meanwhile, the energy expenditure of the heart, lungs, kidneys, brain, and liver is estimated to be 15 to 40 times greater than muscle and 50 to 100 times greater than fat tissue on a pound to pound basis.

Resting metabolism is the calories your body burns at rest and usually accounts for 50 to 75 percent of total calories for the day.

Skeletal muscle tends to makes up about 40 percent of an adult's body weight and is not as metabolically active as the organs just mentioned when we are not moving. Skeletal muscle energy expenditure contributes about 25 percent to our RMR. However, keep in mind that this expenditure takes place when skeletal muscle is not working! In fact, researchers have estimated that the metabolic rate of muscle is about 4½ to 7 calories per pound (muscle) per day or about 10 to 15 calories per kilogram. On the other hand, fat tissue contributes relatively little to our RMR unless a person has a lot of body fat and then it makes a relatively greater contribution.

How Important Is Body Composition to Resting Metabolic Rate?

Since skeletal muscle and body fat typically make up more than half of our body weight it is easy to understand why these two tissues will have a major impact on RMR and daily metabolism. This is especially true since they are the tissues that are most easily manipulated. You can voluntarily gain or lose fat and muscle but you cannot grow more brain or heart. In fact, the ratio of skeletal muscle to body fat is the best predictor of a person's RMR for a given body weight. For example, we would expect an athletic, muscular 200-pound man (91 kilograms) with 12 percent body fat to have a higher RMR than a different man who weighs the same but has 25 percent body fat. Simply put, the more muscular man has a higher muscle to fat ratio, and thus a higher RMR. On a per-weight basis RMR is typically higher in males than in females because men tend to have a higher skeletal muscle to body fat ratio.

How Does Age Impact RMR?

RMR is highest during infancy when considered as calories per pound (or kilogram) of body weight. At this stage resting metabolism not only reflects normal life-sustaining operations of the infant but also must power the building of new tissue. The same can be said for growth spurts in children and teens. Conversely, as we age, our basal metabolism seems to slow down. Some researchers have estimated the slowdown to be on the order of 2 to 3 percent in each decade. This downward progression of RMR in later life can be largely attributed to the loss of fat-free mass caused by physical inactivity. Therefore, while researchers agree that some of this is related to changes in hormones, much of it is reflected in changing body composition. As we age we become less active and thus lose muscle mass and gain fat mass. In fact, when older individuals are placed on an exercise program that includes resistance exercise for muscle development they tend to gain muscle and increase their RMR.

Body composition, specifically the ratio of muscle to body fat, has the greatest impact on a person's RMR.

Can We Determine RMR Based on Muscle Mass?

The equation above is appropriate for inactive adults. However, for leaner, muscle muscular people such as athletes and fitness enthusiasts, estimating RMR based on body composition is more appropriate. The equation below is the Cunningham equation and uses fat free mass (FFM) to estimate RMR:

RMR = 500 + 22 (fat free mass)

Estimating FFM is simple once percentage body fat has been determined (below). Begin by calculating fat mass, which is body weight times percentage body fat. Then subtract fat mass from body weight to determine FFM. Assuming our example man (82 kilograms, 180 cm) from above is also an athlete with 15 percent body fat, let's use the Cunningham equation to estimate his RMR:

step 1—determine %FFM: 100% – 15% = 85% FFM

step 2—determine FFM: 82 kilograms × 0.85 = 70 kilograms FFM

step 3—determine RMR: 500 + 22 (70) = 2,040 calories.

You see that the estimate of RMR is higher for our example man, using the Cunningham equation versus Mifflin–St Jeor equation, since he is more muscular than the average man and the Cunningham equation is based on fat free mass. The difference is largely skeletal muscle mass and condition.

What Is Physical Activity and How Do We Estimate It?

The physical activity factor is the energy used by skeletal muscle activity. Simply stated, the more we contract our skeletal muscle the more calories will be used to power this activity. Physical activity includes everything from every day basic tasks such as showering, loading the dishwasher, and driving to work, to exercise such as running, swimming, and dancing.

You can use the physical activity factors (PAF) presented in Table 8.4 to get a general estimate of total calories burned daily. Let's apply these factors to estimate total calories burned daily for our example man as either an inactive person and as an athlete training most days of the week.

Total energy expenditure = RMR × PAF (daily activities + exercise)

Inactive (PAF = 1.2): 1,775 calories × 1.2 = 2130 calories

Athlete (PAF 1.725): 2,040 calories × 1.725 = 3520 calories.

Table 8.4 Physical Activity Factors (PAFs)

PAF	Class	Description
1.2	Sedentary	Little or no exercise and desk job
1.375	Lightly Active	Light exercise or sports 1–3 days a week
1.55	Moderately Active	Moderate exercise or sports 3–5 days a week
1.725	Very Active	Hard exercise or sports 6–7 days a week
1.9	Extremely Active	Hard daily exercise or sports and physical job

Obesity: A Modern-Day Nutrition Epidemic

In Chapters 9 and 10 we will discuss vitamins and minerals. In doing so our discussion will include symptoms related to deficiencies of these substances. Many of these deficiency disorders, such as goiter, were fairly common as the twentieth century began, and these deficiency diseases are still a concern in many underdeveloped countries. However, embracing the twenty-first century, the greatest nutritional concern worldwide is not one of deficiency but toxicity!

> Obesity is excessive body fatness. Not only does it affect how our body looks and functions but also increases the risk of numerous diseases including heart disease, diabetes, and arthritis.

Obesity is a condition resulting from chronic excessive energy consumption leading to accumulation of excessive body fat. Obesity is considered a disease because it can negatively impact numerous internal operations and the signs and symptoms include high blood pressure, high blood lipids, glucose intolerance, and often complaints of lethargy. Obesity also has an emotional impact as individuals are more likely to experience depression and reduced perception of self worth.

What Are Some Ways to Gauge Body Weight Status?

The term *overweight* is used to describe an individual's body weight relative to a reference or what has been deemed a more ideal body weight. There are several methods used to classify body weight. Today, however, the most globally accepted method is Body Mass Index (BMI). Body Mass Index (BMI) is derived by taking a person's weight and dividing it by his or her height squared (Table 8.5). A BMI under 25 is considered healthier because the risk of body weight related diseases is lower. As BMI climbs above 25 the risk of diseases increases. Recent estimates using BMI suggest that almost two-thirds of American adults and roughly three out of five Canadian adults are overweight.

Table 8.5 Body Mass Index Calculations

$$BMI = \frac{Weight\ (kilograms)}{Height^2\ (meters^2)} \qquad BMI = 703 \times \frac{Weight\ (pounds)}{Height^2\ (inches^2)}$$

BMI categories:

- underweight = less than 18.5
- normal weight = 18.5 to 24.9

- overweight = 25 to 29.9
- obesity = 30 or greater

What Exactly Is Obesity?

Simply stated, obesity is a state of excessive body fat. Based on research using BMI almost one-third of American adults are obese. However, one potential downfall to using BMI as a measure for obesity is that BMI is not sensitive to body composition. Remember, obesity refers to excessive contribution of fat to an individual's body weight, not necessarily total body weight. However, more times than not, the two go hand in hand. One exception is in the case of heavier yet more muscular people. These people would include bodybuilders and other strength athletes who train with weights. The training leads to the development of greater than typical amounts of muscle tissue. Thus, if we merely use body weight to determine the BMI of a 5-feet 10-inch 220-pound man with 12 percent body fat, he would have a BMI over 30 and would be considered obese. Consequently, to accurately identify obesity, we must measure body fatness, not just body weight. A body fat percentage greater than 25 percent for men and 30 percent for women is generally considered obese.

What Health Concerns Are Associated with Obesity?

Time and time again researchers have reported that strong associations exist between obesity and a greater occurrence of various diseases. These diseases include hypertension (high blood pressure), type 2 diabetes mellitus, arthritis, gallstones, heart disease, and various forms of cancer. Furthermore, a greater risk exists of complications during pregnancy and surgery and, sadly, obese people tend to live relatively shorter lives. Furthermore, it seems that the greater the obesity, the greater the risk.

The risk for type 2 diabetes mellitus is particularly disturbing. Roughly 90 percent of the people diagnosed with type 2 diabetes mellitus are obese. What has also become clear is that when these people reduce their body fat, this disease lessens in severity. Whether obesity is a direct cause of type 2 diabetes mellitus remains unclear, but scientists have determined that as fat cells swell during the accumulation of more fat, they release factors that probably make the disease worse.

Is Being Overweight and Obese Due to Genetic Reasons?

This is a difficult question to answer in the manner in which we would like it to be answered. Quite simply, obesity results from an energy (calorie) imbalance whereby more energy is brought into our body than is expended. We store the bulk of excessive energy as body fat and the weight gain also includes supporting materials such as connective tissue, muscle, bone, etc. Certainly that seems simple enough. However, identifying the underlying reasons for the imbalance is a bit more complicated. Is it merely a matter of excessive energy intake, meager energy expenditure, or a combination of both? And, are we genetically programmed to promote the energy imbalance and body fat accumulation?

An argument can easily be made that nearly all aspects of our being have a genetic basis. Thus genetic disposition must be involved in determining body weight and composition. But how? Although "faulty genes" can certainly play a role in establishing a sluggish metabolism in some people, scientists estimate that this may account for only a small percentage of obese individuals. Here the problem may lie in hormonal imbalances, such as lowered thyroid hormone. Scientists also believe that some people are genetically inclined to store body fat and hold on to it once it is stored. In this situation the cause is not hormonal as much as altered activity of the enzymes and other factors involved in storing fat.

> Obesity is caused by excessive calorie intake over time. Genetics can make certain people more susceptible to obesity in a variety of ways.

Can genetics pattern an individual's behavior, thereby rendering him or her more inclined to develop obesity? For example, people who prefer to be less active or favor energy-dense foods are likely candidates for an energy imbalance. If we apply genetics to the incidence of obesity in this manner, we can certainly attribute obesity in many people to a genetic origin of some form. For others, excessive energy consumption may be a manifestation of psychological disturbances. Here, food may serve more as an instrument of comfort or as a way to cope. The role of genetics in promoting obesity will continue to show that there are hundreds of genes that can play a role in the development of obesity; the hard part will be to apply this knowledge to help specific individuals.

Has Modern Day Society Contributed to Obesity?

Regardless of the exact causes for obesity, one thing is certain: the incidence of obesity in many countries has increased dramatically within the past few decades. In fact, in many countries almost everywhere one turns, a soda and/or vending machine can be found. It also seems that most of the commercials on television are for chips, soda, candy, and other energy-dense foods. Furthermore, many modern societies take great pride in developing ways to reduce people's physical activity level. Escalators grace every mall; airports have moving sidewalks; and everywhere you go, you can sit down. All too often roads are constructed without sidewalks or bicycle lanes.

Long ago, even eating itself involved significant energy expenditure. As hunters and gatherers, our ancestors had to spear their fish, hunt and scavenge animals, dig up roots, climb trees for leaves, and pick fruits and vegetables. Today, one simple trip to the convenience store or dialing a phone number yields a bounty of food. Even the act of preparing food, which could take hours even a generation ago has been greatly simplified and requires less expenditure of energy.

Are There Different Kinds of Obesity?

Visually it may indeed seem as if there are different types of obesity. Some people, particularly men, seem to store more fat above the waist in the abdominal region, which is referred to as upper-body obesity. Often this body shaping is described as "apple like." Others, especially women, store more fat below the waist in the buttocks and thighs which is referred to as lower-body obesity. This type of body design has been described as "pear shaped."

People exhibiting the upper-body obesity pattern seem to be at a higher risk for heart disease, stroke, diabetes mellitus, and some types of cancers. In this type of obesity more of the fat is found deeper, surrounding internal organs in the abdomen. This fat tissue is referred to as visceral fat and researchers believe that this fat functions a little differently than fat found under the skin. While the reasons for preferential storage of fat in specific sites are still unclear, hormone levels (such as estrogen) and different levels of activity of fat-storing enzymes in different parts of our body probably play the biggest roles. These enzymes are called lipoprotein lipase (LPL) and hormone-sensitive lipase (HSL).

Body Fat Can Be Assessed Several Ways

How Is Body Fat Assessed?

Some of the more common methods used to estimate body fat percentage include skinfold measurements and bioelectrical impedance assessment (BIA). Skinfold measurements are commonly performed in health clubs by personal trainers. Meanwhile, BIA equipment can be found in clinical settings, health clubs as well as in homes in the form of bathroom scales. Underwater weighing, Bod Pod, and DXA (dual energy X-ray absorptiometry) provide a more accurate and precise estimation of body fat, however, they require specialized equipment and trained personnel. These assessments are usually performed in medical clinics and university research labs.

How Does Skinfold Assessment Work?

Skinfold measurements technique is based on the premise that the layer of fat found beneath the skin, called subcutaneous fat, is a reliable indicator of total body fat. Skinfolds are pinched and measured with calipers from regions ("sites") of the body such as the back of the arm (triceps), mid-back (subscapular), above the hip (suprailiac), abdomen, and thigh. Care must be taken to pinch only the skin and the underlying layer of fat, not the skeletal muscle beneath. The measurements can then be used in an equation to determine body fat percentage. These equations were mostly generated from underwater weighing studies within specific groups of people, such as female college students, male swimmers, women or men ages thirty to fifty, and so forth. Therefore, to be accurate, we need to use the equation most applicable to the person being assessed.

Body fat percentage is commonly assessed by skinfold caliper at health clubs or BIA devices built into bathroom scales or hand-held devices.

The accuracy of skinfold assessment in estimating body fat percentage depends largely on the person doing the assessment. The average of multiple measures should be applied and equations using multiple skinfold sites should be used. A minute or more to allow compressed tissue to recover should separate the multiple measurements at the same site. A pinch should not be held for more than 4 to 5 seconds before taking a measurement. If performed correctly, skinfold measurements can be accurate plus or minus 5 percent. For example, if a person assessed body fat percentage is 20 percent, the 5 percent error range would be 19 to 21 percent.

How Does Bioelectrical Impedance Assessment (BIA) Assess Body Fat?

Bioelectrical impedance assessment or BIA is based on electrical conductance. Electrodes, which transmit and receive electricity, are in contact with two limbs and a tiny electric current is passed from one electrode to the other using our body as a conductor. Body fat will act as an insulating material, while lean tissue such as muscle will serve as a conducting material. This is because muscle contains a lot of water and electrolytes whereas fat tissue contains relatively little. Therefore, the amount of body fat relative to leaner tissue in the body will determine the speed of conduction of the electric current, which in turn is used to estimate body fat.

How Does Underwater Weighing and Bod Pod Work?

Underwater weighing and Bod Pod apply the same general principle of densitometry (density measurement) to estimate body fat. However, to do so, the former uses water and the second uses air displacement to estimate body volume. In both situations a person's weight and volume is used to determine their density (density = mass/volume), which in turn is used to estimate percent body fat.

Underwater weighing has been done at universities for decades and is still considered one of the "gold standards." Since our body is about 60 percent water, this weight would be negated when we are submerged in a tank of water. After removing as much air from the lungs as possible, the remaining body weight underwater is largely attributed to the relative amounts of body fat and nonfat or lean body mass (LBM). A person with a higher percentage of body fat will be less dense and thus a little more buoyant than a leaner person who weighs the same. Thus the person with the higher body fat level would actually weigh less underwater than a leaner individual of the same body weight.

How Does DXA Measure Body Fat?

While dual energy X-ray absorptiometry (DXA, previously DEXA) is most commonly used to assess bone health, it also provides one of the most accurate means for assessing body fat. In fact one of the advantages of DXA is that it also estimates regional body fat, such as in the abdomen, arms, and legs. The name is based on the method. Two X-ray beams with differing energy levels are transmitted at the body. Since the absorption of these beams varies with different tissue, this can used to estimate body fat as well as bone mass. DXA scans are not commonly done for body composition assessment; however, if you are have a DXA scan performed for bone health status be sure to ask for your body composition as well.

> DXA scans for bone health also provide accurate information about body fat percentage and distribution of body fat.

Food and Physical Activity: Sculptors of Body Composition

What Causes Changes in Body Weight and Composition?

Very rapid changes in body weight are usually caused by fluctuations in body water status. For instance, water losses via sweating and/or poor fluid consumption can reduce body weight by 2 pounds (1 kilogram) for each lost liter. This mild dehydration is common and triggers thirst, the principal prompter of fluid consumption. In fact, you might not perceive thirst until your body weight has been reduced by 1 percent from water losses. Also it should be recognized that when a person does not eat for an entire day, more than half of weight loss they experience would be attributable to water loss. On the contrary, there are certainly times when we may hold a little extra water in our tissue. Women certainly know this to be true at certain points in their menstrual cycles.

On the other hand, more significant changes in body weight and composition over time are more attributable to regular over-consumption or under-consumption of calories as well as the type of diet we eat and the exercise we perform. In general, the effects of these factors are relegated to specific hormones and other signals. The handling of energy nutrients being absorbed from the digestive tract is primarily influenced by insulin. In contrast, glucagon, cortisol, and epinephrine largely control the handling of stored body nutrients during fasting or exercise. In addition, serious exercise leads to additional signals in muscle to adapt and possibly get bigger (thus influencing body composition).

How Would Weight Gain from Overeating Affect Body Composition?

When we eat more energy (calories) than we use, much of it will be stored and we will gain weight. Remember, our ability to store carbohydrate (as glycogen) is limited to about 300 to 500 grams and body protein content is based upon the protein needs of our body, not how much protein we eat. This means that the more carbohydrate and protein we eat, the more we will use for energy during the hours that follow and throughout the day. This will decrease our use of fat as a fuel source. In addition, some of the energy in the carbohydrate and protein we eat will be used to make fat. So when we eat too many calories, less body and food fat is used for energy and a little fat is made as well. Subsequently, more and more body fat will accumulate over time.

> More than 80 percent of the weight gain from overeating is fat; the rest is supportive materials such as bone, muscle, and connective tissue.

When We Gain Weight, Is It All Fat?

Not all of weight gain is fat. By virtue of expanding fat cells and of simply being a larger person, the absolute amount of body protein, mineral, and water also increases. For example, if a person's body weight increases by 10 pounds (approximately 4.5 kilograms) because of overeating, the amount of protein in the body may increase by ¼ to ½ pound (approximately ½ to 1 kilogram). The accumulation of non-fat, supportive substances may account for as much as 20 percent of our weight gain from chronic overeating. However, since the increase of these nonfat substances like protein is small relative to the increase in fat, their percentage of our total body weight will still decrease. Body fat percentage can climb upward of 70 percent of total body weight in morbidly obese people. This latter situation would leave only about 30 percent for all other body components.

Will Different Types of Diets Evoke the Same Weight Gain?

The conversion of excess glucose and protein to fat is not a simple process. These substances must engage in chemical reaction pathways, which will require energy to operate. Therefore, our body must expend energy to make fat. This means that a person eating a higher-carbohydrate/protein diet in excess of energy needs will not store quite as much energy in the form of fat in comparison with an individual who eats a high fat diet in excess of energy needs. So, to address the notion that higher-carbohydrate diets make us "fat," the answer is yes, but only when we eat more calories than we burn over time. However, if we eat the same amount of fat calories in excess of expenditure it is easier for our body to store the food fat as body fat.

Are Energy Nutrient Ratios Important in Weight Loss?

Over the past couple of decades several popular diet programs and philosophies were founded on eliminating energy sources or creating energy nutrient ratios. The late 1970s and 1980s seemed to be about removing fat from the diet, while in the past couple of decades we have seen the emergence of *The Zone* and re-emergence of *Dr Atkins' Diet Revolution* and the explosion of *The South Beach Diet*. The Zone is based on a lowered calorie intake and partitioning calories between carbohydrate, protein and fat in a 40:30:30 ratio. Meanwhile, Atkins and South Beach are based on carbohydrate restriction for a period of time followed by reintroduction of some carbohydrate back into the diet.

But what do we really know about energy nutrient ratios and their influence on weight loss, weight gain, and body composition? It does seem that when we eat carbohydrates and protein they are used for energy before fat; there is a hierarchy of food calorie utilization. For instance, if we eat 70 percent carbohydrate, then roughly 70 percent of our energy expenditure will be carbohydrate. This is mostly due to the ability of insulin to promote the use of glucose for energy. If we eat 50 percent protein, then roughly that amount of our daily energy expenditure will be from protein. Meanwhile, if you switch to a high fat diet it will take a week or more before you begin to match the higher fat intake with higher fat used for energy, but you get there.

Research studies have helped health professional understand how different types of diets can help people lose weight and improve body composition. It does seem that in the short run—up to 6 months of dieting—lower carbohydrate intakes allow for a little more weight loss than higher carbohydrate intakes. However extending out longer, both diets do about the same when it comes to weight lost and people aren't able to stick with one diet better than the other. So, in general the most important nutritional factor in determining weight loss is calorie level. However, as we will discuss soon, determining the energy nutrient ratio can be important in controlling hunger and increasing leanness.

Are Certain Nutrients Better for Weight Management Than Others?

Research studies have supported the notion that all calories are not equal when it comes to leading to body fat accumulation. For instance, all foods increase our metabolism to some degree, which scientists refer to as the thermal effect of food. However, when people eat different meals containing the same number of calories but with different nutrient compositions, in some cases they burn more calories in the couple of hours that follow. In particular, foods with more calories from protein and unsaturated fat tend to increase calorie burning more than if those same calories came from carbohydrate and saturated fat. So less of the food calories would be available for fat storage.

> Energy nutrients such as protein and unsaturated fat are not easily converted to fat and are ideal choices to substitute for saturated fat and simple sugars.

Furthermore, certain types of unsaturated fat can play additional roles in influencing our ability to make fat from excessive diet-derived carbohydrate and amino acids. Some studies have shown that eating a diet that derives more of its fat from good sources of omega-3 PUFAs (for example, fish) may actually decrease our ability to make fat from excessive diet-derived carbohydrate and amino acids. This is another good reason to eat a couple of servings of fish weekly or to take a fish oil or an algae omega-3 supplement.

What Happens When We Completely Restrict Calories to Lose Weight for a Day or Two?

If we completely fast for a day or two, weight loss would certainly be rapid and this fact is encouraging for "crash dieters." However, the composition of the weight loss may not be as expected. As much as 60 to 70 percent of that weight loss might be attributable to water loss. Meanwhile, much of the remaining weight loss would be carbohydrate, and to a lesser degree, fat and protein. Keep in mind that glycogen stores bind water. As mentioned earlier, scientists estimate that every gram of glycogen sponges about three grams of water. So during that fasting period when liver glycogen is broken down for energy, water will move out of liver cells into our blood, circulate to our kidneys, and be urinated out. This process makes the scale go down rapidly as the loss of a half of glycogen would lead to about 2 pounds of total weight loss.

What Happens If We Continue to Fast for Longer Periods?

As the fast continues beyond a day or two, liver glycogen is no longer a major energy storage resource. Body fat breakdown is in high gear and becomes the major fuel source. Keep in mind that because all cells in the body have at least a minimal need for glucose at all times, our liver will need to generate some glucose. Amino acids become the major resource for this process. Most of the amino acids will be derived from skeletal muscle protein at first. Thus, with severe energy restriction you can certainly count on burning body fat, but you will also lose body protein (that is, muscle mass). This is usually not what we want!

How Much Body Protein Would We Lose During Fasting?

Even though your body would be fueled mostly by fat during prolonged fasting, protein would still make a remarkable contribution to your weight loss. The reason lies in the energy density differences between fat and protein. Consider this example: if a man has been fasting for 5 days, on the fifth day he might be deriving about 75 percent of his energy from body fat and the remainder from protein. If he expended 2,000 calories that day, then 1,500 calories would have come from fat and 500 calories from body protein. If we calculate the mass (weight) of the fat and protein used it would be roughly 165 grams of fat and 125 grams of protein. That's roughly one-third of a pound of fat and a quarter pound of protein. Some weight loss from water would be expected due to its association to lost protein.

If starvation were to endure for even longer, less body protein would be broken down on a daily basis and used as energy. This happens for a couple of reasons. First, our brain would require lesser amounts of glucose as it adapts to use more ketone bodies. As we discussed in Chapter 5, ketone bodies are made in our liver during periods of high fat utilization. This is a survival mechanism serving to reduce the rate of loss of body protein. During prolonged starvation, the cause of death is usually related to body protein loss. Amazingly, our brain can replace about half of its glucose requirement with ketone bodies after a week or so of complete starvation. Second, during prolonged energy restriction, the thyroid gland may release less and less thyroid hormone. This slows our RMR and in turn decreases the requirement for protein breakdown.

Rapid weight loss can increase muscle loss which in turn can lower metabolic rate, slow weight loss and make weight regain easier.

What Happens to Our Body Composition During Semi-Starvation?

During extended periods when our energy intake is mildly to moderately restricted and most of the diet energy is derived from carbohydrate and protein, the composition of the weight loss would be different than during complete starvation. Since glycogen stores would be partially restored in response to meals, this would lead to less reliance upon the breakdown of our body protein. Furthermore, our diet will also provide protein to replace some of the amino acids used for energy.

Insulin would promote the rebuilding of body protein, especially muscle, as well as liver and muscle glycogen. Contrary to the complete fast (zero energy) there would not be the early rapid weight loss that is attributable mostly to water. The weight loss experienced during extended periods of a mild to moderate energy restriction will largely be a mixture of fat, some protein, and a little water. However, the relative fat to protein contribution to energy expenditure would be much more favorable versus complete fasting. In addition, resistance training and eating more protein will also help minimize body protein loss.

Some moderate energy-restricted diet plans (1,000 to 1,200 calories) include protein levels that well exceed the RDA. This design is believed to help spare body protein during weight loss. The reason is that the diet protein-derived amino acids can be used for glucose production, thus sparing some body protein from breakdown. Furthermore, if the energy restriction is also limited in carbohydrate (as popular today), amino acids can also stimulate the release of insulin, although to a much lesser degree than carbohydrate. Insulin will help move amino acids into skeletal muscle and dampen the protein breakdown processed. Further still, the branched chain amino acids, particularly leucine, plays a direct role in promoting muscle protein manufacturing.

Can We Lose Only Fat During Weight Loss?

When body weight is reduced, we must expect some obligatory loss in protein, water, and minerals. This only makes sense because these nutrients were important to a person before the weight loss. Even though fat tissue is composed of about 86 percent fat, when fat cells expand, more of the other nutrients are needed to support the new size and metabolism of the larger cells and tissue. For instance, cell membranes of fat cells must expand and more enzymes may be needed. Furthermore, new fat cells may have been made during the accumulation of body fat. On the contrary, when fat is mobilized from fat cells, these cells shrink, thereby decreasing the need for the extra supporting nutrients. When the body was heavier, the amount of skeletal muscle and density of the bones may have been a little greater to support and move the larger body. Researchers usually find that heavier people have denser bones. Thus, as body weight decreases, it is only reasonable that these areas will decrease as well. Excessive skin and some connective tissue would be broken down during weight loss as well; both of these tissues are protein rich.

Moderate calorie restriction coupled with resistance exercise can reduce the loss of muscle during weight loss which can support maintenance.

If you incorporate resistance training in your efforts to change your body composition, it certainly is possible to lose more body fat than without training. Here, the maintenance of body protein, minerals, and water may be necessary as you hold onto as much muscle mass as possible. In fact, it is possible that you might not even lose weight as you lose body fat. This might be indicative for people who are slightly overweight compared with those who are obese.

Weight Loss Employs Smart Planning and Execution

What Do We Need to Know Before Starting a Weight Loss Regimen?

Before engaging in any type of weight loss program, some things must be understood and then tracked moving forward. First, begin by assessing the current situation.

- What is your current body weight and what is a realistic goal weight (including short-term goal weights)?
- What is your body composition, including body fat percentage as well as fat and fat free masses?
- What are your starting tape measurements (waist, hips, chest, shoulders, thigh, arm, leg, etc)?

- What are your starting health risk indicators (blood cholesterol levels, triglycerides, blood pressure, and glucose)?
- What are your emotional and physical goals?
- What is the right calorie level for you?
- What types and amount of exercise will you do?

Be sure to track these measures moving forward. Keep a food and exercise log for at least 2 weeks to get a handle on your calorie balance and compliance to your exercise program.

How Many Calories Should We Eat During Weight Loss?

Most health professionals recommend a much less drastic energy reduction coupled with exercise for weight reduction. Rarely are energy levels restricted below 1,000 to 1,200 calories. You can begin by using the equations provided earlier in the chapter to identify a calorie level that is right for you. Then calculate the calorie level that will allow you 1 to 2 pounds of weight loss per week.

The golden rule of dieting states that to theoretically lose one pound of body-fat tissue, you need to create an energy imbalance of 3,500 calories in the favor of weight loss. Since 1 pound of fat weighs 454 grams and because fat cells are roughly 86 percent fat, to lose a pound of fat it would require about 3,500 calories:

$$454 \text{ grams} \times 0.86 = 390 \text{ grams of fat} \times 9 \text{ calories} = 3,510 \text{ calories.}$$

Therefore to reduce body weight by a pound of fat per week, an individual would need to create an energy imbalance of 3,500 calories per week favoring weight loss. Dividing 3,500 calories by 7 days, one would need to create an average energy deficit of 500 calories daily. To lose two pounds, create a calorie imbalance of 1,000 calories daily.

Increasing physical activity throughout the day as well as exercising can account for a lot of the calorie imbalance. Table 8.6 provides the approximate number of calories expended during various activities and exercises. For example, a 185-pound man walking at a 5 mph pace for 60 minutes would expend about 600 calories of energy.

What Are Plateaus?

The rate of weight loss may not be consistent throughout your efforts. Weight loss rate may be greater earlier on, taper off as the regimen continues and even plateau. First and foremost, this is typical! Periods of plateau can represent your body's adaptation to the energy restriction by slowing down a bit. As a survival mechanism, your metabolism can slow

Table 8.6 Energy Expended During Various Sports

Activity	Approximate Energy Expended (Calories/pound of body weight/ minute)					
	100 lb (45.5 kg)	120 lb (54.5 kg)	140 lb (63.6 kg)	160 lb (72.7 kg)	180 lb (82 kg)	200 lb (90 kg)
Bicycling						
5 mph	1.9	2.3	2.7	3.1	3.5	3.9
10 mph	4.2	5.1	5.9	6.8	7.6	8.5
15 mph	7.3	8.7	10	11.6	13.1	14.5
20 mph	10.7	12.8	14.9	17.1	19.2	21.3
Running						
6 mph	7.2	8.7	10.2	11.7	13.1	14.6
7 mph	8.5	10.2	11.9	13.6	15.4	17.1
8 mph	9.7	11.6	13.6	15.6	17.6	19.5
9 mph	10.8	12.9	15.1	17.3	19.5	21.7
Skiing (downhill)	6.5	7.8	9.2	10.5	11.9	13.2
Skiing (cross country)						
2.5 mph	5	6	7	8	9	10
4.0 mph	6.5	7.8	9.2	10.5	11.9	13.2
5.0 mph	7.7	9.2	10.8	12.3	13.9	15.4
Soccer	5.9	7.2	8.4	9.6	10.8	12
Tennis	5	6	7	8	9	10
Walking						
3 mph	2.7	3.3	3.8	4.4	4.9	5.4
4 mph	4.2	5.1	5.9	6.8	7.6	8.5
5 mph	5.4	6.5	7.7	8.7	9.8	10.9
Weightlifting	5.2	6	7.3	8.3	9.4	10.5

down to accommodate imbalances in energy intake. Some of this will be hormonal (for example, thyroid hormone) while the bulk of it is due to the loss of body tissue, especially muscle. This is one of the most important reasons to do some resistance exercise during weight loss. This will help your body hold on to as much muscle as possible as you lose weight and minimize the reduction of RMR.

> Weight loss plateaus happen and should be used to re-evaluate your calorie level and exercise program to make adjustments.

Keep in mind that changes in body weight do not always reflect changes in body composition. This is why it is important to monitor body composition with body weight. Furthermore, make note of changes in "fatty" regions of the body such as the waist, face, and chin. Your clothes may begin to fit differently and you may feel less jiggling when climbing stairs. Your exercise program can lead to tape measurements of different body parts as your body composition changes and you redistribute your weight. Furthermore, health risk measures can continue to change as you stick with your program. So even though the scale isn't moving you are probably still making progress. This is a good time to start weighing yourself less frequently and focus on other measures.

Can Drugs Help People Lose Weight?

The short answer is more than likely. There are a couple of ways for substances such as these to work. Approved weight-loss drugs target appetite suppression (Sibutramine and Rimonibant) or reducing fat digestion (Orlistat). Amphetamines (for example, fenfluramine (Pondimin) and dexfenfluramine (Redux), which increase energy expenditure, were taking off the market in the 1990s because of risk of serious cardiovascular side effects. See the FAQ Highlight "Weight Loss Drugs and Supplements" at the end of the chapter for more details.

Can Nutrition Supplements Help People Lose Weight and Body Fat?

Numerous nutrition supplements are available that tout weight loss, increased fat breakdown and/or burning or appetite suppression. The most common ingredients or origin include caffeine (and related molecules), guarana, green tea, conjugated linoleic acid (CLA), citrus auranteum, hydroxy citric acid (HCA), and Hoodia. Among these the best scientific support is with caffeine which is why caffeine or similar molecules (theobromine, theophylline) or natural sources such as guarana, teas, and cocoa are typically the foundation of weight loss supplements. See "FAQ Highlight: Weight Loss Drugs and Supplements" at the end of the chapter for more details.

> Supplements and drugs offer some hope to controlling body weight, however people need to know how they work and possible side effects.

Can Frequent Dieting Have Derogatory Effects?

Many people are on a dieting roller coaster. Some starve or semi-starve themselves for several days to weeks and then eat excessively for a period of time. This is sometimes called *yo-yo dieting*. During the period of drastic energy restriction, the body will deplete its glycogen stores and rely heavily upon stored fat and protein to power metabolic activities. Since protein is largely derived from lean body tissue, such as skeletal muscle, this practice tends to reduce muscle mass and in turn decrease basal metabolism. This can result in a decrease in RMR calories and a greater likelihood of gaining weight when we return to eating an unrestricted amount of energy. Furthermore, it may be that the activity of some of the enzymes involved in making fat from excessive carbohydrates and amino acids may be slightly higher once we begin to eat again. There-fore, we have ultimately set ourselves up for a potentially quick return of body weight, especially body fat.

Is It Possible to Be Too Lean?

It is not healthy to be excessively lean as it increases the risk for various diseases as well as malnutrition. An excessively lean male would have less than 5 percent body fat, while an excessively lean female would have less than 10 to 12 percent body fat. Do not forget that 0 percent body fat cannot be a goal, as not all body fat is stored in adipose tissue, which is classically called "fat." Some fat is stored in bone marrow and other vital places. Excessively lean girls often fail to produce adequate sex hormones (such as estrogens), a condition which is associated with irregular or halted menstrual cycles, which promotes the loss of bone mineral, setting them up for bone disorders such as osteoporosis.

FAQ Highlight

Weight Loss Drugs and Supplements

The mainstream use of prescription drugs for weight loss extends back to the start of the 20th century. Since then several drugs including thyroid hormone and more recently *phen-fen* have been offered to patients to help shed those unwanted pounds. Today only a few options are available for weight loss and the mode of action is either appetite suppression or lipase inhibition.

What Are Appetite Suppressants?

Sibutramine (Meridia) and phentermine (for example, Adipex-P, Fastin, Ionamin, Oby-trim, Pro-Fast, Zantrylare) are the most commonly pre-scribed appetite suppressants in the US. Appetite suppressants support weight loss by decreasing appetite and/or promoting satiety (sense of feeling full). In order to do so these drugs must increase one or more chemicals in the brain that affect appetite, namely serotonin. Phen-fen coupled phentermine with fenfluramine, an amphetamine which was removed from the market in 1996 because of an increased risk of cardio-vascular complications. Side effects of sibutramine can include mild increases in blood pressure and heart rate, headache, dry mouth, consti-pation, and insomnia. Phentermine along with other appetite suppres-sants (phendimetrazine (Bontril, Plegine, Prelu-2, X-Trozine, Adipost) and diethylpropion (Tenuate, Tenuate dospan) can cause sleeplessness and nervousness.

Rimonabant is also an appetite suppressant and it works by blocking a brain cell receptor called a cannabinoid-1 receptor. Blocking this receptor has been shown to reduce appetite which can decrease long-term calorie intake and lead to weight loss.

What Are Lipase Inhibitors?

Orlistat (Xenical) is a lipase inhibitor that decreases fat digestion in the small intestine by blocking the action of lipase coming from the pancreas. This in turn decreases fat absorption which can support weight loss. However, the decreased fat absorption means that more ends up in the large intestine and thus in feces as well as acted upon by the bacteria in the colon. Side effects can include frequent oily bowel movements, diar-rhea, bloating, and abdominal pain. *Alli* is the dietary supplement version of Orlistat and provides the same active ingredient but at half the level of Orlistat. It was released to market in mid 2007 with guidance to con-sumers to use a low-fat diet to reduce the risk of undesirable side effects.

What Is Alli?

Alli hit the shelves of stores that sell supplements in 2007. Alli contains the same ingredients as the drug Orlistat, but at half the dosage level. Thus like Orlistat, the primary function of Alli is to block the enzyme that digests fat in the digestive tract, which in turn would lead to less fat absorbed in the body. The undigested fat would continue into the colon and become part of feces. However, the fat can be metabolized by bac-teria leading to some unpleasant side effects including gas, incontinence, and oily spotting.

What Is Ephedra and Ma Huang?

Ma huang is a Chinese herb that has been used for thousands of years to treat asthma and other conditions as it contains ephedra alkaloids. Ephedra alkaloids are a stimulate and are able to stimulate to cardiovascular system as well as promote the breakdown of fat. In the 1980s and 1990s, ephedra was found in numerous weight-loss products; however, safety issues motivated the FDA to ban sales of ephedra and extract with ephedra (such as ma huang) in 2004.

Can Caffeine Help Us Lose Weight?

Caffeine can be found in some plant leafs, nuts, and seeds, such as the coffee bean, tea leafs (for example, green, black, oolong), kola nut, cacao seed, and certain herbal extracts (such as yerbe maté, guarana) shrubs. An average cup of coffee may contain 50 to 150 milligrams of caffeine, while a cup of tea may contain 50 milligrams. A 12-ounce (355 milliliters) can of soda can contain about 35 milligrams. Although chocolate contains some caffeine, most of its caffeine-like potency comes from a similar substance called theobromine, while tea contains more theophylline.

Caffeine can promote wakefulness and alertness, which in turn can promote more activity and more calories burned. Caffeine seems to do this by competing with the neurotransmitter adenosine in the brain. Adenosine seems to be more of a relaxing substance, as it appears to decrease the activity of the brain. However, to counter the effects of caffeine competition, the brain adapts by producing more and more receptors for adenosine. So adenosine can overcome the presence of caffeine. This means that we will begin to need to ingest more caffeine to feel the same stimulating effects. This also explains why we feel especially groggy and "washed out" when we do not have the usual morning coffee.

Caffeine also can have cardiovascular stimulatory effects and possibly increase the use of fat as an energy source in the body. In fat cells caffeine promotes the breakdown of fat from stores and the release of fat into the blood. If muscle and the liver are using fat as a principal fuel source, such as in-between meals and during exercise, this can help optimize fat utilization during those times.

In general the research performed on caffeine suggests that it can play a supportive role in weight loss efforts by increasing energy expenditure (thermogenic) slightly above normal. Over the long term this could lead to additional weight loss in conjunction with a caloric imbalance favoring weight loss.

Does Green Tea Extract Promote Weight Loss?

All teas, such as white, black, green, and oolong are made by processing the leaves or buds of the tea bush (*Camellia sinensis*) and differ in their degree of processing after harvest. Teas and extracts can support weight loss efforts by providing caffeine and other potentially beneficial factors called catechins. Research supports the notion that caffeine can raise metabolism slightly, which over time could add up to weight loss if an individual consumes a calorie level that does not counterbalance this effect.

Catechins include the highly touted EGCG (epigallocatechin gallate) which in some research has been shown to positively influence some of the events involved in the accumulation of body fat as well as the reduction of existing body fat. Since by and large this research was performed on tissue samples and rodents it is difficult at this time to apply the finding to people.

Can Red Peppers Assist in Weight Loss?

When red peppers are part of a meal, the calories a person burns is typically greater than if the same meal was consumed without peppers. Thus red peppers seem to be thermogenic. However, the limited amount of research involving people and weight loss has not clearly shown that red peppers by themselves or as an extract, promote weight loss or help block the regain of weight once it is lost by dieting. Based on the research information to date, red peppers or extracts seem to be a viable addition to a weight loss plan.

9   Vitamins Are Vital Molecules in Food

Almost a century ago a scientist coined the term *vitamine* when describing a vital nitrogen (amine)-containing component of food. Vitamine was a condensed word for a *vital amine*-containing substance. However, as more and more vitamins were discovered, researchers observed that many did not contain nitrogen, so eventually the "e" was dropped from vitamine, converting it to the more familiar term *vitamin*.

Vitamin Basics

What Are Vitamins?

For a substance to be added to the highly dignified list of vitamins, it must be recognized as an essential player in at least one necessary chemical reaction or process in the body. Vitamins are non-caloric substances and are required in very small amounts, typically micrograms (µg) to milligram (mg) quantities. A microgram and a milligram are one-millionth and one-thousandth of a gram, respectively. Vitamins either can't be made in the body or are not made in sufficient quantities to meet our needs. We will discuss two vitamins (niacin and vitamin D) that can be made in the body, and two others (vitamin K and biotin) that are made by the bacteria inhabiting the large intestine. However, they are still considered vitamins, which will be explained shortly.

What Is the Basic Difference Between Fat-Soluble and Water-Soluble Vitamins?

Because the basis of the body is water, it only makes sense that vitamins are grouped together based upon their ability to dissolve in water. There are ten water-soluble and four fat-soluble vitamins (Table 9.1). Some general assumptions regarding the two different classes of vitamins can be made. For instance, water-soluble vitamins generally have limited storage ability in the body and are more susceptible to removal from the body in the urine (with the exception of vitamin B_{12}). Therefore, it is logical to

Table 9.1 Vitamins

Water-Soluble Vitamins		Fat-Soluble Vitamins
Vitamin C	Vitamin B_{12}	Vitamin A
Thiamin (B_1)	Folate	Vitamin D
Riboflavin (B_2)	Pantothenic acid	Vitamin E
Niacin (B_3)	Biotin	Vitamin K
Vitamin B_6	Choline	

think that signs of a deficiency of a water-soluble vitamin may appear more rapidly than would fat-soluble vitamins' symptoms when they are lacking from the diet.

Are There Special Considerations for Fat-Soluble Vitamins in the Digestive Tract?

Fat-soluble vitamins are very dependent upon the processes of normal lipid digestion and absorption, such as the presence of bile and the construction of chylomicrons in the cells lining our small intestine. Thus, any situation in which there is decreased bile production and/or delivery to our small intestine would greatly decrease fat-soluble vitamin absorption into our body. Because the presence of fat in the diet is the most powerful stimulus for bile delivery to the small intestine, it only makes sense that a nutrition supplement containing fat-soluble vitamins should be taken with a fat-containing food or meal.

What Are B-Complex Vitamins?

Decades ago researchers knew there was a complex of factors involved in proper energy metabolism in the cells. They called this the B complex. Soon researchers were able to identify the specific individual factors involved in the B complex. Hence, the classification of vitamins B_1, B_2, B_3, B_6, and B_{12}. Folate, biotin, and pantothenic acid are also involved in the processing of energy nutrients and are thus included in the B-complex family. Vitamin C and choline are not included in the B-complex family with its water-soluble brethren because it is not directly involved in the chemical reaction pathways that either break down or build energy nutrients.

Water-Soluble Vitamins

The water-soluble vitamins include the B-complex vitamins and vitamins C and choline. DRI recommendations for water-soluble vitamin intake is in the range of micrograms to milligrams and those levels are provided in Chapter 3. In addition to foods, supplements make a significant contribution to many people's intake.

Vitamin C

What Is Vitamin C?

Vitamin C is the common name for ascorbic acid. People, along with other primates, guinea pigs, and birds, are unable to make vitamin C. Other animals and plants can make their own vitamin C from glucose. Vitamin C has long enjoyed popularity as a nutrition supplement and continues to be one of the most recognizable and sought after nutrients.

What Are Food and Supplement Sources of Vitamin C?

When we think of good sources of vitamin C, citrus fruits instantly come to mind. However, other fruits and some vegetables such as strawberries, tomatoes, and broccoli can make a significant contribution to our vitamin C intake (Table 9.2). Ascorbic acid (L-ascorbic acid) is a popular nutrition supplement and there isn't an advantage to supplementing vitamin C extracted from plants or synthetic (laboratory made) forms. Supplement makers often manufacture ascorbic acid–mineral combinations (for example, sodium ascorbate and calcium ascorbate) that are less acidic than ascorbic acid. These forms can help people who find ascorbic acid irritating to their stomach.

Table 9.2 Vitamin C Content of Select Fresh Foods

Food	Vitamin C (mg)	Food	Vitamin C (mg)
Fruits		*Vegetables*	
Orange juice (1 cup)	124	Green peppers (½ cup)	95
Kiwi (1)	108	Cauliflower, raw (½ cup)	75
Grapefruit juice (1 cup)	94	Broccoli (½ cup)	70
Cranberry juice cocktail (1 cup)	90	Brussels sprouts (½ cup)	65
		Collard greens (½ cup)	48
Orange (1)	85	Cauliflower, cooked (½ cup)	30
Strawberries (1 cup)	84	Potato (1)	29
Cantaloupe (¼)	63	Tomato (1)	23
Grapefruit (1)	51		
Raspberries (1 cup)	31		
Watermelon (1 cup)	15		

*Does Vitamin C Break Down After Fruit/Vegetable Harvest and
During Cooking?*

Vitamin C is susceptible to breakdown during certain cooking, processing, and storage procedures (that is, heat or cooking in neutral or basic
mediums). For instance, potatoes can lose nearly half of their vitamin C
by boiling. Spinach can lose nearly all its vitamin C if stored for 2 to 3
days at room temperature. Thus, for practical purposes, citrus fruits
and other vitamin C-containing fruits and vegetables usually are better
dietary sources of vitamin C as they are generally eaten uncooked and
shortly after harvest.

How Much Vitamin C Is Absorbed?

Vitamin C is fairly well absorbed from our digestive tract when consumed
in typical dietary amounts. However, as the amount of vitamin C
increases in our diet its absorption efficiency decreases. For example, a
vitamin C intake of 180 milligrams (two times the RDA for an adult man)
is about 80 to 90 percent absorbed, while for an intake approximating
5 grams, only about one quarter is absorbed. However, 25 percent
absorption of 5 gram is still about 1.2 gram of vitamin C. Much of
this excessive vitamin C will be quickly removed from the body in the
urine.

How Much Vitamin C Do We Need?

The Recommended Dietary Allowance (RDA) for vitamin C for adult
men and women is 90 and 75 milligrams, respectively. During pregnancy
and lactation the RDA increases to 85 and 120 milligrams for adult
women. This is the level of vitamin C that will provide for good blood
and organ vitamin C status for most adults. Meanwhile an intake of
400 milligrams for healthy adults is recommended by many nutritionists
to ensure that the levels in the blood and cells are optimal.

Where Is Vitamin C Found in Our Body?

Vitamin C is found in most of the tissue throughout the body with greater
concentrations in the heart, brain, pancreas, adrenal glands, thymus, and
lungs. Two of the most vitamin C-dense regions in the body are the pituitary gland and the lens of the eye. Vitamin C status in the body is typically
assessed by measuring serum levels as well as the level of white blood
cells. The former is more reflective of recent dietary intake while the latter
is a better indicator of tissue stores. As vitamin C circulates in the blood it
is vulnerable to kidney filtration and subsequent loss in the urine either as
ascorbic acid or derivatives (metabolites) such as oxalates.

What Roles Does Vitamin C Play in Our Body?

The activity of vitamin C is realized in its ability to either donate or accept electrons. In doing so it participates in many metabolic processes. Perhaps its most famous role is its involvement in the production of collagen. However, vitamin C plays a role in the production of other vitamin molecules including carnitine, norepinephrine, and bile acids.

> Vitamin C is a potent antioxidant and supports the production of bile, collagen, carnitine, and norepinephrine.

Collagen is a connective tissue protein and is found in teeth, bone, tendons, ligaments, cartilage, and arteries. Vitamin C is fundamentally involved in modifying specific amino acids in the collagen protein which ultimately affects collagen's structure and function. Without vitamin C, the collagen that is made is relatively worthless.

Norepinephrine functions as a neurotransmitter in the brain and in organs to regulate their function as well as a hormone released from the adrenal glands during exercise and fasting. Among other operations norepinephrine is involved in the "fight or flight" response which helps us deal with stressful and threatening situations. Norepinephrine is made from the amino acid tyrosine and vitamin C plays a role in the conversion process.

Carnitine is needed to use longer chain length fatty acids for energy, as it basically chaperones these fatty acids into the mitochondria of our cells where they can be broken down for ATP production. The making of carnitine in the liver requires vitamin C among other substances.

Bile acids are produced in the liver and are vital for efficient fat digestion and absorption. Since bile acids are derived from cholesterol, which in turn decreases the amount of cholesterol that circulates, vitamin C plays a role in lowering the risk of heart disease.

Vitamin C is also an antihistamine factor and an immune function potentiator, and is involved in the making of thyroid hormone, serotonin, and steroid hormones.

Vitamin C enhances iron absorption from our digestive tract. This means that both iron and vitamin C would need to be part of the same meal for this to occur.

Is Vitamin C a Potent Antioxidant?

One role of vitamin C, which is receiving more and more attention today, is that of antioxidant. Antioxidants serve as lines of protection against free radicals, as discussed in Chapter 1. Antioxidants provide protection against free-radical activity that can lead to heart disease, cancers, and other medical concerns, so this role of vitamin C is more of a nutraceutical role. Not only does vitamin C serve as potent antioxidant it can also reactivate other antioxidants, namely vitamin E.

What Happens If We Don't Get Enough Vitamin C?

Poor consumption of fruits and vegetable sources of vitamin C, as well as smoking can reduce vitamin C status in the body. This in turn can lower antioxidant protection and over time could reduce the efficiency of other vitamin C roles in the body. Meanwhile, true vitamin C deficiency syndrome is referred to as *scurvy*. For adults, scurvy will appear approximately 1 to 3 months after discontinuing vitamin C consumption. Medical signs and symptoms include impaired wound healing, fluid buildup in ankles and wrists (edema), swollen, bleeding gums with tooth loss, fatigue, lethargy, and joint pain. In infants who are not breast-fed, deficiency can be recognized at around 6 months of age when the vitamin C stores transferred from the mother during pregnancy have been exhausted. Medical signs of this syndrome (Moeller-Barlow disease) include abnormal bone character and development, severe joint pain, anemia, and fever. The abnormalities in bone are directly related to vitamin C's involvement in the proper manufacturing of collagen.

What Happens If Too Much Vitamin C Is Consumed?

If you set out to increase your vitamin C intake through the use of supplements, a couple of possible side effects and a practical issue should be considered. First, as discussed, as vitamin C intake increases, the efficiency of absorption decreases. This still leads to more vitamin C absorbed per day, but a proportionate increase in urinary loss of vitamin C and its metabolites also occurs. Perhaps one of the biggest concerns associated with consuming gram-size doses ("gram dosing") is gastrointestinal discomfort since it is an acid. Furthermore, large concentrated doses can promote diarrhea. Otherwise supplementation of a couple grams of vitamin C daily is pretty safe. The latest DRI Upper Limit is set at 2 grams for adults.

Can Vitamin C Prevent or Treat Colds?

As an antioxidant and also an immune function potentiator, vitamin C has been suggested for use in decreasing the incidence and severity of the common cold. Research to date suggests that vitamin C supplementation probably won't decrease the incidence of colds; however it might lessen the severity, especially for some athletic populations. However, starting vitamin C supplementation at the onset of symptoms does little to decrease the severity.

Thiamin (Vitamin B₁)

What Is Thiamin?

Thiamin is classically known as vitamin B_1 and sometimes aneurine. It was identified in the 1930s and was one of the first substances to be classified as a vitamin. Along with the other water-soluble vitamins (except vitamin C and choline), thiamin is a B-complex vitamin. The most salient role of B-complex vitamins is their involvement in energy metabolism.

What Foods Have Thiamin and Which Form Is Found in Supplements?

Thiamin is found widely distributed in foods, although most contain low concentrations. Brewer's yeast, pork, and whole grain and enriched grain products are good sources of thiamin (Table 9.3). Thiamin is found is nutritional supplements and for fortification as thiamin hydrochloride and thiamin nitrate (for example, thiamin mononitrate).

How Much Thiamin Do We Need?

The RDA for men and women is 1.2 and 1 milligrams of thiamin respectively. Meanwhile the RDA for pregnant and lactating women is 1.4 milligrams. Because thiamin is important in energy operations it might be more appropriate to express thiamin recommendations based on level of additional calories burned during exercise and sport training/ competition. Here recommendations of 0.5 milligrams of thiamin would be recommended for every 1,000 calories expended daily. Thus athletes

Table 9.3 Thiamin Content of Select Foods

Food	Thiamin (mg)	Food	Thiamin (mg)
Meats		*Grains*	
Pork roast (3 ounces)	0.8	Bran flakes (1 cup)	0.6
Beef (3 ounces)	0.4	Macaroni (½ cup)	0.1
Ham (3 ounces)	0.4	Rice (½ cup)	0.1
Liver (3 ounces)	0.2	Bread (1 slice)	0.1
Nuts and seeds		*Vegetables*	
Sunflower seeds (¼ cup)	0.7	Peas (½ cup)	0.3
Peanuts (¼ cup)	0.1	Lima beans (½ cup)	0.2
Almonds (¼ cup)		Corn (½ cup)	0.1
Fruits		Broccoli (½ cup)	0.1
Orange juice (1 cup)	0.2	Potato (1)	0.1
Orange (1)	0.1		
Avocado (½)	0.1		

expending 3,000 to 6,000 calories daily would have a recommendation of 1.5 and 3 milligrams. See Table 3.2 for recommended levels for children and teens.

Does Thiamin Break Down During Cooking?

Similar to vitamin C, thiamin is not very stable during cooking processes. Convection cooking of meat may result in destruction of roughly half of its thiamin content. The baking of breads and the pasteurization of milk may result in destruction of approximately 25 percent and 15 percent of thiamin content, respectively. In light of its water-soluble nature, some thiamin may also be washed away in the thaw drip. The thaw drip is the watery fluid that drains from thawing meats. In addition, certain fish and shellfish contain natural *thiaminases*, which are enzymes that break down thiamin. Fortunately, cooking inactivates these enzymes.

Where Is Thiamin Found in Our Body?

Most of the thiamin that we eat is absorbed in the small intestine. Once in the body, thiamin does not seem to have a primary organ of storage, however, the brain, kidneys, liver, and skeletal muscle seem to have higher concentrations. In fact, because of its high energy demands, the brain accounts for as much as one-half of the total thiamin in the body. Thiamin circulates around primarily aboard red blood cells (RBCs) and the activity of a thiamin-associated enzyme is used to gauge thiamin status. Thiamin and its metabolites are subject to removal from the body in urine.

What Does Thiamin Do in Our Body?

Thiamin serves as a coenzyme in many key reactions in the cells. A coenzyme is a substance that will interact directly with an enzyme; together the two allow a chemical reaction to proceed. The enzyme will not function optimally without the presence of the coenzyme. Many water-soluble vitamins function as coenzymes. Thiamin is active in the form of thiamin pyrophosphate (TPP) which is a coenzyme for a couple of enzymes involved in energy pathways. As a co-enzyme, thiamin is involved in complete carbohydrate, protein, and fat breakdown for energy (Figure 9.1).

Thiamin is involved in energy metabolism, DNA, and ATP formation as well as proper functioning of muscle and the brain.

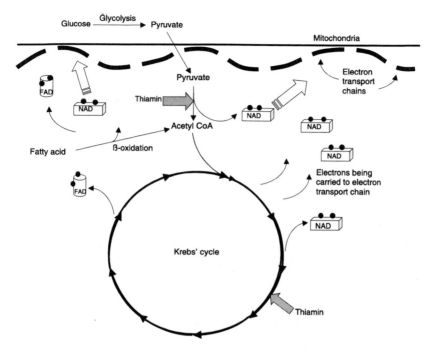

Figure 9.1 Chemical reaction pathways in our mitochondria allow for electrons (black dots) to be removed from involved molecules and they are carried to electron transport chains found in the mitochondria membrane (inner). The carriers are niacin and riboflavin based.

Thiamin is also involved in converting glucose to ribose in the cells. Ribose, and a slightly modified form, deoxyribose, are key components of deoxyribonucleic acids (DNA) and ribonucleic acids (RNA). You will remember that DNA provides the instructions or blueprints for making cells, while RNA is involved in translating the blueprints into the construction of proteins.

What Does Thiamin Do in the Brain and Muscle?

Without question thiamin is crucial to the proper functioning of the brain, nerves, and muscle. However, the exact involvement of thiamin may not be easily explained within the confines of thiamin's classic energy-support functions. Thiamin appears to have the ability to increase the efficiency of the electrical events that allow nerves and muscle to function properly. Interestingly, when thiamin is deficient in the diet the brain tends to hold on to its thiamin more vigorously than other tissues do. This suggests that a very special relationship exists between the brain and thiamin. We will discuss thiamin's role in the aging brain and conditions such as Alzheimer's disease in Chapter 12.

What Happens If Too Little Thiamin Is Consumed?

If thiamin is deficient from our diet for several weeks, symptoms will begin to appear. Classic thiamin deficiency has been termed *beriberi*, which is often separated into two types. *Wet* and *dry* beriberi describe the effects of thiamin deficiency with special reference to the presence of fluid buildup in tissue (edema). Enlargement of the heart sometimes occurs and appears to be more prevalent in those individuals with the fluid buildup (wet beriberi). Muscular weakness, loss of appetite, and atrophy of legs are also characteristic symptoms of thiamin deficiency. Beriberi is said to mean "I can't, I can't," which probably refers to the deficits in voluntary movement that accompany thiamin deficiency.

An infant who is breast-fed by a thiamin-deficient mother is also at risk of thiamin deficiency. This situation, called infantile beriberi, typically occurs between 2 and 6 months of age, and these infants may lose their desire to eat, may regurgitate milk, and may also experience vomiting and diarrhea. A rapid heart rate and a bluish tint to the skin may also develop.

Can Alcohol Consumption Affect Thiamin Status?

Mild alcohol consumption doesn't impact thiamin status in the body. However, the heavy, chronic alcohol consumption of an alcoholic increases the risk for thiamin deficiency for a couple of reasons. Diet in alcoholism is typically low in thiamin along with other essential nutrients. Furthermore, there appears to be a reduced ability to absorb thiamin in the digestive tract of alcoholic people, with an accompanying increase in metabolic need for this vitamin.

Can Too Much Thiamin Be Consumed?

Because much of excessive thiamin will be rapidly removed from the body in the urine, excessive consumption of thiamin appears relatively safe. In fact, the current DRIs do not include a Tolerable Upper Limit for thiamin. However, long-term thiamin intake of greater than 100 times the RDA (1,200 milligrams) has been associated with headaches, convulsions, weakness, allergic reactions, and irregular heart rhythms.

Riboflavin (Vitamin B₂)

What Is Riboflavin?

Riboflavin has long been called vitamin B_2 and is a B-complex vitamin meaning that it plays a key role in energy metabolism. The name riboflavin refers both to a component of its molecular structure and also its yellow color: *ribo-* with respect to the ribose (a simple sugar) portion of the molecule and *flavin* from the Latin word for yellow, *flavus.*

What Foods Have Riboflavin?

Sources of riboflavin include rapidly growing, green leafy vegetables, beef liver, beef, and dairy products (Table 9.4). About one-fourth to one-half of the riboflavin Americans consume is provided by milk and milk products. Meats are also a primary supplier of dietary riboflavin along with fortified and enriched foods (breads and breakfast cereals, for example).

Is Riboflavin Stable During Cooking and Storage?

Riboflavin appears to be more stable than vitamin C and thiamin with regard to cooking and storage. However, significant riboflavin losses in foods are experienced when foods are exposed directly to light (for example, sunlight). This was a bigger concern back when milk was packaged in clear glass bottles and delivered to your doorstep usually before people got out of bed. The milk would then be exposed to the morning sunlight until it was brought in the house. As most milk producers no longer package their product in clear containers such as glass bottles this helps milk retain most of its riboflavin. Sun drying and cooking foods in an open pot can lead to significant riboflavin losses as well. Furthermore, like other water-soluble vitamins, riboflavin can be washed away during boiling and thawing (thaw drip).

Table 9.4 Riboflavin Content of Select Foods

Food	Riboflavin (mg)	Food	Riboflavin (mg)
Milk and milk products		*Meats*	
Milk, whole (1 cup)	0.5	Liver (3 ounces)	3.6
Milk, 2% (1 cup)	0.5	Pork chop (3 ounces)	0.3
Yogurt, low-fat (1 cup)	0.5	Beef (3 ounces)	0.2
Milk, skim (1 cup)	0.4	Tuna (3 ounces)	0.1
Yogurt (1 cup)	0.1	*Vegetables*	
Cheese, american (1 ounce)	0.1	Collard greens (½ cup)	0.3
Cheese, cheddar (1 ounce)	0.1	Broccoli (½ cup)	0.2
Grains		Spinach, cooked (½ cup)	0.1
Macaroni (½ cup)	0.1	*Eggs*	
Bread (1 slice)	0.1	Egg (1)	0.2

How Much Riboflavin Do We Need?

The RDA for adults is 1.1 to 1.3 milligrams of riboflavin for adult women and men. Meanwhile the RDA for pregnant and lactating women is 1.4 and 1.6 milligrams respectively. Because riboflavin is important in energy operations it might be more appropriate to express recommendations for more athletic people based on level of additional calories burned during exercise and sport training/competition. Here, 0.6 grams of riboflavin would be recommended for every 1,000 calories expended daily. Thus athletes expending 3,000 to 6,000 calories daily would have a recommendation of 1.8 and 3.6 milligrams. See Table 3.2 for recommended levels for children and teens.

Where Is Riboflavin in Our Body?

Riboflavin in foods is well absorbed from our digestive tract. Although riboflavin is found in most cells in the body, higher concentrations will be found in very active tissue, such as the heart, liver, and kidneys. This makes sense due to riboflavin's heavy involvement with aerobic energy metabolism. Riboflavin status is typically assessed by taking a sample of blood and assessing the activity of process that requires riboflavin to operate efficiently. Because of its water solubility, riboflavin is lost from the body in urine, which is visually obvious as urine turns a bright yellow a short time after ingesting riboflavin supplements.

What Does Riboflavin Do in the Body?

Riboflavin functions in the cells as an essential component of two coenzymes, *FAD* and *FMN*, which are often referred to as *flavins*. With regard to energy metabolism, FAD (flavin adenine dinucleotide) serves as one of the electron carriers mentioned in our discussion of aerobic energy metabolism in Chapter 8. FAD transfers electrons from reactions in the Krebs' cycle and also the breakdown of fatty acids, a pathway that researchers call β-oxidation (see Figure 9.1).

> Riboflavin is involved in several operations that help convert food and stored energy to ATP to power cell activities.

FMN (flavin mononucleotide), on the other hand, also functions in electron transfer as a key component of the electron-transport chain in the mitochondria in our cells. Beyond energy metabolism, FAD and FMN are used in many of our cell systems such as amino acid and steroid hormone metabolism. As you might have guessed, these and other riboflavin-requiring cell activities involve the transfer of electrons from one molecule to another. That is what riboflavin-based co-enzymes do: they transfer electrons.

What Happens If Too Little or Too Much Riboflavin Is Consumed?

Deficiency of riboflavin rarely occurs by itself. However, if a diet contains very little riboflavin, a person would begin to show deficiency signs after a couple of months, such as inflammation of the mouth and tongue. Other signs of riboflavin deficiency include dryness and cracking at the corners of the mouth, lesions on the lips, accumulation of fluid in tissue (edema), anemia, and neurological disorders, as well as mental confusion. On the other hand, there does not appear to be great concern regarding riboflavin toxicity because of its rapid removal from the body in urine.

Niacin (Vitamin B₃)

What Is Niacin?

Niacin is more commonly recognized as vitamin B_3 and is part of the B-complex vitamins. Niacin in its two forms, nicotinic acid and nicotinamide, is active in the body as part of co-enzyme structures that participate in many bodily activities. In addition to niacin's fundamental role in nutrition, higher levels of niacin can be used therapeutically to lower blood cholesterol levels.

What Foods Contain Niacin and What Is the Supplemented Form?

Niacin is found well distributed throughout most foods. Brewer's yeast and most fish, pork, beef, poultry, mushrooms, and potatoes offer higher niacin content (Table 9.5). Niacin in foods appears to be stable in most forms of cooking and storage while some losses may occur during the boiling of foods as well as during the thaw drip. In these cases some niacin can dissolve into the water that eventually is drained from the food. Both nicotinamide or nicotinic acid can be used in formulating nutrition supplements, however nicotinamide is the form typically used as well as in food fortification.

How Much Niacin Do We Need?

The adult RDA is 14 and 16 mg or niacin equivalents (NE) for women and men respectively, to prevent deficiency and provide for good status. During pregnancy and lactation the recommendation increases for

Table 9.5 Niacin Content of Select Foods

Food	Niacin (mg)	Food	Niacin (mg)
Meats		*Vegetables*	
Liver (3 ounces)	14.0	Asparagus (½ cup)	1.5
Tuna (3 ounces)	10.3	*Grains*	
Turkey (3 ounces)	9.5	Wheat germ (1 ounce)	1.5
Chicken (3 ounces)	7.9	Rice, brown (½ cup)	1.2
Salmon (3 ounces)	6.9	Noodles, enriched (½ cup)	1.0
Veal (3 ounces)	5.2	Rice, white, enriched (½ cup)	1.0
Beef, round steak (3 ounces)	5.1	Bread, enriched (1 slice)	0.7
Pork (3 ounces)	4.5	*Milk and milk products:*	
Haddock (3 ounces)	2.7	Milk (1 cup)	1.9
Scallops (3 ounces)	1.1	Cheese, cottage (½ cup)	2.6
Nuts and Seeds			
Peanuts (1 ounce)	4.9		

Note: Niacin recommendations are often stated in niacin equivalents (NE) whereby 1 NE = 1 mg of niacin = 60 mg tryptophan.

women to 18 and 17 mg respectively. Because niacin is important in energy operations it is more appropriate to express recommendations for more athletic people based on level of additional calories burned during exercise and sport training/competition. Here, 6.6 grams of niacin would be recommended for every 1,000 calories expended daily. Thus athletes expending 3,000 to 5,000 calories daily would have a recommendation of 20 to 35 milligrams. See Table 3.2 for recommended levels for children and teens.

Where Is Niacin Found in Our Body?

The niacin in foods is well absorbed from our small intestine and is found in all of our cells. Like riboflavin we can expect to find higher concentrations of niacin in more metabolically active tissue, or those tissues with higher energy demands such as the heart, brain, liver, and skeletal muscle. Niacin will be lost from the body mostly as part of our urine.

What Does Niacin Do in the Body?

Like riboflavin, niacin imparts coenzyme activity to our cells. In fact, hundreds of chemical reactions depend upon niacin to proceed. Like riboflavin in the form of FAD, niacin in the form of NAD (nicotinamide dinucleotide) is a carrier of electrons from energy pathways to the electron-transport chain during aerobic energy metabolism (see Figure 9.1).

> Niacin is involved in energy-generating processes in the body as well as the production of cholesterol and fat.

Niacin is also part of another electron-transferring molecule called *NADP* (nicotinamide dinucleotide phosphate). NADP also transfers electrons between molecules and is vitally important in making cholesterol and fatty acids.

Can We Make Niacin in Our Body?

Some niacin can be made in the body starting with the essential amino acid tryptophan. However, the conversion is very inefficient and it requires about 60 milligrams of tryptophan to produce 1 milligram of niacin. Since daily niacin needs are 13 to 20 milligrams for adults, it is unrealistic to rely upon the conversion of tryptophan to niacin, especially since tryptophan is not one of the most abundant amino acids in our diet and serves critical roles beyond protein production. Nevertheless, since some niacin can be made from tryptophan, the RDA is stated as niacin equivalents (NE) where 1 NE is equal to 1 milligram of niacin or 60 milligrams of tryptophan.

What Happens If Too Much Niacin Is Consumed?

Ingesting more than 100 milligrams of niacin as nicotinic acid can result in an uncomfortable feeling. Headache and itching are common, accompanied by an increased blood flow to our skin ("flushing"). On the other hand, physicians often prescribe niacin (2 to 5 grams/day) as a means of reducing blood cholesterol. Because gram doses of niacin can have a pharmaceutical effect, this practice is not suggested unless under medical supervision. Furthermore a tolerable upper limit is set at 35 milligrams/day.

What Happens in Niacin Deficiency?

Based on the many roles of niacin in energy processes, poor niacin status can reduce the efficiency of energy systems. Some of the earlier symptoms of a niacin deficiency include a decreased appetite, weight loss, and a general feeling of weakness. More severe niacin deficiency can result in a severe disease syndrome called *pellagra*, which is characterized by the three "D's" (dermatitis, diarrhea, dementia) possibly leading to the fourth "D" (death).

Biotin

What Is Biotin?

Biotin is a B-complex vitamin based on its basic role in energy metabolism. However, because biotin deficiency has been associated with hair (fur) loss in animal studies, it is often marketed in products to improve hair.

What Foods Contain Biotin and What Forms are Used in Supplements?

Biotin is widely dispersed throughout the foods we eat, although its concentration is somewhat limited. Liver, oatmeal, almonds, roasted peanuts, wheat bran, brewer's yeast, and molasses are good sources. While milk and milk products contain only mediocre amounts of biotin, they actually are some of the best providers of biotin in our diet because of their popularity. Eggs offer a respectable amount of biotin, however, egg whites contain a protein called *avidin* that will bind to biotin in our digestive tract and decrease its absorption. Fortunately, avidin's ability to bind biotin is diminished when eggs, or their whites, are cooked. In addition to preventing salmonella infection, this is another reason to avoid uncooked eggs (or egg whites) as well as egg-based products that have not been pasteurized.

Can Some Biotin Be Made in Our Body?

The bacteria living in the colon can produce biotin, and some of this biotin can be absorbed. This seems to make a respectable contribution toward meeting our biotin needs, however it is not enough to be relied upon exclusively. Furthermore, since it is bacterial cells and not our own cells that make biotin, it should not really be viewed as a vitamin that the human body can make. Therefore, biotin indisputably maintains its place on the list of vitamins.

How Much Biotin Do We Need?

The AI for biotin for adults is 30 micrograms daily. The recommendation remains the same during pregnancy and is increased to 35 micrograms during lactation. Because biotin is important in energy operations it is extremely important that more active people get at least the recommended level and perhaps more appropriately 50 to 60 micrograms daily. See Table 3.2 for recommended levels for children and teens.

What Does Biotin Do in Our Body?

Similar to thiamin, riboflavin, and niacin, biotin also provides vital assistance to energy operations and is found in higher concentrations in the brain, muscle, and liver. Serving as a coenzyme, biotin is pivotal in making glucose from other substances such as amino acids and lactate to help maintain blood glucose levels during fasting and prolonged exercise. Biotin is also necessary to make fatty acids from excessive glucose and certain amino acids. Lastly, biotin is necessary for the pathways that help break down certain fatty acids (odd-chain length) and amino acids for energy.

Can Too Much or Too Little Biotin Be Consumed?

Because biotin is widely available in foods and is also derived from the bacteria in our intestinal tract, deficiency is very uncommon. However, some of the rare cases of biotin deficiency include hospital patients fed a biotin-deficient solution intravenously (IV) or in infants fed a lot of egg whites as a protein supplement. On the other hand, biotin seems to be relatively nontoxic.

Pantothenic Acid

What Is Pantothenic Acid?

Pantothenic acid was once known as vitamin B_5. The term pantothenic acid is derived from the Greek word pantothen which means "from every side." This name was given to imply pantothenic acid's widespread availability in foods. Although crucial in energy metabolism, recent research suggests that a derivative of pantothenic acid called pantothenine might help regulate blood cholesterol levels (see Chapter 13.)

What Foods Provide Pantothenic Acid and What Forms are Used in Nutrition Supplements?

Good sources of pantothenic acid include egg yolk, animal tissue, whole grain products, legumes, broccoli, milk, sweet potatoes, and molasses. Some losses of pantothenic acid can be expected in cooking and during the thawing of foods. Supplement manufacturers typically use calcium and sodium pantothenate.

What Are the Recommended Intake Levels of Pantothenic Acid?

The adult AI is 5 milligrams regardless of age and gender. During pregnancy and lactation, the recommendation increases for women to 6 and

7 milligrams respectively. Because pantothenic acid is essential in energy operations, it is important that people who exercise seriously and athletes get at least 10 milligrams of pantothenic acid daily. See Table 3.2 for recommended levels for children and teens.

What Does Pantothenic Acid Do in the Body?

Pantothenic acid is part of two very special molecules that impact carbohydrate, protein, and fat metabolism. These molecules are called *coenzyme A* (CoA) and *acyl carrier protein* (ACP). We have mentioned CoA a few times already in regard to acetyl CoA, the "feed in" molecule for the Krebs' cycle. Furthermore, CoA is also utilized in a chemical reaction in the Krebs' cycle, as well as during the breakdown of fatty acids for ATP production. In these situations, CoA is attached to specific molecules, which enhances their metabolism tremendously. CoA is also necessary for cholesterol and derived steroid hormone (testosterone, estrogens) production as well as melatonin, hemoglobin, and acetylcholine.

Pantothenic acid is involved in energy metabolism as well as the production of fat and cholesterol in cells.

ACP is also indispensable but for different reasons than CoA. Where CoA is fundamental in the processes that help generate ATP from energy molecules, ACP is fundamental in a preliminary step whereby fatty acids are made from excessive carbohydrates and amino acids. Here pantothenic acid, as part of ACP, is essential for storing energy in the form of fat in our body.

Can Too Little or Too Much Pantothenic Acid Be Consumed?

Even though foods will experience some loss of pantothenic acid during cooking and thawing, a deficiency is still unlikely. In fact, there have been no cases of a "real-world" pantothenic acid deficiency alone. Just as a deficiency has not been documented, neither has a toxicity of pantothenic acid. However, there have been reports that large doses of pantothenic acid do cause diarrhea.

Vitamin B₆

What Is Vitamin B₆?

Vitamin B_6 is the general term for the six compounds, namely pyridoxal (PL), pyridoxine (PN), pyridoxamine (PM), and their phosphate derivatives including pyridoxal 5'-phosphate (PLP), pyridoxine 5'-phosphate (PNP), and pyridoxamine 5'-phosphate (PMP). It is the PLP form that is the most significant in human operations. Although long recognized for its pivotal role in the processing of amino acids, vitamin B_6 has received attention for its role in homocysteine metabolism and in reducing cardiovascular disease risk.

What Foods Provide Vitamin B_6 and What Form Is Found in Supplements?

One form of vitamin B_6 is pyridoxine, which is mostly found in plant foods, with good sources being bananas, navy beans, and walnuts. The remaining four forms of vitamin B_6 are found mostly in animal foods with good sources being meats, fish, and poultry (Table 9.6). Vitamin B_6 is fairly well absorbed from the small intestine but vitamin B_6 from animal sources may be better absorbed than B_6 from plant sources. In addition, vitamin B_6 is fairly stable in cooking processes; however, some losses are experienced with prolonged exposure to heat, light, or alkaline conditions. Vitamin B_6 is available primarily as pyridoxine hydrochloride in multivitamin, vitamin B-complex, and vitamin B_6 supplements.

Vitamin B_6 is crucial for amino acid metabolism and how much a person needs can be based on their protein intake.

Table 9.6 Vitamin B_6 Content of Select Foods

Foods	Vitamin B_6 (mg)	Foods	Vitamin B_6 (mg)
Meats		*Legumes*	
Liver (3 ounces)	0.8	Split peas (½ cup)	0.6
Salmon (3 ounces)	0.7	Beans, cooked (½ cup)	0.4
Chicken (3 ounces)	0.4	*Fruits*	
Ham (3 ounces)	0.4	Banana (1)	0.6
Hamburger (3 ounces)	0.4	Avocado (½)	0.4
Veal (3 ounces)	0.4	Watermelon (1 cup)	0.3
Pork (3 ounces)	0.3	*Vegetables*	
Beef (3 ounces)	0.2	Brussels sprouts (½ cup)	0.4
Eggs		Potato (1)	0.2
Egg (1)	0.3	Sweet potato (½ cup)	0.2
		Carrots (½ cup)	0.2
		Peas (½ cup)	0.1

What Does Vitamin B₆ Do in the Body?

Vitamin B$_6$ can be found in nearly if not all cells throughout the body with higher concentrations found in muscle and liver tissue. Similar to most of its water-soluble vitamin siblings, vitamin B$_6$ is primarily lost from the body in urine. Once inside the cells, vitamin B$_6$ forms can be converted to the active forms of vitamin B$_6$, *PLP* (pyridoxal phosphate) and *PMP* (pyridoxamine phosphate). PLP and PMP are key participants in many cell reactions. By and large the most significant roles of vitamin B$_6$ are as follows.

- *Amino acid metabolism*—Vitamin B$_6$ is crucial for the processing of amino acids including the production of nonessential amino acids made from other amino acids. During this process, the nitrogen-containing *amine* portion of an amino acid is transferred to a specific molecule (Figure 9.2), which creates a nonessential amino acid. In fact, if an individual developed a vitamin B$_6$ deficiency, most of the nonessential amino acids would actually become dietary essentials.
- *Glycogen breakdown*—Glycogen breakdown in muscle requires vitamin B$_6$. Glycogen is stored glucose and the breakdown of this complex provides invaluable fuel during exercise and work.
- *Neurotransmitter production*—Vitamin B$_6$ is also necessary to convert certain amino acids into the neurotransmitters gamma-amino-butyric acid (GABA) and serotonin.
- *Hemoglobin*—Vitamin B$_6$ is crucial for the normal production of hemoglobin, the oxygen-carrying protein found in RBCs.
- *Immunity*—In addition, vitamin B$_6$ is essential in the formation of hemoglobin and white blood cells. Finally, vitamin B$_6$ also seems to be necessary to break down glycogen stores during exercise and fasting.

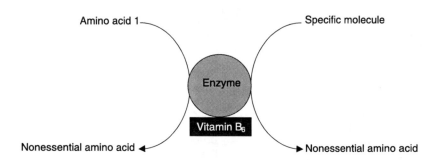

Figure 9.2 Some nonessential amino acids can be made by transferring the nitrogen contain amine group from an existing amino acid to another molecule thereby creating a nonessential amino acid.

What Are the Recommended Intake Levels of Vitamin B₆?

The adult RDA is 1.3 milligrams of vitamin B_6 for women and men 18 to 50 years of age. After 50 the recommendation increases to 1.5 and 1.7 milligrams daily for women and men respectively. During pregnancy and lactation the recommendation increases for women to 1.9 and 2.0 milligrams of vitamin B_6 respectively. The bottom line is that the metabolism of every amino acid at some point or another will encounter a chemical reaction requiring vitamin B_6 as a coenzyme. In fact, vitamin B_6 is so deeply rooted in the metabolism of amino acids that the RDA is based on the typical protein content of the American diet. Approximately 0.016 milligrams of vitamin B_6 is apportioned per gram of protein in our diet. Therefore, since the typical daily protein intake of an American adult has been estimated to be 100 to 125 grams of protein, this translates to about 1.6 to 2 milligrams of vitamin B_6. For athletes consuming more protein and with higher glycogen stores, more vitamin B_6 is warranted and accounted for if vitamin B_6 intake is based on grams of protein intake. See Table 3.2 for recommended levels of vitamin B_6 for people of all ages.

What Happens If Too Little Vitamin B₆ Is Consumed?

Deficiency of vitamin B_6 is unlikely due to the popularity of meat, fish, and poultry as components of the American diet. However, if a deficiency occurred, amino acid metabolism would be greatly restrained, leading to poor protein synthesis. The production of hemoglobin, white blood cells, and many neurotransmitters would also be greatly hindered. Therefore the signs of a vitamin B_6 deficiency would significantly affect human body functions at many levels, including growth, immunity, and reproduction.

Can Vitamin B₆ Be Toxic?

The Tolerable Upper Limit has been set at 100 milligrams daily for both men and women with lower levels for children and during pregnancy and early lactation. If vitamin B_6 is consumed in gram doses (2 to 6 grams) over many months, it can affect nervous function and possibly lead to irreversible damage to nervous tissue. At one time, vitamin B_6 was considered a possible treatment for premenstrual syndrome (PMS), but this concept has since been abandoned and should not be pursued due to lack of promising supportive research and the potential for toxicity.

Folate (Folic Acid)

What Is Folate?

The name folate, as well as the other names associated with this vitamin (folacin and folic acid), suggests its food sources. Folium is Latin for foliage or forage.

What Foods in the Diet Contribute Folate?

As its name suggests, good food sources of folate include green, leafy vegetables such as spinach, turnip greens, and asparagus (Table 9.7). Other vegetables and many fruits, juices, and organ meats also are good contributors of folate. Folate's molecular structure is somewhat unstable when it is heated, making fresh, uncooked fruits and vegetables better sources than cooked foods. The RDA for adults is 400 micrograms of folate daily.

What Does Folate Do in the Body?

Earlier we mentioned that when most molecules are made in the body they are constructed from smaller molecules or parts of other molecules. Folate, functioning as a coenzyme, is dedicated to transferring small, single carbon atom-containing molecules to the processes involved in making some pretty special molecules (Figure 9.3). Key roles for folate include:

- *DNA production*—Before cells can reproduce they must make a copy of their DNA. The necessity of folate is particularly realized in cells that rapidly reproduce. This includes cells associated with the body

Table 9.7 Folate Content of Select Foods

Food	Folate (µg)	Food	Folate (µg)
Vegetables		*Fruits*	
Asparagus (½ cup)	120	Cantaloupe (¼)	100
Brussels sprouts (½ cup)	116	Orange juice (1 cup)	87
Black-eyed peas (½ cup)	102	Orange (1)	59
Spinach, cooked (½ cup)	99	*Grains*	
Lettuce, romaine (1 cup)	86	Oatmeal (½ cup)	97
Lima beans (½ cup)	71	Wild rice (½ cup)	37
Peas (½ cup)	70	Wheat germ (1 tablespoon)	20
Sweet potato (½ cup)	43		
Broccoli (½ cup)	43		

surfaces (skin, hair, and digestive, urinary, and reproductive tracts) as well as blood cells and certain liver cells. Cells of these tissues must constantly be replaced or turned over to guarantee proper function and integrity. However, in order for these cells to reproduce they must first make a duplicate copy of their DNA so that when the cell divides into two cells, both will get a complete set of DNA.

• *Amino acid metabolism*—Folate is also involved in transferring single-carbon molecules in the metabolism of certain amino acids as well. For instance, folate helps convert homocysteine to methionine.

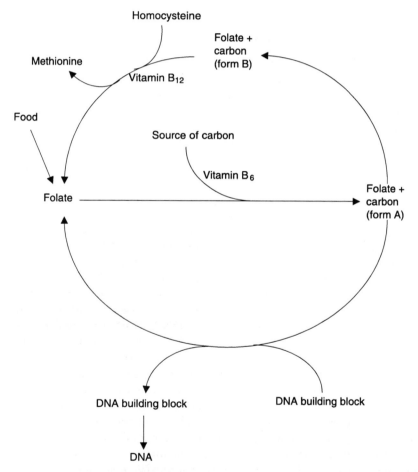

Figure 9.3 Folate passes a single carbon building block to the construction of various molecules such as nucleic acids. In the process folate is converted to an nonreusable form. Vitamin B_{12} can convert folate back to an active form.

- *Homocysteine metabolism*—Recently a link has been made between homocysteine levels and heart disease. When folate transfers a carbon molecule to homocysteine it is converted to methionine (see Figure 9.3). The conversion requires the help of vitamin B_{12} as well. Therefore, a deficiency of folate and/or vitamin B_{12} can allow for homocysteine levels to become elevated. Vitamin B_6 is also important because it helps folate pick up the carbon unit that will be added to homocysteine to form methionine.

> Folate is needed for DNA production as well as the metabolism of homocysteine, which has been linked to heart disease.

How Important Is Folate During Pregnancy?

Because folate is fundamentally involved in DNA production and thus the reproduction of cells, periods of life when rapid growth occurs demand a higher folate intake. During pregnancy a woman's diet must include extra folate to assist in the rapid reproduction of cells of the unborn infant and herself (for example, blood cells, placenta). Chapter 12 provides more details to what can happen if folate status is inadequate during pregnancy. Most prenatal vitamin supplements include folate to help meet a pregnant woman's increased needs.

What Happens If Too Little Folate Is Consumed?

Folate deficiency can result in several problems including anemia. Red blood cells (RBCs) have a life span of about 4 months and are constantly reproducing (two million RBCs per second) in bone marrow to compensate for their normal destruction. Although RBCs do not contain a nucleus (with its DNA), there is a time in its development when each new RBC is created from the division of another cell. Before that cell divided into two new cells, it needed to copy its DNA. During folate deficiency, the original cell cannot properly copy its DNA because folate is not present to help construct the building blocks of DNA. This results in the development of large and immature RBCs, which then enter the blood and are readily noticeable with a microscope. Furthermore, fewer and fewer normal RBCs are produced, resulting in anemia. Anemia is a significant reduction in the level of hemoglobin in the blood. Remember: hemoglobin is found in RBCs, so a reduction in RBC concentration in our blood results in less hemoglobin. The anemia that results from folate deficiency is clinically referred to as *macrocytic megaloblastic anemia.* *Macrocytic* means big cell and *megaloblast* is the name for the pre-RBC form, which still has its nucleus. These changes in RBCs can be observed as early as a few months after consuming a folate-deficient diet.

Can Folate Be Toxic?

Folate toxicity is rare for two principal reasons. First, it is difficult to consume too much folate through normal consumption of foods. Second, the folate content of nutrition supplements is limited by the government. The limitation in supplements is due to an overlap between folate metabolism and vitamin B_{12} function. Vitamin B_{12} is fundamentally involved in folate metabolism in cells as it keeps folate in a form that can be used over and over again in cells (folate recycling). This means that a deficiency in vitamin B_{12} can in turn decrease folate recycling, resulting in the development of the anemia mentioned previously. Therefore, signs of a folate deficiency can actually help physicians identify a vitamin B_{12} deficiency. By taking higher dosages of folate (supplements) we can overcome the need for vitamin B_{12} in the recycling of existing folate in the cells. This is good for folate, but the vitamin B_{12} deficiency still remains and may go undetected. Thus, folate supplementation has eliminated an early warning sign (anemia) of vitamin B_{12} deficiency. If the vitamin B_{12} deficiency progresses it can lead to paralysis and death.

Vitamin B_{12}

What Is Vitamin B_{12}?

Tucked away in the central part of the vitamin B_{12} molecule is an atom of cobalt. Therefore molecules that have vitamin B_{12} activity have been named the *cobalamins*. Because vitamin B_{12} plays a role in activities that process energy nutrients, it holds its place on the roster of B-complex vitamins.

What Foods Provide Vitamin B_{12}?

In the human diet, vitamin B_{12} is only found in foods of animal origin. Unlike animals, plants do not have a functional role for vitamin B_{12} and therefore do not make it. Interestingly, animals do not seem to make vitamin B_{12} either and rely instead upon their intestinal bacteria to make it. Vitamin B_{12} is then absorbed into that animal's body from its digestive tract. The best sources of vitamin B_{12} are meats, fish, poultry, shellfish, eggs, milk, and milk products (Table 9.8). The vitamin B_{12} content in these foods is modest but compatible with our needs.

How Much Vitamin B_{12} Do We Need?

The RDA for adults is 2.4 micrograms regardless of age and gender. During pregnancy and lactation the recommendation increases for women to 2.6 and 2.8 micrograms respectively. See Table 3.2 for recommended levels for children and teens.

Table 9.8 Vitamin B$_{12}$ Content of Select Foods

Food	Vitamin B$_{12}$ (μg)	Food	Vitamin B$_{12}$ (μg)
Meats		*Eggs*	
Liver (3 ounces)	6.8	Egg (1)	0.6
Trout (3 ounces)	3.6	*Milk and milk products*	
Beef (3 ounces)	2.2	Milk, skim (1 cup)	1.0
Clams (3 ounces)	2.0	Milk, whole (1 cup)	0.9
Crab (3 ounces)	1.8	Yogurt (1 cup)	0.8
Lamb (3 ounces)	1.8	Cottage cheese (½ cup)	0.7
Tuna (3 ounces)	1.8	Cheese, american (1 ounce)	0.2
Veal (3 ounces)	1.7	Cheese, cheddar (1 ounce)	0.2
Hamburger (3 ounces)	1.5		

Are There Special Factors Involved in the Absorption of Vitamin B$_{12}$?

The absorption of vitamin B$_{12}$ needs a little help. Special proteins called *R proteins* and *intrinsic factor* produced by the stomach must interact with vitamin B$_{12}$ both in the stomach and small intestine to facilitate its absorption. A lack of these proteins can reduce vitamin B$_{12}$ absorption dramatically. This might be a concern for people who lack a properly functioning stomach, such as people who have had their stomach stapled or part (or all) of the stomach removed (gastroplasty).

How Much Vitamin B$_{12}$ Is Lost from the Body Daily?

Once vitamin B$_{12}$ is in the body it stays there for a while. Very little amounts of this vitamin are actually lost from the body on a daily basis, barring abnormalities. Contrary to the other water-soluble vitamins, the primary route of vitamin B$_{12}$ loss from the body is not by way of the urine but rather in feces. The liver mixes a little vitamin B$_{12}$ in with bile, which carries it to the digestive tract. A small portion of this vitamin B$_{12}$ is not reabsorbed and becomes part of feces.

What Does Vitamin B$_{12}$ Do in the Body?

Vitamin B$_{12}$ is directly involved in the proper metabolism of folate. In fact, a deficiency of vitamin B$_{12}$ can impact folate metabolism to the point that signs of a folate deficiency appear. When folate is used to make molecules it is rendered "unusable," for lack of a better description. Vitamin B$_{12}$ is involved in converting folate back to a usable form. Said another way, vitamin B$_{12}$ is involved in folate recycling. This dramatically reduces the amount of folate we need to eat daily to have optimal levels of usable folate in our cells.

Vitamin B_{12} is also required for the breakdown of certain amino acids and fatty acids that have an odd chain length (for example, three carbons) for ATP production. Finally, vitamin B_{12} appears to be vital in maintaining the special wrapping around nerve cells called *myelin*. Myelin serves as insulation, which increases the velocity of a nerve impulse traveling from one part of the body to another.

What Happens If Too Little Vitamin B_{12} Is Consumed?

Contrary to other water-soluble vitamins, vitamin B_{12} losses from the body are small and occur primarily through the feces. Small quantities of vitamin B_{12} enter the digestive tract daily as part of bile released during meals. Most of this vitamin B_{12} is reabsorbed from the digestive tract while some is lost through feces. It has been estimated that we lose only about 0.1 percent of vitamin B_{12} stores daily through this process. Therefore, provided that there is optimal vitamin B_{12} reabsorption from the digestive tract, a person with good vitamin B_{12} stores could eat a diet lacking vitamin B_{12} for years before showing signs of deficiency—at least in theory.

Deficiency of vitamin B_{12} will result in a form of anemia in which red blood cells appear large and immature (macrocytic megaloblastic anemia, see above). About 150 years ago, English physicians recognized that people with this type of anemia often died. They called this illness *pernicious anemia*, as pernicious means "leading to death." This anemia is usually related to the involvement of vitamin B_{12} in folate metabolism and DNA production. People who are vitamin B_{12} deficient also show destruction of nerve myelin, which can lead to nerve impulse conduction disturbances, paralysis, and ultimately death.

What Situations Can Result in Vitamin B_{12} Deficiency?

There are a couple of situations that can lead to a deficiency of vitamin B_{12}.

- *Strict vegetarianism*—Eating only plant-derived foods (vegan) without vitamin B_{12} supplementation will eventually lead to deficiency. Individuals who became a vegetarian later in life may not show signs of a vitamin B_{12} deficiency for a long time but for children the onset of deficiency will be shorter. In either case the time to deficiency depends on the level of body B_{12} stores prior to conversion.
- *Absorption/digestion conditions*—Factors that affect vitamin B_{12} digestion and absorption are more likely to cause vitamin B_{12} deficiency than insufficient dietary intake. Diseases and surgical manipulation of the stomach (removal and stapling) can affect its ability to make and release adequate intrinsic factor and R proteins. This can result in a dramatic decrease in vitamin B_{12} absorption. These

proteins are very important in absorbing vitamin B_{12} in food and also reabsorbing the vitamin B_{12} entering the small intestine as part of bile.

- *Aging*—Older people are at increased risk of a vitamin B_{12} deficiency as their stomachs lose the ability to make sufficient acid with age. Stomach acid helps liberate the vitamin B_{12} in food so that it can interact with R proteins and intrinsic factor. Beyond anemia, other signs of a vitamin B_{12} deficiency include weakness, back pain, apathy, and a tingling in the extremities. These signs and symptoms usually appear before significant nerve damage occurs.

Vitamins A, D, E, and K Are Vital Lipids

Vitamin A

What Is Vitamin A?

Vitamin A in foods includes members of two chemical families, the *retinoids* such as retinol, retinal, and retinoic acid, and the *carotenoids* such as α-carotene, β-carotene, and other carotenes. However, in order for a carotenoid to have vitamin A activity it must first be converted to a retinoid in the body. Therefore, carotenoids are often referred to as *provitamin A*. Although there are hundreds of carotenoids found in nature, only about fifty may be converted to vitamin A. Furthermore, only about a half dozen of those carotenoids are found in the human diet in appreciable amounts. Because of its availability in the diet and relatively efficient conversion to a vitamin A, β-carotene may be the most significant carotenoid with regard to conversion to vitamin A.

What Foods Provide Vitamin A?

Vitamin A in the retinoid form is found in animal products with the best sources being liver, fish oils, eggs, and vitamin A-fortified milk and milk products (Table 9.9). Meanwhile, carotenoids are found in plant sources— mainly in orange and dark green vegetables and some fruits (squash, carrots, spinach, broccoli, papaya, sweet potatoes, pumpkin, cantaloupe, and apricots). In fact, the term *carotenoid* is derived from the species name for carrots. Nutrition supplements tend to provide vitamin A in the form of retinyl acetate or retinyl palmitate or as β-carotene.

> Vitamin A is found naturally in some foods and can be made in our body by converting carotenoids from fruits and vegetables.

Table 9.9 Vitamin A Content of Select Foods

Food	Vitamin A (μg or RE)	Food	Vitamin A (μg or RE)
Vegetables		*Meats*	
Pumpkin, canned (½ cup)	2712	Liver (3 ounces)	9124
Sweet potato, canned (½ cup)	1935	Salmon (3 ounces)	53
		Tuna (3 ounces)	14
Carrots, raw (½ cup)	1913	*Eggs*	
Spinach, cooked (½ cup)	739	Egg (1)	84
Broccoli, cooked (½ cup)	109	*Milk and milk products**	
Winter squash (½ cup)	53	Milk, skim (1 cup)	149
Green peppers (½ cup)	40	Milk, 2% (1 cup)	139
Fruits		Cheese, American (1 ounce)	82
Cantaloupe (¼ whole)	430		
Apricots, canned (½ cup)	210	Cheese, Swiss (1 ounce)	65
Nectarine (1)	101	*Fats*	
Watermelon (1 cup)	59	Margarine* (1 teaspoon)	46
Peaches, canned (½ cup)	47	Butter (1 teaspoon)	38
Papaya (½ cup)	20		

RE = retinol equivalents.
* Fortified.

What Does Vitamin A Do in the Body?

Vitamin A is crucial to growth, health and maintenance for many reasons.

- *Eye health*—Within the eye lies a complex neural/sensory processes that allow us to see. Vitamin A is fundamentally involved in this process and is also involved in maintaining the health of the cornea, which is the clear outer window of the eye. Because of this relationship, poor vitamin A status in the human body is often recognized by changes in vision, as will be discussed.
- *Maintenance of mucus-producing tissue*—Vitamin A is also indispensable for the maintenance and regulation of growth of many types of cells in the body. Cells that produce mucus, a lubricating and protecting substance, are particularly sensitive to vitamin A status. These types of cells are found lining the digestive tract and lungs and also in the eye's cornea.
- *Growth of body*—Vitamin A is also essential for normal growth and development of the human body as a whole. It is now clear that vitamin A acts in certain cells throughout the body at the genetic level. This means that some of the function of vitamin A is related to its ability to interact with DNA and affect the manufacturing of certain proteins. This seems to be very important in the proper development and maintenance of various tissues throughout the body.

Do Carotenoids Have a Role in Health Without Being Converted to Vitamin A?

Not all of the β-carotene eaten will be converted to vitamin A. Much of it, along with other carotenoids, will go unchanged and have different functions in the body. For instance, β-carotene and other carotenoids such as lutein and lycopene can function as antioxidants. In this capacity, the carotenoids function more as nutraceuticals helping to protect the body's cells against free radicals. Thus, eating a diet rich in fruits and vegetables will not only support vitamin A intake but also provide carotenoids that help protect us from disease.

How Much Vitamin A Do We Need?

The RDA for vitamin A is 700 and 900 micrograms for women and men, respectively. During pregnancy and lactation the RDA increases to 770 and 1,300 micrograms respectively. Table 3.2 provides recommended levels for children and teens. In Table 9.9 you will see that the vitamin A content of foods is listed as micrograms and *retinol equivalents* (RE). Retinol Equivalents are used because we derive vitamin A from retinoids and carotenoids and REs and the level of activity is not the same for the various forms. For instance, carotenoids are absorbed from the digestive tract with about half the efficiency of the retinoids. Once inside the body, they must be converted to a retinoid, a process that varies in efficiency from one carotenoid to another. In order to account for the inherent differences in obtaining vitamin A activity from retinoids versus the carotenoids, vitamin A is listed in REs. One microgram of retinol equals 1 RE, whereas it takes 12 micrograms of β-carotene to equal 1 RE and 24 micrograms of other carotenes to equal 1 RE. In addition, International Units (IU) are an older method of expressing vitamin activity and are still used on some packaging. One IU is equal to 0.3 micrograms of retinol.

What Happens If Too Little Vitamin A Is Consumed?

When vitamin A is deficient from the diet for many months the body's internal stores are decreased and deficiency is revealed in the form of:

- *Night blindness*—Night blindness is an inability to adapt to dim lighting and is usually accompanied by a prolonged transition from dim to bright light.
- *Xerophthalmia*—Occurs when the mucus-producing cells of the cornea deteriorate and no longer produce mucus; a hard protein called keratin is produced instead. Keratin in combination with a decreased presence of mucus will dry out and harden the cornea of the eye. Xerophthalmia means dry, hard eyes.

- *Drying of body linings—* Inadequate mucus secretion of cells lining the respiratory, digestive, urinary, and reproductive tracts will greatly affect the function and health of these tissues as well. They are subject to drying and infection. Dry, hard skin is an observable sign of a vitamin A deficiency.

How Common Is Vitamin A Deficiency?

Vitamin A deficiency is one of the more recognized nutrient deficiencies worldwide, as roughly two million children in developing countries go blind each year as a result of vitamin A deficiency. International relief efforts to improve health conditions in these countries are attempting to correct this deficiency by giving children large amounts of vitamin A a couple of times per year. It is hoped that the doses are large enough to provide adequate vitamin A storage to last until the next treatment.

Can Vitamin A Become Toxic?

Toxicity of vitamin A is seemingly just as severe as a deficiency. If a person consumes as little as ten times the RDA for vitamin A for several months, signs and symptoms such as bone pain, hair loss, dryness of the skin, and liver complications may develop. If toxicity persists it can eventually result in death. The risk of vitamin A toxicity from eating a balanced diet is low. Even those of us eating very large amounts of carotenoid-containing fruits and vegetables are not at significant risk of toxicity. This is due to the much lower rate of digestive absorption and conversion of carotenoids to vitamin A. Most people who develop vitamin A toxicity seem to do so through use of supplements. Recently, research has revealed that retinol intakes exceeding 5,000 International Units daily might increase the risk of osteoporosis. Furthermore, vitamin A toxicity during pregnancy can result in birth defects. We will look more closely at this situation in Chapter 12.

Vitamin D

What Is Vitamin D?

Vitamin D is a fat-soluble vitamin and is somewhat unique in relation to the other vitamins because the body can produce it in adequate amounts with the assistance of the sun. In fact, many researchers feel that since certain cells can produce vitamin D and because it then circulates and affects tissue throughout the body, it might be better classified as a hormone than a vitamin. However, the body's ability to make vitamin D relies upon exposure to sunlight (ultraviolet B light), and not everyone receives adequate exposure. Furthermore, direct exposure to sunlight is not recommended due to the increased risk of skin cancers. For this reason, vitamin D will maintain its position as a vitamin.

What Foods Provide Vitamin D?

There are two possible ways of supplying the body with vitamin D: through diet and exposure to the sunlight. In the human diet, the richest sources of vitamin D are vitamin D-fortified milk and milk products, tuna, salmon, margarine (vitamin D fortified), herring, and vitamin D-fortified cereals (Table 9.10). Vitamin D in foods appears fairly stable in various cooking and storing procedures. Vitamin is available in nutrition supplements in the form of cholecalciferol. International Units are often used to express vitamin D levels on packaging whereby 1 microgram is equal to 40 IU of vitamin D. Thus 10 micrograms would be equal to 400 IU which is commonly used in supplements and provides 100 percent of the Daily Value (DV).

How Much Vitamin D Do We Need?

The RDA for adults 50 years of age and younger as well as pregnant women is 5 micrograms (200 IU) of vitamin D daily. One microgram is the equivalent of 40 IU of vitamin D. For adults over the age of 50 and 70 the RDA increases to 10 and 15 micrograms (400 IU) daily. See Table 3.2 for recommended levels for children and teens.

How Much Sunlight Is Required to Make Vitamin D?

People with lighter skin color require as little as 10 minutes of sun exposure to make adequate amounts of vitamin D. However this requires direct sunlight exposure to skin during midday. However, sunscreen with SPF 8 or higher significantly reduces the process. Also the necessary

Table 9.10 Vitamin D Content of Select Foods

Food	Vitamin D (µg)	Food	Vitamin D (µg)
Milk		*Fish and seafood*	
Milk (1 cup)	2.5	Salmon (3 ounces)	8.5
Meats		Tuna (3 ounces)	3.7
Beef liver (3 ounces)	1.0	Shrimp (3 ounces)	3.1
Eggs			
Egg (1)	0.7		

exposure is increased for people with darker skin color and in a manner relative to the degree of darkness. This also means that a person will make less and less vitamin D as they tan longer or over several days, such as vacationing at the beach. This helps to protect people from potentially making too much vitamin D. Interestingly, the ability to make vitamin D appears to be stronger during youth and decreases as humans get older. For this reason, the need for vitamin D from food and or supplements increases as we get older (50+).

What Processes Are Involved in Making Vitamin D?

The process of making vitamin D can be simplified to three primary locations within the body. First, within the skin a derivative of cholesterol called 7-dehydrocholesterol is converted to another substance called *cholecalciferol*. In order for this to occur, 7-dehydrocholesterol must be exposed to ultraviolet radiation from the sun or other sources such as tanning beds. As mentioned, the efficiency of this conversion appears to decrease as ultraviolet light exposure time increases.

Once cholecalciferol has been produced it leaves the skin and circulates in the blood with the help of a transport protein called vitamin D binding protein (DBP). In the cholecalciferol form, vitamin D is only minimally active in the body. The activity of vitamin D depends on its ability to be recognized by vitamin D receptors in specific cells. In order for cholecalciferol to become more attractive to the vitamin D receptor, it must undergo more changes in its molecular design. The first change takes place in the liver as circulating cholecalciferol is removed and modified to become 25-hydroxycholecalciferol. This form of vitamin D is released by the liver and re-enters the blood. This form of vitamin D is a little more attractive to vitamin D receptors and some of the effects of vitamin D are realized. 25-Dihydroxycholecalciferol can circulate to the kidneys and be modified further to the most potent form of vitamin D called 1,25-dihydroxycholecalciferol or calcitriol, which is released back into circulation (Figure 9.4). In this form, vitamin D is exceptionally attractive to vitamin D receptors strategically located within certain cells in the body.

Does the Vitamin D in Foods Need to Be Processed in the Body?

The vitamin D in foods is fairly well absorbed across the wall of the small intestine. Because this form of vitamin D is fat soluble (water insoluble), it will require the same digestive and absorptive assistance as other lipid substances. This includes the presence of bile and the incorporation into chylomicrons. This vitamin D will eventually make it to the liver and must also undergo the same modifications in the liver and kidney as did the vitamin D made from cholesterol in the skin.

What Does Vitamin D Do in the Body?

In order for a cell to be influenced by vitamin D it must possess the vitamin D receptor which is located in the nucleus. This further strengthens the argument that vitamin D is more like a hormone than a vitamin. Remember that a hormone must bind with a specific receptor in order to be active. While researchers continue to discover vitamin D receptors in various tissues throughout the body, most of the attention has centered on the bone, kidneys, and intestines. Vitamin D is classically recognized as being principally involved in bone and calcium metabolism although newer functions of vitamin D are being added to the list.

Vitamin D functions include:

- *Calcium balance*—Vitamin D is principally involved in maintaining blood calcium levels. About 99 percent of the body's calcium is found in bone, it serves as a reservoir for blood calcium, the concentration of which is tightly regulated. When blood calcium levels begin to fall below normal levels, the parathyroid gland releases *parathyroid hormone* (PTH) into circulation. PTH is dedicated to re-establishing normal blood calcium levels. One of its activities is to increase the conversion of vitamin D in the kidneys to its most active form. Vitamin D can then work to promote an increase in calcium absorption from the digestive tract and to also decrease the amount of calcium lost from the body in urine. Researchers believe that vitamin D promotes the production and activity of proteins that help transport calcium across the wall of the small intestine.

> Vitamin D is crucial to bone health by increasing calcium absorption as well reducing calcium loss in the urine.

- *Normal cell development*—All cells are derived from reproduction of existing cells. This occurs daily and is ramped up during growth, pregnancy and wound healing. However these cells are immature and lack the final, specialized design and function to do the job they are intended to do. Vitamin D is pivotal in the proper development of cells to their mature and productive form.
- *Immunity*—The active form of vitamin D is a potent stimulator of the immune system. In fact, several cells involved in immune responses including T cells have vitamin D receptors. In addition, other cells involved in immune functions produce the enzyme necessary for conversion of vitamin D to its most active form.

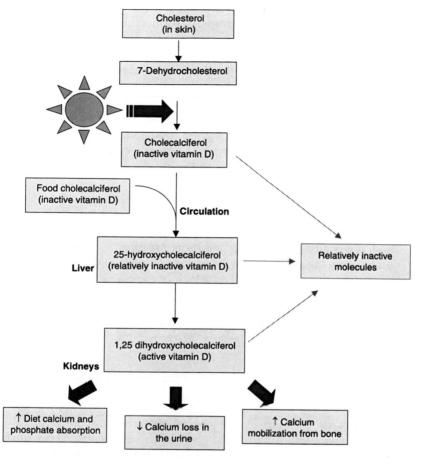

Figure 9.4 Sunlight (ultraviolet light) can convert a cholesterol derivative (7-dehydrocholesterol) to cholecalciferol. Cholecalciferol (from food or sunlight exposure) can be converted to active vitamin D by conversion in our liver and then kidneys. Vitamin D will increase available calcium in our body by increasing absorption from our diet and decreasing urine losses. Also vitamin D can promote the mobilization of calcium from our bone, which can become significant when dietary calcium is lacking.

What Happens If Too Little Vitamin D Is Consumed?

Deficiency of vitamin D can occur when a combination of factors is present. If vitamin D intake and/or absorption is low and an individual does not receive adequate exposure to sunlight, the potential for a vitamin D deficiency is present. Depending on the stage in life, vitamin D deficiency can results in:

- *Rickets*—In children, vitamin D deficiency results in *rickets*, a condition wherein bones are not properly formed and mineralized. Thin, pliable bones of the legs bow under the weight of a child's body. Bowed legs are often accompanied by an enlarged head, rib cage, and joints, which are considered the classic signs of rickets. It is important to remember that milk, whether it is from a human or from another mammal (such as cow or goat), is not a naturally rich source of vitamin D. However, most milk bought in a store is fortified with vitamin D thereby making it a good food source. Infants will be at greater risk of developing vitamin D deficiency if they do not receive periodical exposure to the sun and/or infant foods or a supplement containing vitamin D.
- *Osteomalacia*—The adult form of rickets is medically referred to as *osteomalacia*. This name literally means "bad bones." In osteomalacia bones gradually lose their mineral content, become less dense and physically weaker, and are more susceptible to fracture. The underlying cause of osteomalacia may be related directly to a lack of dietary vitamin D as well as a lack of exposure to sunlight. Or it may be related to internal disease in a vitamin D-metabolizing organ, such as the liver and/or kidneys, or organs involved in digestion and absorption of vitamin D, such as the pancreas, gallbladder, liver, and small intestine. Osteomalacia and a seemingly similar disorder (osteoporosis) are discussed in Chapter 12.

Can Too Much Vitamin D Be Consumed?

Of the vitamins, vitamin D has one of the lowest levels of intakes above recommendations that could give rise to side effects. Many of the manifestations appear to be related to vitamin D's calcium absorption, which in turn results in too much calcium in the blood. Prolonged hypercalcemia (elevated blood calcium) can affect muscle cell activity, which includes the heart, and can induce nausea, vomiting, mental confusion, and lead to calcium deposition in various tissues throughout the body. While the Tolerable Upper Limit has been set at five times the AI for adults, more recent research suggests that the threshold for potential side effects of excessive intake could indeed be at double that level.

Luckily, as exposure to sunlight increases the body's ability to make vitamin D decreases. In addition, as the level of active vitamin D increases, kidney cells produce less and less of the converting enzyme needed to make more active vitamin D. These mechanisms attempt to decrease the potential for toxicity. That's because we may be more sensitive to vitamin D toxicity than other vitamins when looking at the intake level associated with signs and symptoms.

Vitamin E

What Is Vitamin E?

Similar to many other vitamins, vitamin E is not necessarily a single molecule but is a class of similar molecules accomplishing related activities. There are about eight or so vitamin E molecules that can be subdivided into two major classes, *tocopherols* and *tocotrienols*, which themselves can be subdivided and given the Greek descriptors α, β, δ, or γ).

What Foods Are Good Sources of Vitamin E?

Good food sources of vitamin E include plant oils, margarine, and some fruits and vegetables, such as peaches and asparagus (Table 9.11). The average adult intake of vitamin E approximates the RDA, which is 15 α-TE daily (see below for an explanation of TE). More common supplement forms of vitamin E include α-tocopherol succinate and α-tocopherol acetate. In addition, α-tocopherol phosphate, which has the same nutritional value of the succinate and acetate forms, is also available, as are mixed tocopherols and γ-tocopherol versions. Furthermore, α-tocopherol supplements from natural sources (often labeled *dl-α-tocopherol*) will have more of the usable form of vitamin E than synthetic vitamin E, which can contain forms of α-tocopherol that our body can't use.

Table 9.11 Vitamin E (α-TE) Content of Select Foods

Food	Vitamin E (mg)	Food	Vitamin E (mg)
Oils/fats		*Vegetables*	
Oil (1 tablespoon)	6.7	Sweet potato (½ cup)	6.9
Mayonnaise (1 tablespoon)	3.4	Collard greens (½ cup)	3.1
Margarine (1 tablespoon)	2.7	Asparagus (½ cup)	2.1
Nuts and seeds		Spinach, raw (1 cup)	1.5
Sunflower seeds (¼ cup)	27.1	*Grains*	
Almonds (¼ cup)	12.7	Wheat germ	2.1
Peanuts (¼ cup)	4.9	(1 tablespoon)	
Cashews (¼ cup)	0.7	Bread, whole wheat	2.4
Seafood		(1 slice)	
Crab (3 ounces)	4.5	Bread, white (1 slice)	1.2
Shrimp (3 ounces)	3.7		
Fish (3 ounces)	2.4		

α-TE = α-tocopherol equivalents.

How Is Vitamin E Handled in the Body?

Vitamin E shows a fair absorption (25 to 50 percent) from the small intestine. Factors such as an increased need or low stores of vitamin E may certainly increase the absorption percentage. Like other fat-soluble vitamins, vitamin E needs the assistance of lipid digestive and absorptive processes (for example, chylomicrons). Much of the absorbed vitamin E will end up in the liver as chylomicron remnants are removed from the blood. The liver can then add vitamin E to VLDLs, which are then released into circulation where they can be delivered to most cells. By and large this is vitamin E in the form of α-tocopherol which means that it is the most significant form found in the blood as well as throughout our body.

Vitamin E is a powerful antioxidant and most of its activity in the body comes from α-tocopherol.

Because vitamin E is not very water soluble, very little is lost in urine; however, large intakes of vitamin E will result in a proportionate increase in urinary losses. The primary means for vitamin E loss from the body appears to be through the feces. The liver incorporates vitamin E into bile, which is dumped into the digestive tract. Some of this vitamin E, along with vitamin E from dietary sources, is not absorbed and becomes part of feces.

What Does Vitamin E Do in the Body?

By and large vitamin E functions as an antioxidant protecting cells from free radicals and most of its activity is attributable to α-tocopherol. As vitamin E is a lipid-soluble molecule it is logical to think that vitamin E would be most active in lipid-rich areas of our cells. This appears to be the case, as vitamin E's antioxidant activities are recognized mostly in regard to protecting the lipid-rich cell membranes. Cell membranes contain a tremendous amount of phospholipids, each of which contain two fatty acids. Furthermore, double bonds within some of these fatty acids seem to be very vulnerable to free-radical attack. Vitamin E appears to protect fatty acids by donating one of its own electrons to a free radical. This pacifies the free radical and also spares the fatty acids in cell membranes.

Since lipoproteins provide a primary means of shuttling vitamin E throughout the body, researchers have speculated that vitamin E may be involved in the prevention of heart disease. Some evidence suggests that vitamin E helps protect LDL from oxidation. Oxidized LDL is believed to be a strong risk factor for atherosclerosis. This is discussed in more detail in Chapter 13.

How Much Vitamin E Do We Need Daily?

The RDA for men and women of all ages is 15 milligrams (or 22.5 IU) of vitamin E daily. This is also the recommended level during pregnancy while the RDA is increased to 19 milligrams during lactation. See Table 3.2 for recommended levels for children and teens.

What Are α-Tocopherol Equivalents?

Among the vitamin E molecules, α-tocopherol is the most prevalent, popular, and probably potent in the body. For this reason the RDA for vitamin E is provided in α-tocopherol equivalents (α-TE). Here, 1 α-TE unit has the activity of 1 milligram of α-tocopherol. Since other forms of vitamin E are not as potent, the α-TE unit amount bestowed to a food is based on the amount of α-tocopherol as well as the potential vitamin E activity contributions made by the other forms. For example, if a food contained 25 milligrams of α-tocopherol and 50 milligrams of another form of vitamin E which is only 50 percent as potent as α-tocopherol, the food is said to contain 50 α-TE (25 milligrams of α-tocopherol + 25 milligrams [50 percent of 50 milligrams] of other vitamin E form).

What Happens If Too Little Vitamin E Is Consumed?

Vitamin E deficiency is somewhat rare in adults with the exception of those who have medical conditions that impact the normal digestion of lipids. Any situation in which normal fat digestion and absorption are hindered can ultimately reduce the amount of vitamin E absorbed from the digestive tract. A deficiency may take many months or years to show itself through medical symptoms such as red blood cell fragility and neurological abnormalities. Usually the medical condition is treated long before vitamin E deficiency signs are recognized. However, children with cystic fibrosis are a special concern, as the pancreas produces inadequate amounts of digestive enzymes in those with this disease.

Can Vitamin E Become Toxic?

Compared with the fat-soluble vitamins discussed so far, vitamin E is relatively nontoxic. However, studies on people eating fifty to one hundred times the RDA have demonstrated that these amounts can result in nausea, diarrhea, and headaches, while some individuals complained of general weakness and fatigue. It should be recognized that excessive vitamin E supplementation may interfere with vitamin K's activity in blood clotting.

Vitamin K

What Is Vitamin K?

Vitamin K is a general name for a few related compounds that possess vitamin K activity. *Phylloquinone* is the form of vitamin K found naturally in plants; *menaquinones* are the form of vitamin K derived from bacteria; and *menadione*, which is not natural, is the synthetic (laboratory derived) form of vitamin K.

What Foods Provide Vitamin K?

Humans receive vitamin K not only from various foods but also from bacteria in the colon. Good sources of vitamin K include broccoli, spinach, cabbage, Brussels sprouts, turnip greens, cauliflower, beef liver, and asparagus. Foods lower in vitamin K such as cheeses, eggs, corn oil, sunflower oil, and butter also make a respectable contribution to our vitamin K intake because of their frequency of consumption.

How Much Vitamin K Do We Need?

The RDA for men and women is 120 and 90 micrograms of vitamin K daily. The RDA for pregnant and lactating women over the age of 18 is the same as non-pregnant adult women, however, for pregnant females 18 and younger the recommendation is only 75 micrograms daily. See Table 3.2 for recommended levels for children and teens.

It has been estimated that as much as one-half of the vitamin K absorbed from the digestive tract was originally made by intestinal bacteria. Being a fat-soluble substance, vitamin K relies somewhat upon the activities of normal lipid digestion for optimal absorption. Vitamin K must also be transported from the intestines by way of chylomicrons, which ultimately reach the liver. Once in the liver, vitamin K can be packaged into VLDL and carried throughout the body.

What Does Vitamin K Do in the Body?

For years the only recognized activity of vitamin K was its involvement in proper normal blood clotting. In fact, rumor has it that vitamin K was so named by Danish researchers with respect to blood *coagulation*, a word spelled with a "K" in Danish. The liver is responsible for making the proteins, or *clotting factors*, that circulate in the blood. These proteins are activated when there is a hemorrhage and allow blood to clot at that site.

When clotting factors are initially made by liver cells, but before they are released into circulation, several of these proteins are modified by vitamin K. The modification occurs only in few amino acids; however, it changes the design and function of the proteins significantly. With this slightly modified design, these and other clotting factors are released into circulation. Once in circulation, these proteins await the signal to initiate clot formation. The signal is a tear in a blood vessel wall producing a hemorrhage. In light of vitamin K's involvement with blood clotting, the vitamin K status of a patient is typically determined prior to any surgical procedure.

Vitamin K also seems to be active in other tissue besides the liver. In bone, muscles, and kidneys, vitamin K appears to be necessary for activities similar to those in the liver. At least two proteins in bone and one in the kidneys have been identified as needing modification by vitamin K to function properly.

Can Too Little or Too Much Vitamin K Be Consumed?

Unlike other fat-soluble vitamins, vitamin K is not stored very well in the body and appreciable amounts are lost in urine and feces every day. This certainly presents the opportunity for a more rapid onset to deficiency. However, since vitamin K is abundant in the human diet and vitamin K is produced by bacteria in the digestive tract, vitamin K deficiency is uncommon in adults. The typical American adult may eat five to six times the RDA daily.

Opportunities for vitamin K deficiency do arise during infancy. There does not seem to be an appreciable transfer of vitamin K from the mother to the infant prior to birth. Thus newborns enter the world with very limited stores of vitamin K. Furthermore, a newborn's digestive tract is sterile and will not develop a mature bacterial population for a couple of months. Further, maternal breast milk is not a good source of vitamin K. All of these factors place infants at greater risk for developing vitamin K deficiency, which can lead to poor blood clotting and hemorrhage, among other considerations. With these concerns in mind, newborns are commonly provided with vitamin K shortly after birth.

One other situation may raise concern regarding the development of a vitamin K deficiency. People using antibiotics for long periods of time are at a greater risk for vitamin K deficiency. Certain antibiotics can reduce the number of vitamin K-producing bacteria from the colon which puts someone at a greater risk of deficiency, especially if a person eats a low vitamin K diet and/or is experiencing problems with lipid digestion. But the combination of these factors is indeed rare.

Vitamin K is relatively nontoxic in natural forms; however, there have been situations of toxicity from chronic use of excessive vitamin K in the synthetic menadione form.

FAQ Highlight

Antioxidant Teams

Do We Need More Vitamin E If We Eat More Unsaturated Fat Sources?

As unsaturated fatty acids are more prone to free-radical attack, many researchers contend that diets containing more unsaturated fatty acids will increase the need for vitamin E. One fate of diet-derived fatty acids is to become part of phospholipids in cell membranes. In fact, the more unsaturated fatty acids found in the diet, the more unsaturated fatty acids found in cell membrane phospholipids. They argue that as we shift our fatty acid intake to more unsaturated fatty acids, such as the poly-unsaturated ω-3 and ω-6 fatty acids, we may need to provide these fatty acids with adequate antioxidant escorts (for example, vitamin E). Other antioxidants such as vitamin C are not as impressive in directly protecting unsaturated fatty acids. This is because their water solubility keeps them more involved in the watery intracellular fluid rather than the lipid portion of cell membranes.

The choice of unsaturated fatty acid sources, such as plant oils or fish (oil in fish), differs in regard to vitamin E contribution. Plant oils contain vitamin E while fish oils do not. Some researchers believe that if we derive most of our unsaturated fatty acids from fish sources those foods should be complemented with foods higher in vitamin E or a supplement containing vitamin E. The idea seems logical and awaits further study.

Does Vitamin E Work with Other Antioxidants in a Team-Like Manner?

It should be recognized that other antioxidant-like compounds such as vitamin C and selenium can support vitamin E's efforts. After vitamin E concedes an electron to a free radical it can be restocked with another electron from vitamin C. Thus vitamin C helps keep vitamin E equipped in its battle against free radicals. This helps to recycle vitamin E. The mineral selenium, as part of the enzyme glutathione peroxidase, seems to have a beneficial effect upon vitamin E status. It has been suggested that like vitamin C, glutathione peroxidase also helps to recycle vitamin E by restocking it with an electron. Furthermore, glutathione peroxidase helps inactivate free radicals such as peroxides, which ultimately reduces the workload of vitamin E.

10 The Minerals of Our Body

Minerals represent about 5 to 6 percent to total body weight in humans and function in many different ways. Some minerals such as sodium, potassium, and chloride function as electrolytes, while other minerals, such as copper, zinc, iron, chromium, selenium, and manganese can be incorporated into enzyme molecules. Some minerals such as calcium, phosphorus, and fluoride can play a vital structural role in strengthening bones and teeth. After water, minerals are the primary inorganic component of the body; by and large they're the left-over (ash) after cremation of a body, as they will not combust like most organic molecules or evaporate like water.

Minerals can be broken into two broad groups based on their contribution to body weight (Table 10.1). If a mineral accounts for more than one-thousandth of human body weight it is considered a *major mineral*. When a mineral accounts for less than one-thousandth of body weight it is called a *minor mineral* or *trace mineral*. Another way to designate the difference between major and minor minerals is through dietary need. The recommended dietary intake for major minerals is greater than 100 milligrams, while the recommendations for minor minerals are less than 100 milligrams. The term *mineral* is often used

Table 10.1 The Minerals of Humans

Major Minerals	Minor or Trace Minerals	
Calcium	Iron	Copper
Phosphorus	Chromium	Boron
Sulfur	Selenium	Manganese
Potassium	Zinc	Molybdenum
Sodium	Iodine	Fluoride
Chloride	Nickel	Vanadium
Magnesium	Arsenic	Silicon
	Cobalt*	Cadmium*
	Lithium*	Tin*

* Dietary essentiality questionable despite presence in body.

interchangeably with *element*, thereby indicating that all minerals are elements.

Major Minerals Include Calcium, Phosphorus, and Electrolytes

The major minerals make up most of the mineral in our body by weight. Because of this our dietary needs are higher than minor minerals. In addition to foods, supplements make a significant contribution to many people's intake. For instance, calcium-based supplements are among the most popular with consumers who take them primarily for bone support.

Calcium (Ca)

What Is Calcium?

Without question calcium is one of the most recognizable and popular minerals. Perhaps this is well deserved, as calcium is about 40 percent of total body mineral weight and about 1.5 percent of total body weight. Furthermore, calcium tends to be portrayed as a hero for protecting the human body from osteoporosis. However, most people really do not understand how calcium functions. Calcium is found in foods and the body as an atom with a +2 charge (Ca^{++} or Ca^{2+}). Calcium atoms, therefore, are most stable after they have given up two electrons (see Chapter 1). Because of this heavy positive charge, calcium strongly interacts with substances bearing a negative charge. This allows it to form mineral complexes found in bone and teeth as well as interact with proteins to make things happen in certain cells.

> Calcium is a large, charged atom and is the most abundant mineral in our body.

What Foods Provide Calcium to Our Diet?

Without question, dairy products are the greatest contributors of calcium to the diet. Perhaps more than 55 percent of the calcium in the American diet comes from dairy products. For instance, a cup of milk or yogurt or 1.5 oz of cheddar cheese supplies about 300 milligrams of calcium (Table 10.2). Other good or reasonable calcium sources include sardines, oysters, clams, tofu, red and pinto beans, almonds, calcium-fortified foods, and dark green leafy vegetables such as broccoli, kale, collards,

Table 10.2 Calcium Content of Select Foods

Food	Calcium (mg)	Food	Calcium (mg)
Milk and Milk Products		*Vegetables*	
Yogurt low-fat (1 cup)	448	Collard greens (½ cup)	110
Milk, skim (1 cup)	301	Spinach (½ cup)	90
Cheese, Swiss (1 ounce)	272	Broccoli (½ cup)	70
Ice cream (1 cup)	180	*Legumes and products*	
Ice milk (1 cup)	180	Tofu (½ cup)	155
Custard (½ cup)	150	Dried beans (½ cup)	50
Cottage cheese (½ cup)	70	Lima beans (½ cup)	40

mustard greens, and turnip greens. Other vegetables such as spinach, rhubarb, chard, and beet greens contain respectable amounts of calcium. Calcium has also become a popular nutrient for fortification in foods such as bread.

What Forms of Calcium Are Common in Nutrition Supplements?

Most calcium supplements contain calcium carbonate or calcium citrate. Other forms of common calcium supplements include calcium gluconate, calcium acetate, and calcium lactate. Of all of the forms of calcium supplements, calcium carbonate supplies the most calcium (by weight); this form also possesses a slightly greater efficiency of absorption for most people when taken with food. Calcium citrate malate (CCM) is found in some supplements and research suggests that it is better absorbed than the forms above. However, using CCM results in a more expensive supplement so manufacturers tend to either not use it or use it in combination with other calcium forms.

Calcium supplements should be taken with a meal unless the meal contains fiber-rich foods which often contain phytate and oxalates. Calcium carbonate is the form found in many antacids. Meanwhile, calcium citrate is itself an acid and therefore may be better suited for people lacking the ability to produce adequate stomach acid. Recently, supplements containing hydroxyapatite have also begun to appear on the shelves.

Several forms of calcium exist in supplements including calcium carbonate, citrate and citrate malate.

What Dietary Factors Can Influence Calcium Absorption?

Plants can contain substances called oxalates and phytate, which can bind to calcium in the digestive tract and decrease its absorption (Table 10.3). It is estimated that as little as 5 percent of the calcium is absorbed from spinach because of the presence of inhibiting substances in the digestive tract.

In addition, factors such as normal stomach acidity and the presence of certain amino acids in the small intestine seem to increase the efficiency of calcium absorption. Because of this calcium supplements should be taken with a meal and the one with the least amount of vegetables. Furthermore, a diet having a higher phosphorus-to-calcium ratio may reduce calcium absorption and the ratio of phosphorus to calcium in the diet should not exceed 2:1.

What Are the Recommendations for Calcium Intake?

The recommended intake for calcium is the highest among the nonenergy providing essential nutrients with the only exceptions being phosphorus and water, the latter of which does not have a RDA. The Adequate Intake (AI) for adults (including pregnant and lactating women) is 1,000 milligrams of calcium daily until the age of 51 then the AI increases to 1,200 milligrams. Pregnant or lactating females 18 years old or younger the AI for calcium is 1,300 milligrams daily. Recommendations for calcium takes into consideration daily losses of calcium from the body by way of urine, skin, and feces along with an absorption rate of about 20 to 40 percent for adults and up to 75 percent for children and during pregnancy.

Where Is Calcium Found in the Body?

About 99 percent of the calcium in the body can be found in the bones and teeth. Only a small portion of the body's calcium (1 percent) is found outside bone and teeth and is distributed in tissue throughout the body such as muscle, glands, and nerves. This calcium is found in the blood as

Table 10.3 Influence of Various Factors on Calcium Absorption

Calcium Absorption Increased	*Calcium Absorption Decreased*
Vitamin D and PTH	Vitamin D and PTH
Lactose during same meal	Phytate, fiber, and oxalates during same meal
Need (growth, pregnancy, lactation)	Need

PTH = parathyroid hormone.

well as distributed in other tissues throughout the body including muscles, nerves, and glands. However, despite the relatively smaller quantity, it is this portion of calcium that is more important to human existence on a millisecond-to-millisecond, second-to-second, minute-to-minute basis. That's because this calcium will play a role in the beating of the heart, muscle action, blood clotting, and nerve and hormone activity.

What Is Calcium's Role in Bone and Teeth?

Without question the most recognizable function of calcium is to make the bones and teeth hard. The two major calcium-containing complexes in these tissues are calcium phosphate $[Ca_3(PO_4)_2]$ and hydroxyapatite $[Ca_{10}(PO_4)_6OH_2]$ with the latter being the most abundant. Hydroxyapatite crystals have a structure somewhat similar to flagstone: they are basically long and flat. This design allows hydroxyapatite to lie on top of collagen fibers in bones and teeth, thereby complementing the strength of collagen with hardness and rigidity (Figure 10.1). Calcium phosphate is a little different from hydroxyapatite in that it is broken down more readily than hydroxyapatite, which allows it to serve as a resource of both calcium and phosphate to help maintain blood levels of these minerals. Furthermore, calcium phosphate can be used to make hydroxyapatite in bones and teeth.

What Role Does Calcium Play in the Heart and Skeletal Muscle?

Calcium is involved in the function of excitable tissue (muscle and nerves). Before the heart can "beat," special cells in a region of the heart called the sinoatrial node (SA node) must spontaneously initiate an electrical impulse. This impulse then stimulates the rest of the heart to contract. Calcium is fundamentally involved in initiating that impulse in the SA node. Calcium is also involved in the contraction of heart muscle,

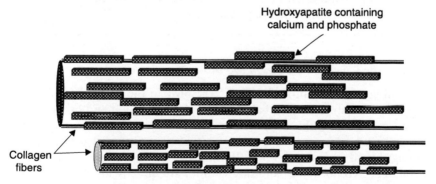

Hydroxyapatite containing
calcium and phosphate

Collagen
fibers

Figure 10.1 Sheets of hydroxyapatite (calcium and phosphate crystals) coating collagen fibers in bone.

as well as contraction of skeletal muscle. In doing so calcium is the factor that initiates the physical action of heart beats and muscle movement.

What Role Does Calcium Play in Nerves and Hormone Action?

Neurotransmitters and hormones are the means by which cells in the body can communicate with each other. However, in order for these substances to provide this service efficiently, they must be released from glands and nerve cells at appropriate times. Calcium is involved in the release of several of these substances. Furthermore, calcium is essential for certain hormones to have an impact upon certain cells. This means that when some hormones interact with their receptors, the result is an increase in the calcium concentration in that cell. As the level of calcium increases in these cells it will then interact with specific proteins and evoke the desired effect in that cell. Calcium sometimes can act as a middleman or intermediate factor as hormones cause things to happen. Scientists sometimes call this a "second messenger" role, whereby the first messenger was the hormone itself.

How Is Calcium Involved in Blood Clotting?

Calcium is also involved in proper blood clotting. When a hemorrhage occurs, clotting factors in the blood become activated and ultimately a clot is formed at the site of the hemorrhage. A clot is somewhat analogous to a bicycle tire patch that is placed specifically to seal off a hole. The clotting process consists of many steps, some which require calcium to proceed. Calcium binds to the clotting factors and allows them to become more active. Therefore, with a less than optimal amount of calcium in the blood, it might take longer to stop a hemorrhage.

> Besides providing hardness to bone, calcium is involved in blood clotting and muscle and hormone action.

How Is the Level of Calcium in the Blood Regulated?

One thing is for certain: calcium is very busy in the body. Again, on an instant-to-instant basis, the calcium found in the blood and other tissues is more vital than the calcium complexes in bones and teeth. As we alluded to, bones serve as a reservoir for calcium to safeguard against falling blood calcium levels. Blood calcium levels are very tightly regulated; two hormones and one vitamin are directly involved in blood calcium status. Parathyroid hormone (PTH), calcitonin, and vitamin D all function with blood calcium levels in mind.

PTH is released into circulation from the parathyroid gland when blood calcium levels begin to decline. PTH increases the activation of vitamin D in the kidneys and, along with vitamin D, PTH decreases the loss of calcium in urine. Vitamin D and PTH also increase the release of calcium from bone into the blood as well as increase the efficiency of calcium absorption from the small intestine. The net result is an increase in the level of calcium in the blood, thus returning it to normal (8.8 to 10.8 milligrams/100 milliliters of blood). On the contrary, the level of the hormone calcitonin in the blood increases when calcium levels increase above the normal range. Calcitonin is made by the thyroid gland and generally works opposite to PTH and vitamin D. Calcitonin decreases bone release of calcium and with the help of urinary loss of calcium promotes a reduction in blood calcium, thus returning it to the more optimal range.

How Does a Calcium Deficiency Impact Bone Health?

A deficiency of calcium results in bone abnormalities. If the deficiency occurs during growing years, poor bone mineralization will occur. Bones become soft and pliable due to a lack of mineralization. As bowed legs are often seen as a result of calcium deficiency during childhood, this disorder seems similar to rickets, which results from a vitamin D deficiency. If a calcium deficiency develops later in life, the result is a loss of mineral that renders bone less dense and more susceptible to fracture. This process is referred to as osteomalacia, which is often confused with osteoporosis. The differences will be explored in Chapter 12.

Can Blood Calcium Levels Be Used to Assess Body Calcium Status?

It is important to keep in mind that poor calcium intake may not be reflected by reductions in blood calcium. This is because the level of calcium in the blood is more influenced by the hormones mentioned previously in the short run (over a period of days and weeks). However, if calcium intake remains poor for longer periods of time, such as months, blood calcium levels can indeed begin to decrease. Therefore, an assessment of blood calcium levels is somewhat incomplete without an assessment of the hormones that regulate blood calcium levels.

Is Calcium Toxic in Large Amounts?

Today, it is fairly common for people to take in more calcium than years gone by because of supplementation practices and the large number of calcium-fortified foods. Based on this it is possible for people to exceed the AI. Although the efficiency of calcium absorption decreases as more is ingested and body calcium status is optimal, this can still lead to increased entry of calcium into the body. The Upper Limit (UL) has been set at 2,500 milligrams for children and adults, a level that is usually only achieved with the assistance of supplementation. Beyond this intake level the risk of undesirable effects increases, and can include loss of appetite, nausea, vomiting, constipation, abdominal pain, dry mouth, thirst, and frequent urination. In addition, since most forms of kidney stones are calcium oxalate, higher levels of calcium in the urine can increase the risk of kidney stones in people prone to them. Very high intakes of calcium from supplements and usually in combination with calcium-containing antacids, over time, can lead to increased calcium content in tissues such as muscle (including our heart), blood vessels, and lungs. This will affect the activity of the tissues by making them more rigid.

Phosphorus (P)

What Is Phosphorus?

Phosphorus in food or in the body is usually in the form of phosphate (PO_4). Thus, phosphorus and phosphate are often used interchangeably. After calcium, phosphate is the most abundant mineral in our body. Similar to calcium, phosphate bears a strong charge; only in this case it is negative. Calcium and phosphate therefore interact with each other nicely in bone and teeth because of their strong, opposite charges. Approximately 85 percent of the phosphorus found in the body is in the skeleton and teeth and is found in every cell in the body serving a vital role in energy operations.

What Foods Provide Phosphorus?

Those foods with a higher content of phosphorus include meat, poultry, fish, eggs, milk and milk products, cereals, legumes, grains, and chocolate (Table 10.4). Coffee and tea contains some phosphate as do many soft drinks contain phosphorus in the form of phosphoric acid. On the other hand, aluminum-containing substances ingested with a meal can decrease phosphorus absorption. Aluminum hydroxide and magnesium hydroxide are common ingredients in antacids.

Phosphate is important to bone strength as well as cell structure and energy systems.

Table 10.4 Phosphorus Content of Select Foods

Food	Phosphorus (mg)	Food	Phosphorus (mg)
Milk and milk products		*Grains*	
Yogurt (1 cup)	327	Bran flakes (1 cup)	180
Milk (1 cup)	250	Bread, whole wheat (1 slice)	52
Cheese, American (1 ounce)	130	Noodles, cooked (½ cup)	47
Meat and alternatives		Rice, cooked (½ cup)	29
Pork (3 ounces)	275	Bread, white (1 slice)	24
Hamburger (3 ounces)	165	*Vegetables*	
Tuna (3 ounces)	162	Potato (1)	101
Lobster (3 ounces)	125	Corn (½ cup)	73
Chicken (3 ounces)	120	Peas (½ cup)	70
Nuts and seeds		Broccoli (½ cup)	54
Sunflower seeds (¼ cup)	319	*Other*	
Peanuts (¼ cup)	141	Milk chocolate (1 ounce)	66
Peanut butter (1 tablespoon)	61	Cola (12 ounces)	51
		Diet cola (12 ounces)	45

What Are the Recommendations for Phosphorus Intake?

The recommended intake for phosphorus is similar to those for calcium and even exceeds one gram daily for teens. The Recommended Daily Allowance (RDA) for adults is 700 milligrams including pregnant and lactating women. However, for pregnant or lactating females 18 years old or younger the RDA for phosphorus is 1,250 milligrams daily matching recommendations for teens and pre-teens.

What Role Does Phosphorus (Phosphate) Play in Bone and Teeth?

Phosphorus found in the body is in the skeleton and teeth as a component of calcium phosphate $[Ca_3(PO_4)_2]$ and hydroxyapatite $[Ca_{10}(PO_4)_6OH_2]$. These complexes function to make bone and teeth hard. In addition, the phosphate found in bone can serve as a resource of this mineral to help maintain adequate amounts of phosphate in other tissues.

What Role Does Phosphorus Play in Energy System?

Phosphate is also vital to the processes that allow our cells to capture the energy released in the breakdown of carbohydrates, protein, fat, and alcohol. As mentioned several times, when energy is released from carbohydrates, protein, fat, and alcohol some of it is trapped in chemical bonds involving phosphate of special molecules such as ATP (adenosine triphosphate). Other phosphate-containing energy molecules are creatine phosphate (CP) and guanosine triphosphate (GTP). It is important to keep in mind that while carbohydrates, protein, fat, and alcohol are endowed with energy, the body's cells cannot directly use that energy. Thus, these substances are broken down as needed to produce ATP and GTP, which then can be used to power cell operations.

What Other Roles Does Phosphate Play in Our Body?

Phosphate is used by the cells to help regulate the activity of key enzymes. For instance, a key enzyme involved in the breakdown of glycogen stores is activated when a phosphate is attached to it. It is like an on/off switch for that enzyme as well as others. In addition, phosphate is a vital component of phospholipids in cell membranes and also nucleic acids (RNA and DNA). Phospholipids are the primary structural components of cell membranes, while DNA serves as the instruction manuals for building proteins in cells.

Can Too Little or Too Much Phosphorus Be Consumed?

Because most foods contain phosphorus, a deficiency is somewhat rare under normal circumstances. Toxicity is also rare perhaps with the exception of infants who receive a high phosphorus-containing formula. However, most commercially available infant formulas are not a threat in regard to their phosphorus content.

Sodium (Na)

What Is Sodium?

Sodium is one of the most abundant minerals on Earth. The sodium atom is most comfortable when it gives up an electron. Thus, sodium in foods as well as in the body will have a positive charge (Na^+). In light of the involvement of sodium in the electrical events of the body, we often refer to sodium, along with chloride and potassium, as electrolytes. Again, an electrolyte is a substance that when dissolved into a body of water will increase the speed of the electrical conduction of the water.

What Foods and Other Substances Contribute to Our Sodium Intake?

The adult diet can include 3 to 7 grams of sodium daily, which is a lot compared with other minerals. Oddly, the natural sodium content of

Table 10.5 Sodium Content of Select Foods

Food	Sodium (mg)	Food	Sodium (mg)
Meat and alternatives		*Other*	
Corned beef (3 ounces)	808	Salt (1 tablespoon)	2132
Ham (3 ounces)	800	Pickle, dill (1)	1930
Fish, canned (3 ounces)	735	Broth, chicken (1 cup)	1571
Sausage (3 ounces)	483	Ravioli, canned (1 cup)	1065
Hot dog (1)	477	Broth, beef (1 cup)	782
Bologna (1 ounce)	370	Gravy (¼ cup)	720
Milk and milk products		Italian dressing (2 tablespoons)	720
Cream soup (1 cup)	1070	Pretzels (salted), thin (5)	500
Cottage cheese (½ cup)	455	Olives, green (5)	465
Cheese, American (1 ounce)	405	Pizza, cheese (1 slice)	455
Cheese, Parmesan (1 ounce)	247	Soy sauce (1 tablespoon)	444
Milk, skim (1 cup)	125	Bacon (3 slices)	303
Milk, whole (1 cup)	120	French dressing (2 tablespoons)	220
Grains		Potato chips (10)	200
Bran flakes (1 cup)	363	Catsup (1 tablespoons)	155
Corn flakes (1 cup)	325	Bagel (1)	260
English muffin (1)	203		
Bread, white (1 slice)	130		
Bread, whole wheat (1 slice)	130		
Crackers, saltines (4 squares)	125		

most foods is very low. Typically, more than half of the sodium consumed is added to foods by food manufacturers for taste or preservation purposes (Table 10.5). Some of the foods having higher sodium content are snack foods (such as chips), luncheon meats, gravies, cheeses, and pickles. Sodium is also added in the kitchen during cooking and by "salting" foods at the table. The sodium occurring naturally in foods such as eggs, milk, meats, and vegetables may provide less than one-fourth of the total sodium people consume. Drinking water can also contribute to sodium intake along with certain medicines.

> Most of the sodium we consume comes from processed foods and snacks.

Within the past few decades many people have become concerned about how sodium in their diet might impact their health. This has applied pressure upon food companies to reduce the sodium content of some of their products. In order for a product label to make certain sodium-related

Table 10.6 Labeling Guidelines for Sodium Content

Label Claim	Sodium Content (per serving)
"Sodium free"	Must contain less than 5 milligrams per serving
"Very low sodium"	Must contain 35 milligrams sodium per serving or less
"Low sodium"	Must contain 145 milligrams sodium per serving or less
"Reduced sodium"	75% Reduction in sodium content
"Unsalted"	No salt added to the recipe
"No added salt"	No salt added to the recipe

claims, it must meet the criteria listed in Table 10.6. We will take a closer look at the relationship between sodium and various diseases and disorders such as high blood pressure, cancers and so forth later on.

How Much Sodium Do We Need Daily?

The AI for sodium is 1.5 grams for younger adults and teens which includes pregnancy and lactation. Since sodium is a key component of sweat, people who sweat profusely such as athletes, may need a little more sodium which is easily provided in foods. The AI decreases to 1.3 for people over 51 and then 1.2 grams over the age of 70.

What Does Sodium Do in the Body?

Sodium is very well absorbed (about 95 percent) from the digestive tract. Therefore the primary means of regulating body sodium content is through urinary loss. Sodium is the predominant positively charged electrolyte dissolved in extracellular fluid. This, of course, includes the blood. Because of its abundance in the body, sodium is perfect for serving fundamental roles in the electrical activity of excitable cells such as muscle and neurons as explained in Chapter 2.

Sodium is also involved in regulating body water content as water is naturally attracted to sodium. Water will always move from one area to another in an effort to balance the total concentration of dissolved substances in both areas. This process is called *osmosis* and is a fundamental law of nature. Under certain circumstances the body will lessen the amount of sodium lost in the urine to decrease the amount of urinary water loss. This may occur as an adaptive measure during dehydration or a reduction in blood pressure such as after significant blood loss. *Aldosterone* is the principal hormone that governs the amount of sodium in urine.

Can Sodium Deficiency Develop?

Unlike most essential nutrients whereby aberrations resulting from a diet deficiency can take weeks, months, or even years to develop, electrolyte imbalances can lead to alterations much more rapidly. A reduced level of sodium in the body would result in alterations in the activity of excitable tissue, which certainly includes the brain, nerves, and muscle. This can occur within a day or two.

Because of the abundance of sodium in the human diet, the potential for a deficiency is somewhat low. However, certain situations may place some people at a greater risk. These include eating a very low-sodium diet in conjunction with excessive sweating and/or chronic diarrhea. Still, even under these conditions deficiency is very rare. Excessive sweating makes us thirsty and beverages would probably include some sodium. Furthermore, since the sodium concentration in our sweat is lower than in our blood it would take the loss of a couple of pounds of body weight in the form of sweat before any distress would occur.

Can Sodium Be Toxic?

Provided that the kidneys are operating efficiently, humans can rapidly remove excessive diet-derived sodium from the body without concern. However, individuals eating a very salty diet should include more water in their diet. Since water is attracted to sodium, more water will be urinated along with the excessive sodium. For people experiencing significantly decreased kidney performance, sodium becomes more of a concern. Dialysis may be necessary to remove excessive sodium and other substances from their body fluid.

Ingesting salt tablets on a hot day used to be a common practice, especially for athletes. However, this practice is no longer recommended for several reasons. First, it can cause intestinal discomfort and possibly diarrhea. Second, it would add more sodium to the body than is lost in sweat. To correct the elevated sodium concentration in the blood, more urine would have to be produced. This would lead to more water loss from the body, which during athletic performance could be a problem.

Potassium (K)

What Is Potassium?

Similar to sodium, potassium atoms are most comfortable when they concede an electron and exist as a positively charged atom (K^+). Potassium is one of the most important electrolytes in human body fluid; it is concentrated in the fluids inside of cells while sodium exists mainly outside of cells. The symbol for potassium is a K because of its Latin name *(kalium)*.

What Foods Contribute to Potassium Intake?

Unlike sodium, potassium is not routinely added to foods. Therefore, foods naturally containing potassium must be eaten to meet the body's needs. Luckily, potassium is found in most natural foods in the human diet (Table 10.7). Many vegetables and fruits and their juices rank among the best sources of potassium. In fact, some athletes refer to bananas as "potassium sticks" with respect to their potassium content, although their potassium content really is not that outstanding compared with other fruits and vegetables. Along with fruits and vegetables, milk, meats, whole grains, coffee, and tea are among the most significant contributors to daily potassium intake.

How Much Potassium Do We Need Daily?

Recommendations for potassium are the highest among the minerals. The AI for potassium is 4.7 grams for teens and adults, even during pregnancy. The AI is increased to 5.1 grams during lactation.

Potassium is mostly found dissolved in the fluid within cells.

Table 10.7 Potassium Content of Select Foods

Food	Potassium (mg)	Food	Potassium (mg)
Vegetables		*Meats*	
Potato (1)	780	Fish (3 ounces)	500
Squash, winter (½ cup)	327	Hamburger (3 ounces)	480
Tomato (1 medium)	300	Lamb (3 ounces)	382
Celery (1 stalk)	270	Pork (3 ounces)	335
Carrots (1)	245	Chicken (3 ounces)	208
Broccoli (½ cup)	205	*Grains*	
Fruit		Bran buds (1 cup)	1080
Avocado (½)	680	Bran flakes (1 cup)	248
Orange juice (1 cup)	469	Raisin bran (1 cup)	242
Banana (1)	440	Wheat flakes (1 cup)	96
Raisins (¼ cup)	370	*Milk and milk products*	
Prunes (4)	300	Yogurt (1 cup)	531
Watermelon (1 cup)	158	Milk, skim (1 cup)	400

What Does Potassium Do in the Body?

Most of the potassium we ingest is absorbed by the digestive tract. So, like sodium, the amount of potassium in the body will need to be regulated by the kidneys. Unlike sodium (and chloride) though, about 98 percent of the potassium is located within the cells, making it the major positively charged electrolyte dissolved in the fluid within the cells. Therefore, potassium is extremely important in the electrical activity of excitable cells in the body as detailed in Chapter 2.

Can Too Little or Too Much Potassium Be Consumed?

Although dietary potassium intake is by and large adequate to meet human needs, situations can place the body at risk for potassium deficiency. Persistent use of laxatives can result in a lowered body potassium level by decreasing the amount of potassium absorbed from the digestive tract. Furthermore, chronic use of certain diuretics used to control blood pressure may also result in increased urinary loss of potassium. Physicians will routinely monitor the potassium levels of patients following either of these prescribed protocols. People who frequently vomit after a meal, either involuntarily or voluntarily, can reduce potassium absorption. Finally, people following a very low calorie diet (VLCD) for extended periods of time need to be concerned about their potassium consumption along with levels of other nutrients as well.

Is It Possible to Develop Potassium Toxicity?

Potassium toxicity is not necessarily a concern provided that the kidneys are functioning appropriately. However, if the blood potassium level does become elevated (hyperkalemia) it would certainly affect the proper functioning of the excitable tissue, especially the heart and brain. The heart may actually fail to beat if hyperkalemia is severe and prolonged. Together with sodium, blood potassium levels are monitored closely in people diagnosed with diseases affecting their kidneys.

Chloride (Cl)

What Is Chloride?

Chloride is the ion name for chlorine. Chlorine is an atom that is most comfortable when it removes an electron from another atom and as a result takes on a negative charge (Cl^-). Sodium and potassium as electrolytes often overshadow chloride, but chloride should not be underestimated in importance. Furthermore, chloride is involved in some interesting aspects of protein digestion as well as carbon dioxide elimination from the body.

What Foods Provide Chloride in the Diet?

Although some fruits and vegetables contain respectable amounts of chloride, the natural content of this mineral in most foods is naturally low. Chloride, as part of sodium chloride (table salt) added to foods, is the major contributor of chloride in our diet. Sodium chloride is 60 percent chloride by weight, thus 1 gram of table salt is 600 milligrams chloride. The minimum requirement for chloride for an adult is about 700 milligrams per day, yet the average American diet contains about six times this amount.

How Much Chloride Do We Need Daily?

The AI for chloride is 2.3 grams for younger adults and teens which includes pregnancy and lactation. Since chloride is a key component of sweat, people who sweat profusely such as athletes, may need a little more sodium which is easily provided in foods. The AI for chloride decreases to 2.0 grams for people over 51 and then 1.8 grams over the age of 70.

What Does Chloride Do in the Body?

Similar to sodium and potassium, chloride functions as an electrolyte. In fact, chloride is the major negatively charged electrolyte in human extracellular fluid, which includes the blood. Chloride is important in the optimal functioning of excitable cells, which once again are nervous tissue and muscle as detailed in Chapter 2. It is also part of hydrochloric acid (HCl), which is a key component of stomach juice.

> Chloride is an important component of stomach acid and in ridding our body of carbon dioxide.

Furthermore, chloride is important in helping the body to remove carbon dioxide. This process is very complex and involves changing carbon dioxide into a substance called *carbonate* that will dissolve more easily into the blood. Remember, gases such as oxygen and carbon dioxide do not dissolve very well in watery human blood. Therefore, the blood either carries them on hemoglobin (mostly oxygen) or converts carbon dioxide to a more water-soluble substance. This allows for more and more carbon dioxide to be circulated to the lungs and breathed out of the body.

What Happens If Too Little or Too Much Chloride Is Consumed?

In light of Americans' heavy use of salt in food manufacturing, processing, and seasoning in the kitchen and at the table, chloride deficiencies are very rare. As mentioned, Western diets contain many times the estimated minimum requirement for chloride. Thus the potential for deficiency is believed to be rather low and is rarely seen. However, heavy, prolonged sweating can cause excessive loss of chloride which in turn could impact the activity of muscle and the nervous system. However the consumption of food and beverages will recover lost chloride. Sport drinks and related products provide chloride for endurance athletes.

On the other hand, like sodium and potassium, chloride is almost entirely absorbed from the digestive tract. Therefore, the responsibility of body chloride regulation is placed upon the kidneys. Provided that the kidneys are functioning properly, the risk of chloride toxicity is not necessarily a major concern either. However, if the kidneys are not functioning optimally this can result in elevations in the chloride in body fluid along with the other electrolytes. This then would most obviously affect the proper functioning of excitable cells in the body, although all cells would become compromised.

Magnesium (Mg)

What Is Magnesium?

Magnesium, like calcium, is most comfortable in nature when it gives up two electrons and takes on a double positive charge (Mg^{2+}). Therefore, like calcium, you may be thinking that magnesium may provide at least some of its function by electrically interacting with other substances. This is certainly the case as is discussed next.

What Foods Provide Magnesium?

Magnesium is found in a variety of foods; better sources include whole grain cereals, nuts, legumes, spices, seafood, coffee, tea, and cocoa (see Table 10.8). Certain processing techniques such as the milling of wheat and the polishing of rice may result in significant losses of magnesium from grains and other foods. Furthermore, some magnesium can dissolve into cooking water during boiling, which results in some cooking loss as well.

What Are the Recommendations for Magnesium Intake?

The RDA for magnesium varies depending on age gender and condition. For instance, the RDA for 19 to 30 year old women and men is 310 and

Table 10.8 Magnesium Content of Select Foods

Food	Magnesium (mg)	Food	Magnesium (mg)
Legumes		*Vegetables*	
Lentils, cooked (½ cup)	134	Bean sprouts (½ cup)	98
Split peas, cooked (½ cup)	134	Black eyed peas(½ cup)	58
Tofu (½ cup)	130	Spinach, cooked (½ cup)	48
Nuts		Lima beans (½ cup)	32
Peanuts (1/3 cup)	95	*Milk and Milk Products*	
Cashews (1/3 cup)	140	Milk (1 cup)	30
Almonds (1/3 cup)	145	Cheddar cheese (1 ounce)	8
Grains		American cheese	6
Bran buds (1 cup)	240	(1 ounce)	
Rice, wild, cooked	119	*Meats*	
(½ cup)		Chicken (3 ounces)	25
Wheat germ	45	Beef (3 ounces)	20
(2 tablespoons)		Pork (3 ounces)	20

400 milligrams. However after the age of 30 the RDA bumps up to 320 and 420 milligrams, respectively.

What Does Magnesium Do in the Body?

Roughly 60 percent of the magnesium in the body is located in the bones. The remaining magnesium is found mostly in the intracellular fluid of cells throughout the body. Only a small percentage of magnesium is found in extracellular fluid. Magnesium in the bone can interact with calcium and phosphates to help increase the integrity of bones. The bones also serve as a reservoir or storage site for magnesium.

> Magnesium is found in bone and all cells within our body as it is crucial for efficient energy processing.

One thing that magnesium seems to do is to interact with the phosphates of ATP (Figure 10.2). This adds stability to ATP and improves the ability of ATP to power cell operations. Many chemical reactions require the splitting of an ATP molecule to release the energy necessary to drive the reaction or cell activity. In fact, magnesium seems to be a vital factor in the proper functioning of more than three hundred chemical reaction systems.

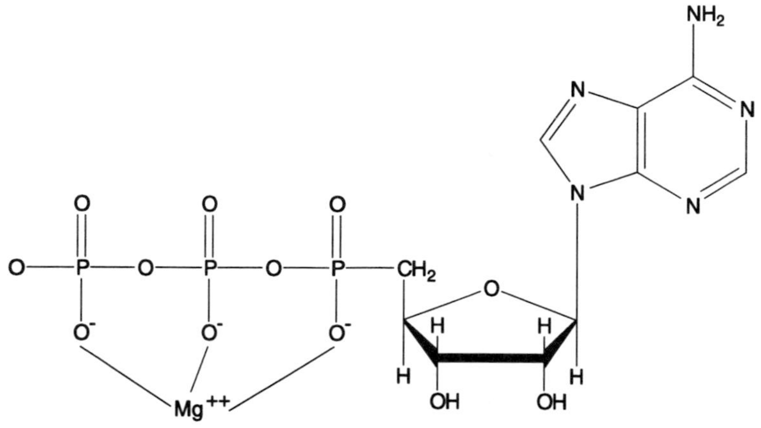

Figure 10.2 Because of its positive charge, magnesium (Mg) has the ability to electrically interact with the phosphate tail of ATP (negative charge). This stabilizes ATP and allows it to be used more efficiently by cells.

What Happens If Too Little or Too Much Magnesium Is Consumed?

Magnesium absorption from the digestive tract is fair (25 to 50 percent) with several factors being able to influence this efficiency. For example, a low body magnesium status results in a higher percentage of absorption. On the other hand, a high magnesium diet or excessive dietary calcium, phosphate, or phytate can decrease the efficiency of magnesium absorption.

Subtle alterations in blood magnesium content can affect the release of parathyroid hormone (PTH) and its activity. Further, a magnesium deficiency can negatively influence the ability of the cell membranes to maintain optimal sodium and potassium concentration differences across membranes. This is largely because magnesium is needed to stabilize ATP, which is the power source for pumping these ions across cell membranes. Thus, the proper function of excitable and other cells is jeopardized during magnesium deficiency. On the other hand, toxicity induced by a high dietary intake of magnesium can be thwarted by appropriately functioning kidneys.

Sulfur (S)

Sulfur is not really an essential nutrient but rather a vital component of essential nutrients. These nutrients include the amino acid methionine as well as biotin and thiamin. Therefore, the presence and actions of sulfur in the body is more of a reflection of what is going on with these substances rather than sulfur as an independent essential nutrient. Sulfur is also part of several food additives.

Minor Minerals Function as Components of Proteins and Other Molecules

The minor minerals account for less than 1 percent of our body by weight and are needed in much smaller levels than the major minerals. However, lower presence in the body and dietary requirements should not be associated with importance. For instance, deficiency of several minor minerals can lead to severe disorders and death. For zinc, selenium, copper and other trace minerals, the amount of these nutrients in natural foods is directly related to the conditions in which the plants were grown and/or animals raised. Soil rich in minor minerals will lead to higher concentrations of these nutrients in plants that are grown there. This also means that animals grazing on those plants will consume plants rich in these nutrients. Further still, minor mineral soil and rocks typically leads to higher levels in neighboring streams, rivers and lakes which in turn can increase the content of these nutrients in the fish and other marine life.

Iron (Fe)

What Is Iron?

Iron is one of the most recognizable minerals in the body, although an adult may have a little less than a teaspoon's amount in his or her body. However, quantity should not be associated with importance as the effects of iron deficiency are tragic and severe. In humans, as well as other animals, iron is found as the central component of a very important molecule called *heme*. Heme is part of larger protein complexes that rank among the most important in the human body. One aspect that makes animals different from plants is the presence of heme. Plants do not have it.

> Heme iron, which is derived from animal foods, is better absorbed than nonheme iron.

What Foods Provide Iron and What Influences Its Absorption?

Iron is part of both animal and plant foods (Table 10.9). The iron found in these foods exists in the form of either heme iron or nonheme iron. Animal foods (meats) contain both heme and nonheme iron. Good animal sources include beef, chicken (dark meat), oysters, tuna, and shrimp. Meanwhile, plants and plant-derived foods contain only

Table 10.9 Iron Content of Select Foods

Food	Iron (mg)	Food	Iron (mg)
Meat and alternatives		*Grains*	
Liver (3 ounces)	7.5	Breakfast cereal (1 cup)*	4–18
Round steak (3 ounces)	3	Oatmeal (2 cups)*	8
Hamburger, lean (3 ounces)	3	Bagel (1)	1.7
Baked beans (½ cup)	3	English muffin (1)	1.6
Pork (3 ounces)	2.7	Bread, rye (1 slice)	1
White beans (½ cup)	2.7	Bread, whole wheat (1 slice)	0.8
Soybeans (½ cup)	2.5	Bread, white (1 slice)	0.6
Fish (3 ounces)	1	*Vegetables*	
Chicken (3 ounces)	1	Spinach (½ cup)	2.3
Fruits		Lima beans (½ cup)	2.2
Prune juice (½ cup)	4.5	Peas, black-eyed (½ cup)	1.7
Apricots, dried (½ cup)	2.5	Peas (½ cup)	1.6
Prunes (5 medium)	2	Asparagus (½ cup)	1.5
Raisins (¼ cup)	1.3		
Plums (3 medium)	1.1		

* Iron-fortified.

nonheme iron. Good plant sources include raisins, tofu, molasses, lentils, potatoes, and kidney beans.

What Factors Influence Iron Absorption?

The importance in the difference of these two forms of iron is largely in their efficiency of absorption. Nonheme iron is absorbed less efficiently (2 to 20 percent) in comparison with heme iron (25 to 35 percent). However, if the nonheme iron is part of a meal containing vitamin C, meat, fish, or poultry or organic acids such as citric acid, malic acid, tartaric acid, and lactic acid, its absorption can increase. Conversely, the presence of phytates and oxalates in some plant foods (vegetables) can interact with nonheme iron in the digestive tract and decrease its absorption (Table 10.10). Soy protein and polyphenols in some

Table 10.10 Factors Influencing the Efficiency of Iron Absorption

Increased Absorption of Iron	Decreased Absorption of Iron
Vitamin C at the same meal	Phytate, oxalates from plants
Normal stomach acid production	Tannins such as from tea
Increased iron need (growth, pregnancy, poor status)	Decreased stomach acid production or the use of antacid medication
Meat, fish, poultry at same meal	

fruits, vegetables, coffee, and tea can also decrease non-heme iron absorption. Many nutritionists recommend that those people taking an iron-containing supplement should do so with a meal that has the least raw plant foods. For many people that meal is breakfast, which may also include citrus juice whose vitamin C may increase the absorption of nonheme iron.

Since the absorption efficiency of both forms of iron is low, it seems likely that the iron content of the body is primarily regulated at the point of absorption. This idea is reinforced by the fact that the efficiency of iron absorption increases during times of greater iron need, such as when iron stores are low. The efficiency of iron absorption also increases during periods of growth and pregnancy.

What Are the Levels of Recommended Intake for Iron?

The RDA for iron varies depending on age gender and condition. For instance, the RDA for adult men is 8 milligrams while the RDA for women aged 19 to 50 is 18 milligrams daily. The recommendation for younger women is dramatically higher than for men to compensate for menstrual losses of iron. Meanwhile the RDA drops to 8 milligrams for women after the age 50.

What Is the Difference Between Heme and Non-Heme Iron in Our Body?

As with other animals, iron is found in the cells as a part of heme and nonheme molecules. As mentioned, heme is an interesting molecule with iron situated at its core. In fact, iron seems to hold the whole molecule together (Figure 10.3). One of the most recognizable heme-based molecules is hemoglobin in RBCs and myoglobin in muscle. Iron that is not part of heme is found as part of a few enzymes and stored in molecular iron containers, namely ferritin and hemosiderin.

What Are Some Non-Heme Iron-Containing Components of Our Body?

Iron serves many roles in the body including:

- *Hemoglobin*—Hemoglobin is a protein found in RBCs that binds oxygen so that it can be transported throughout the body in the blood. A RBC may contain about 250 million hemoglobin molecules, each with the ability to bind four oxygen, a single RBC could carry roughly one billion oxygen molecules.
- *Myoglobin*—Myoglobin is found in muscle tissue and like hemoglobin, it binds oxygen. This allows myoglobin to act as an oxygen

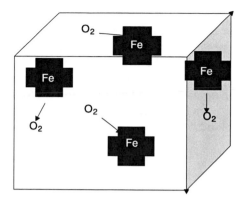

Figure 10.3 Red blood cells contain a lot of hemoglobin. There are four iron (Fe) containing heme units found in hemoglobin. Iron holds the heme together as well as attaches it to the protein. In addition the iron also binds oxygen.

reservoir in muscle fibers, which becomes readily available during exercise. When meat is eaten, which is just skeletal muscle of other mammals, much of the iron is derived from myoglobin.

- *Aerobic energy production*—Iron is part of heme-containing molecules called *cytochromes* that help form the electron-transport chain in mitochondria. Therefore not only is iron important in delivering oxygen (hemoglobin) to cells for aerobic energy metabolism, it is also a key component of much of the aerobic ATP manufacturing machinery itself.
- *Antioxidant protection*—Iron has an antioxidant role as part of an antioxidant enzyme called *catalase* found in many tissue. Catalase can metabolize hydrogen peroxide to water and oxygen.
- *Immunity*—Iron is also fundamental in proper immune function.

What Happens If Too Little Iron Is Consumed?

A poor iron intake over time will result in a reduction of blood hemoglobin levels. *Anemia* is the medical term used to describe a condition whereby hemoglobin levels fall well below normal levels. Normal hemoglobin levels for men and women are less than 14 and 12 milligrams per 100 milliliters of blood, respectively. In an anemic state (less than 7 to 9 milligrams per 100 milliliters), there is a decrease in the oxygen-carrying capability of our blood. Less oxygen is able to reach cells and anemic people will often complain of lethargy as well as early fatigue when they exercise. Beyond oxygen transport in the blood, iron deficiency decreases the ability of cells to make ATP by aerobic means.

How Can Our Body Iron Status Be Assessed?

Lower levels of iron in the body are indicated several ways. For the longest time we assessed hemoglobin levels and hematocrit (percent of blood that is RBCs) and used these as indicators of iron status. However, today we know that reductions in hemoglobin and hematocrit levels tend to occur later on as the body's iron status becomes more severely compromised. There are three additional ways to assess body iron status from a sample of blood.

- *Transferrin*—This is an iron transport protein and has the capacity to pick up iron from tissues throughout the body. Each transferrin molecule can carry multiple atoms of iron much like a bus can carry multiple passengers.
- *Total iron binding capacity (TIBC)*—TIBC indicates the potential for iron transport above what is currently being transported on transferrin. For instance, if transferrin levels are somewhat normal yet the capacity to bind iron (TIBC) is relatively high, this suggests poor iron status. This is similar to having plenty of buses driving around but carrying fewer people than normal. The total people-carrying capacity would be high, indicating that the buses are people deficient.
- *Ferritin*—Perhaps the most sensitive indicator of iron status is the level of ferritin in our blood. Ferritin is a large complex that stores iron in cells, such as in the liver. Therefore, the more iron in the tissues the more ferritin in the body. Now and then, some of the ferritin seems to leak into the blood and can be used to gauge iron status in the body as it reflects tissue iron content. High levels of ferritin in the blood implies that more iron is in the body.

Can Too Much Iron Be Consumed?

Recently, a fair amount of attention has been focused on what happens when there is too much iron in the body. For instance, researchers reported that men in Finland who have higher levels of ferritin in their blood were more likely to experience heart attacks in comparison with men with lower levels.

In more extreme examples of having excessive body iron, people in certain sub-Saharan countries noted for drinking beer with a high iron content seem to develop cirrhosis of the liver beyond what would be expected from excessive alcohol consumption alone. Further evidence is genetic-based disorders in which iron absorption is dramatically enhanced. This can lead to excessive body iron content in these people. The disorder is referred to as genetic-based *hemochromatosis* and is apparent in as many as 12 of every 1,000 people of European descent. This disorder is associated with severe liver disease and early death.

Zinc (Zn)

What Is Zinc?

Zinc is one of the most active minerals in the body as it influences the functioning of hundreds of different enzymes. Although often overshadowed in the popular press by the likes of iron and chromium, lately zinc has been thrust into the limelight. Zinc supplements have been purported to reduce the length and severity of the common cold, which will be discussed.

What Foods Provide Zinc?

In living things, zinc is more associated with amino acids and proteins. Therefore, it is logical to presume that animal foods, with their higher protein content, would be better zinc sources than plant foods. This is true. The best sources of zinc include organ meats, other red meats, and seafood (especially oysters and mollusks). Poultry, pork, milk and milk products, whole grains (especially germ and bran), and leafy and root vegetables are also respectable contributors of zinc (Table 10.11).

> Zinc is found in higher amounts in animal foods such as meats and oysters as well as the germ and bran of grains.

Table 10.11 Zinc Content of Select Foods

Foods	Zinc (mg)	Food	Zinc (mg)
Meats and Alternatives		*Legumes*	
Liver (3 ounces)	4–5	Dried beans, cooked (½ cup)	1
Beef (3 ounces)	4	Split peas, cooked (½ cup)	1
Crab (½ cup)	3–4	*Nuts and seeds*	
Lamb (3 ounces)	3–4	Pecans (¼ cup)	2
Pork (3 ounces)	2–3	Cashews (¼ cup)	1–2
Chicken (3 ounces)	2	Sunflower seeds (¼ cup)	1–2
Grains		Peanut butter (2 tablespoons)	1
Wheat germ (2 tablespoons)	2–3	*Milk and milk products*	
		Cheddar cheese (1 ounce)	1
Oatmeal, cooked (1 cup)	1	Milk, whole (1 cup)	1
Bran flakes (1 cup)	1	American cheese (1 ounce)	1
Rice, brown, cooked (2 cups)	0.5		
Rice, white (2 cups)	0.5		

What Are the Levels of Recommended Intake for Zinc?

The AI for zinc varies depending on age gender and condition. For instance, the AI for adult women and men is 8 and 11 milligram while that for pregnant and lactating women is 11 and 12 milligrams daily.

What Factors Can Influence Zinc Absorption?

Absorption of zinc from the digestive tract is not well understood. However, it does seem that many factors can influence how efficiently zinc is absorbed. For instance, zinc derived from meat boasts better absorption than zinc from plant sources. Zinc absorption from meat may actually be enhanced by certain amino acids, which would be present during simultaneous protein digestion. On the other hand, the efficiency of zinc absorption from plant foods seems to be lower which may in part be due to the presence of phytate, oxalates, and probably other substances (tannins) also found in many plants. Recommendations for dietary zinc takes into consideration the impact of various substances on zinc absorption.

What Does Zinc Do in the Body?

The distribution of zinc in the body may provide some indication as to its broad and extensive function. Zinc is found in all tissue of the body and is believed to be necessary for more than two hundred different chemical reactions. Zinc largely functions as a necessary component of various enzymes, which would regulate all of those chemical reactions. In fact, the number of enzymes whose optimal function relies upon zinc is probably greater than the total number of enzymes that rely on all of the other trace elements combined. Zinc is involved with enzymes that affect body function:

- antioxidant protection (superoxide dismutase)
- pH (carbonic anhydrase)
- alcohol metabolism (alcohol dehydrogenase)
- bone mineralization (alkaline phosphatase)
- protein digestion (carboxypeptidases)
- protein and nucleic acid metabolism (polymerases)
- heme production
- immunity

What Happens If We Get Too Little Zinc?

Zinc deficiency results in aberrations stemming from a decreased activity of zinc-dependent enzymes. These signs include stunted growth in children, abnormal bone growth and/or mineralization, delayed sexual maturation, decreased immune capacity, and poor wound healing. Because of zinc's widespread function throughout cells, many people feel that zinc supplementation is a necessity.

Can Zinc Become Toxic?

Zinc toxicity would tend to happen only by supplementation. One of the biggest concerns with higher zinc intakes is its relationship to copper. It is possible to reduce copper intake and induce signs of copper deficiency by consuming as little as three to ten times the RDA for zinc over several months. Because of the inverse relationship between dietary zinc and copper absorption, the utilization of high zinc supplements is not recommended unless a physician has recognized a need. This is particularly true for people who use zinc supplements to treat the common cold. These supplements should not be continued beyond 5 to 7 days.

Copper (Cu)

What Is Copper?

Although it brings to mind Abraham Lincoln's profile on the United States penny, copper is a very important mineral in many basic human functions. For instance, copper is needed to make collagen and it is a component of a powerful antioxidant enzyme.

What Foods Contain Copper?

The richest sources of copper include organ meats, shellfish, nuts, seeds, legumes, dried fruits, and certain vegetables such as spinach, peas, and potato varieties (Table 10.12). Similar to the efficiency of absorption of several other minerals, copper absorption is also sensitive to the presence of other substances in the digestive tract. For instance, researchers have shown that substances such as vitamin C, fiber, and bile in excessive amounts can decrease the efficiency of copper absorption. Furthermore, increased consumption of zinc can decrease copper absorption, as mentioned previously.

What Are Current Recommendations for Copper Intake?

The RDA for copper is the same for adult men and women at 900 micrograms daily. However during pregnancy and lactation the RDA increases to 1,000 and 1,300 micrograms daily. However, diet intake surveys have reported that the American population may not be meeting these recommendations.

Table 10.12 Copper Content of Select Foods

Food	Copper (μg)	Food	Copper (μg)
Liver, beef (3 ounces)	1000	Cocoa powder (2 tablespoons)	400
Cashews, dry roasted (¼ cup)	800		
Black-eyed peas (½ cup)	700	Prunes, dried (10)	400
Molasses, blackstrap (2 tablespoons)	600	Salmon, baked (3 ounces)	300
		Pizza, cheese (1 slice)	100
Sunflower seeds (¼ cup)	600	Bread, whole wheat (1 slice)	100
V8® drink (1 cup)	500	Milk chocolate (1 ounce)	100
Tofu, firm (½ cup)	500	Milk, 2% (1 cup)	100
Beans, refried (½ cup)	500		

Copper is part of antioxidant systems, energy metabolism, iron metabolism and collagen formation.

What Does Copper Do in the Body?

Although a little bit of copper may be absorbed across the wall of the stomach, by and large most of the absorption takes place in the small intestine. From there copper is found in most tissue playing a role as an essential component of many enzymes with various roles throughout the body. These enzymes are involved in:

- *Iron metabolism*—As part of the enzyme called ferroxidase, copper in iron is responsible for making sure iron is in the appropriate state to hop aboard its primary transport protein (transferrin) in the blood. Without copper, iron is not efficiently transported to bones, which make RBCs.
- *Antioxidant protection*—Copper is the key mineral in the enzyme superoxide dismutase, which is a key antioxidant enzyme found inside and outside cells.
- *Energy production*—As part of cytochrome c oxidase, a key component of the electron transport chain, iron is vital for aerobic energy generation.
- *Epinephrine/norepinephrine production*—Copper is part of the dopamine β-hydroxylase enzyme which is involved in the formation of epinephrine (adrenaline) and norepinephrine. These substances are called catecholamines and are involved in many of the activities during exercise and exciting situations.
- *Collagen production*—Collagen is a connective tissue protein and

is vital to bone, joints, and tissue in general. Copper is an important component of the enzyme lysyl oxidase, which helps form bone.

What Happens If We Get Too Little Copper?

Because of copper's fundamental role in iron metabolism, copper deficiency can result in anemia. Scientists have also reported alterations in heart muscle tissue and function in animals fed diets low in copper. However, whether the same can be said for humans is not clear. Copper deficiency can alter white blood cell numbers in the blood as well as reduce immune functions.

What Happens If We Get Too Much Copper?

Long-term use of high level copper supplements may induce toxicity wherein the function of the liver, kidneys, and brain may become compromised. In an extreme case, Wilson's disease is a rare genetic form of copper toxicity induced by increased copper storage.

Selenium (Se)

What Is Selenium?

Although seemingly unknown by many for so long, selenium jumped into the spotlight a couple of decades ago when researchers identified that a mysterious type of heart disease in Asia (see below) was actually caused by selenium deficiency—another example of how a small amount of a mineral can have a huge impact on the normal functioning of the body.

What Foods Provide Selenium?

Like many of the trace minerals, the quantity of selenium in natural food sources is often a reflection of the soil content in which plants were grown and the animals grazed. Animal products, including seafood, seem to be better sources of dietary selenium than plants (Table 10.13).

What Are Current Recommendations for Selenium Intake?

The RDA for selenium is the same for adult men and women at 55 micrograms daily. However during pregnancy and lactation the RDA increases to 60 and 70 micrograms daily.

Table 10.13 Selenium Content of Select Foods

Food	Selenium (μg)	Food	Selenium (μg)
Snapper, baked (3 ounces)	148	Sunflower seeds (¼ cup)	25
Halibut, baked (3 ounces)	113	Granola (1 cup)	23
Salmon, baked (3 ounces)	70	Ground beef (3 ounces)	22
Scallops, steamed (3 ounces)	70	Chicken, baked (3 ounces)	17
Clams, steamed (20)	52	Bread, whole wheat (1 slice)	16
Oysters, raw (¼ cup)	35	Egg (1)	12
Molasses, blackstrap (2 tablespoons)	25	Milk, 2% (1 cup)	6

What Does Selenium Do in the Body?

Selenium is absorbed well from our digestive tract. Therefore, absorption may not be the primary site of body selenium regulation. Selenium is a necessary component of a couple of enzymes with the following functions:

- *Antioxidant protection*—As part of the enzyme called *glutathione peroxidase*, selenium helps protect cells from free radical damage. Glutathione peroxidase inactivates free-radical substances such as hydrogen peroxide and organic peroxides. Glutathione peroxidase is a water-soluble molecule, its antioxidant activities will usually take place in the watery portion of the cells rather than in and around cell membranes like vitamin E. However, the peroxides that glutathione peroxidase inactivate typically travel to and assault cell membranes. In fact, selenium and vitamin E have co-protective function against oxidative damage to cells.
- *Thyroid hormone activity*—Selenium also appears to be incorporated into an enzyme (deiodinase) that is involved in iodide metabolism. This function of selenium is still unclear and scientists are currently engaged in trying to understand its function better. It appears that this selenium-containing enzyme helps convert the less potent form of thyroid hormone, thyroxine (T_4), to the more active form, triiodothyronine (T_3), in certain organs.

What Happens If We Get Too Little Selenium?

Mild selenium deficiency can reduce antioxidant capabilities as well as compromise efficient thyroid hormone action. Meanwhile, extreme selenium deficiency has been determined to be the cause of Keshan disease. The major medical problem associated with Keshan disease is an enlargement and abnormal functioning of the heart and eventual heart failure. The disease was observed in discrete regions of Asia where the selenium content of the soil is extremely low. The people within this region relied exclusively on crops and livestock grown in that area for food yet both of these food sources had very low selenium contents. Keshan disease is preventable with selenium supplementation.

Can We Get Too Much Selenium?

Selenium intakes greater than 750 micrograms/day over time can produce toxic alterations such as hair and nail loss, fatigue, nausea and vomiting, and a hindrance of proper protein manufacturing. Selenium toxicity is rare and seems likely only with excessive supplementation.

Manganese (Mn)

What Is Manganese?

Similar to zinc, manganese is also involved in the proper functioning of numerous enzymes. However, manganese still struggles for recognition.

What Foods Provide Manganese?

Whole-grain cereals, fruits and vegetables, legumes, nuts, tea, and leafy vegetables are good food sources of manganese. Animal foods are generally poor contributors of manganese. Additional substances in plants, such as fiber, phytate, and oxalate along with excessive calcium, phosphorus, and iron, can decrease manganese absorption.

What Are Current Recommendations for Manganese Intake?

The AI for manganese is 1.8 and 2.3 milligrams for adult women and men daily. However during pregnancy and lactation the AI increases to 2.0 and 2.6 milligrams daily.

What Does Manganese Do in the Body?

Manganese is involved with several general functions in the cells. First, manganese can interact with specific enzymes to increase their activity. These manganese-activated enzymes are involved in many operations, including protein digestion and the making of glucose from certain amino acids and lactate (gluconeogenesis). Second, manganese is a component of many enzymes. These enzymes are engaged in many activities including urea formation, glucose formation, and antioxidation. Lastly, manganese may be involved in the activity of some hormones.

What Happens If Too Little Manganese Is Consumed?

Manganese deficiency in humans is rare. However, nausea, vomiting, dermatitis, decreased growth of hair and nails, and changes in hair color can result from a deficiency. Manganese toxicity is also rare, although miners inhaling manganese-rich dust can experience Parkinson's-like symptoms.

Iodide (I)

What Is Iodide?

Many people can recall iodine being applied to cuts and scrapes as children. Iodide is like chloride in that it is most comfortable in nature after it has acquired an extra electron and becomes negatively charged (I^-).

What Foods Contain Iodide?

The iodide content of foods is mostly related to the soil content in which plants were grown and/or the iodide content of any fertilizers used to cultivate the soil. Furthermore, the iodide content in drinking water usually reflects the iodide content of the rocks and soils through which the water runs or is maintained. Seafood is typically a better source of iodide than freshwater fish (Table 10.14). Dairy foods may be a fair source of iodide, but the iodide content of cows' milk reflects either the iodide content of the cows' feed and/or the soil content of their grazing region. Iodide deficiency for the most part has been eradicated from many regions of the world including the United States, where iodide is added to salt. Check your salt label for "iodized salt."

What Are Current Recommendations for Iodide Intake?

The RDA for iodide is the same for adult men and women at 150 micrograms daily. However during pregnancy and lactation the RDA increases to 220 and 290 micrograms daily.

Table 10.14 Iodide Content of Select Foods

Food	Iodide (μg)	Food	Iodide (μg)
Salt, iodized (1 tablespoon)	400	Egg (1) Cheddar cheese (1 ounce)	18–26 5–23
Haddock (3 ounces)	104–145	Ground beef (3 ounces)	8
Cottage cheese (½ cup)	26–71		
Shrimp (3 ounces)	21–37		

What Does Iodide Do in the Body?

Iodide is one of the largest atoms found in the body, yet it appears to have only one critical function. Iodide is a key component of thyroid hormone, which is made in the thyroid gland located in the neck. Thyroid hormone is constructed from iodide and the amino acid tyrosine and has two forms thyroxine (T_4) and triiodothyronine (T_3) based on the number of iodide atoms (3 or 4). Thyroid hormone affects most cells in the body, perhaps with the exception of the adult brain, testes, spleen, uterus, and the thyroid gland itself. Thyroid hormone promotes the activities associated with glucose breakdown and general energy metabolism and heat production. Today, thyroid hormone is prescribed mostly to treat hypothyroidism, a condition in which the thyroid gland fails to produce adequate thyroid hormone. During the growing years thyroid hormone is very important because it promotes growth and maturation of the skeleton, the central nervous system, and the reproductive organs.

> Iodide is best known as a component of thyroid hormone which is principally involved in energy metabolism.

What Happens in Iodide Deficiency?

A deficiency of iodide limits the ability of the thyroid gland to make adequate thyroid hormone. During childhood, an iodide deficiency can result in poor growth, poor maturing of organs, and mental deficits. A striking characteristic of iodide deficiency is an enlargement of the thyroid gland which is commonly referred to as *goiter*. Treatment of goiter usually begins with iodide-rich foods including iodized salt, which will shrink the goiter with time but not necessarily correct any developmental problems (growth and mental aptitude) in children. Certain foods contain substances called *goitrogens* that appear to block iodide entry into the thyroid gland. Foods containing goitrogens include broccoli, kale, cauliflower, rutabaga, turnips, Brussels sprouts, and mustard greens. However, we probably do not eat enough of these vegetables to pose a threat. Routine blood tests include T_3 and T_4 concentrations thus providing a screening tool for thyroid deficiency or other thyroid hormone-impacting diseases.

Fluorine (F)

What Is Fluoride?

In nature, the element fluorine exists as a negatively charged atom or ion. Thus, similar to iodide (iodine) and chloride (chlorine), we commonly refer to fluorine as *fluoride* (F⁻). Fluoride salt (NaF) is routinely added to toothpaste.

What Are Fluoride Sources in the Human Diet?

Most foods are poor sources of fluoride and probably should not be used exclusively to meet the human body's needs. However, the process of adding fluoride to drinking water (*fluoridation*) has greatly improved general fluoride consumption. However, the decision to use fluoride is not federal; it is regulated county by county in the United States.

What Are Current Recommendations for Fluoride Intake?

The RDA for fluoride is 3 and 4 milligrams for adult women and men. During pregnancy and lactation the RDA is maintained at 3 milligrams daily.

What Does Fluoride Do in the Body?

Earlier in this century it was recognized that people living in regions of the United States where the fluoride content in their water supply was relatively high had a much lower incidence of dental caries. From this it was realized that fluoride is important to protect the teeth against the development of cavities. Fluoride may function in part by associating with hydroxyapatite in teeth and, to a lesser degree, bone.

What Happens If Too Little Fluoride Is Consumed?

The most obvious concern with getting too little fluoride in the diet is an increased likelihood of dental caries. This has led to the widespread fluoridation of drinking water and in doing so the incidence of dental caries in those regions tends to decrease.

What Happens If Too Much Fluoride Is Consumed?

Fluoride seems to be very efficiently absorbed from the digestive tract regardless of the amount consumed. Even though excessive fluoride in the body is removed in the urine, humans can overwhelm this function by ingesting larger quantities of supplemental fluoride. Fluoride toxicity is called *fluorosis* and problems such as alterations in bones, teeth, and possibly excitable cells may result. Mottling of teeth is evidence of dental fluorosis in children. Taking gram doses of fluoride, 5 to 10 grams of sodium fluoride, can lead to subsequent nausea, vomiting, and a decrease in body pH (acidosis). Furthermore, irregular heart activity and death may also result.

Chromium (Cr)

Chromium has received a considerable amount of attention in recent years as supplemental chromium is purported to increase lean body mass and reduce body fat. Furthermore, chromium supplementation has been suggested as a possible benefit for people diagnosed with diabetes mellitus.

What Are Food and Supplement Sources of Chromium?

Egg yolks, whole grains, and meats are good sources of chromium (Table 10.15). Dairy products are not a particularly good source of chromium. Plants grown in chromium-rich soils may also make a significant contribution to the human diet. Many multivitamin/mineral supplements include chromium typically in the form of chromium picolinate or nicotinate.

What Are Current Recommendations for Chromium Intake?

The AI for chromium is 35 and 30 micrograms for adult men under 50 and over 50 respectively. For women under 50 the AI is 25 micrograms which is then reduced to 20 micrograms after the age of 50. During pregnancy and lactation the AI for adult women is increased to 30 and 45 micrograms.

What Does Chromium Do in the Body?

Chromium is a key component of a molecule or complex of molecules called *glucose tolerance factor* (GTF). As such, chromium is involved

Table 10.15 Chromium Content of Select Foods

Food	Chromium (μg)	Food	Chromium (μg)
Meats		*Fruits and vegetables*	
Turkey ham (3 ounces)	10.4	Broccoli (½ cup)	11.0
Ham (3 ounces)	3.6	Grape juice (½ cup)	7.5
Beef cubes (3 ounces)	2.0	Potatoes mashed (1 cup)	2.7
Chicken (3 ounces)	0.5	Orange juice (1 cup)	2.2
Grain products		Lettuce, shredded (1 cup)	1.8
Waffle (1)	6.7	Apple, unpeeled (1 cup)	1.4
English muffin (1)	3.6		
Bagel, egg (1)	2.5		
Rice, white (1 cup)	1.2		
Bread, whole wheat (1 slice)	1.0		

in the regulation of blood glucose levels as it appears to be necessary to maximize the efficiency of insulin to maintain normal levels of glucose in the blood. Although it is questionable whether chromium may have application to diabetes mellitus in people with good chromium status, poor chromium status may worsen type 2 diabetes mellitus. Therefore, those people diagnosed with type 2 diabetes mellitus should make sure that their diet provides adequate chromium either through foods or a supplement containing chromium.

What Happens During Chromium Deficiency and Toxicity?

Chromium deficiency can result in *glucose intolerance*, which is an inability to reduce blood glucose levels properly after a meal and throughout the day. Conversely, little is known about the toxic effects of chromium in larger doses. Some scientists have reported that supplements of as much as 800 micrograms daily are safe, while others question as to whether excessive chromium consumed chronically would build up in body tissues such as bone, and have milder long-term effects.

> Chromium is important for the efficient processing of glucose in the blood.

Vanadium (V)

What Is Vanadium?

Vanadium is present in trace concentrations in most organs and tissues throughout the body and has long been questioned in regard to essentiality. However, it is important to realize that the presence of a substance in the body does not necessarily indicate essentiality. Nevertheless, researchers have discerned that the absence of vanadium from animal diets reduces their growth rate, infancy survival, and levels of hematocrit, despite the inability of researchers to identify specific functions for vanadium.

What Foods Provide Vanadium?

Although still only containing nanograms to micrograms of vanadium, breakfast cereals, canned fruit juices, fish sticks, shellfish, vegetables (especially mushrooms, parsley, and spinach), sweets, wine, and beer are good sources. A dietary requirement for vanadium has yet to be established, but 10 to 25 micrograms of vanadium per day may be appropriate.

What Does Vanadium Do in the Body?

Vanadium appears to be able to affect glucose metabolism in a manner similar to insulin. Promising research with diabetic animals has suggested that vanadium therapy may control high blood glucose levels (hyperglycemia). However, the application to hyperglycemia in humans is still questionable and supplementation cannot be recommended at this time.

What Do We Know About Vanadium Deficiency and Toxicity?

As mentioned, vanadium deficiency may result in reductions in growth rate, infancy survival, and hematocrit. Further, vanadium deficiency may alter the activity of the thyroid gland and its ability to utilize iodide properly. Signs of vanadium toxicity such as a green tongue, diarrhea, abdominal cramping, and alterations in mental functions have been reported in people ingesting greater than 10 milligrams of vanadium daily for extended periods of time.

Boron (B)

What Foods Provide Boron?

Fruits, leafy vegetables, nuts, and legumes are rich sources of boron, while meats are among the poorer sources. Beer and wine also make a respectable contribution to boron intake. Although not established to date, human requirement for boron is probably about 1 milligram daily.

What Does Boron Do in the Body?

In the human body boron is found in relatively greater concentration in bone. Although its exact involvement remains a mystery at this time, boron seems to affect certain factors that impact calcium metabolism. This is an area that has been receiving more and more attention as scientists attempt to better understand bone diseases.

What Happens During Boron Deficiency and Toxicity?

Boron deficiency results in an increased urinary loss of calcium and magnesium, assumedly derived from storage primarily in bone. Conversely, taking large amounts of boron may induce nausea, vomiting, lethargy, and an increased loss of riboflavin.

Molybdenum (Mo)

What Foods Provide Molybdenum in the Human Diet?

Most of the foods humans eat contain a respectable amount of molybdenum, which ultimately reflects the soil content in which the plants were grown. Organ and other meats, legumes, cereals, and grains are among better sources of molybdenum. Diets high in molybdenum decrease copper absorption and also increase copper loss in the urine. The RDA for adults is 45 micrograms of molybdenum daily.

What Does Molybdenum Do in the Body?

Molybdenum seems to be active in the cells as part of a molecule that interacts with a few specific enzymes and makes them active. These enzymes are involved in the metabolism of the sulfur-containing amino acids (methionine and cysteine) and the metabolism of pyrimidine and purines which are building blocks for nucleic acids (that is, DNA and RNA).

What Happens If Too Much or Too Little Molybdenum Is Consumed?

Because of molybdenum's widespread availability in the human diet, a deficiency is somewhat unlikely. However, people receiving intravenous (IV) feedings for several months are at risk. In contrast, molybdenum is fairly nontoxic. Molybdenum is involved in the breakdown of purines to a waste product called uric acid. Uric acid is removed from the body in urine, and theoretically there is a greater risk for developing kidney stones formed by excessive uric acid. Excessive uric acid production may also increase the risk of developing *gout*, which is characterized by recurrent inflammation of joint regions and deposition of uric acid in those areas.

Nickel (Ni)

What Foods Contribute Nickel to the Diet?

In general, plants are more concentrated sources of nickel than are animal sources. Nuts are the most concentrated sources while grains, cured meats, and vegetables offer respectable amounts. Fish, milk, and eggs are recognized as poorer sources of nickel. The absorption of nickel from the digestive tract is probably affected by varying the amounts of copper, iron, and zinc, and perhaps vice versa. Adult requirements for nickel are most likely about 35 micrograms daily although the RDA has yet to be established.

What Does Nickel Do in the Body?

The possible essentiality of nickel was not seriously considered until about 20 years ago. Defining exact roles for nickel in the body remains somewhat elusive. However, nickel does seem to be involved in the breakdown of the amino acids leucine, valine, and isoleucine (branch-chain amino acids) and odd chain length fatty acids. Nickel research is relatively young and more clear-cut roles for nickel will probably emerge in the next decade.

Arsenic (Ar)

What Foods Are a Source of Arsenic?

As a natural constituent of the earth's crust, arsenic can be found in most soils and is taken up by plants grown in that area. However, the arsenic content of foods can also be affected by the arsenic in pesticides and airborne pollutants. Among the most concentrated sources of arsenic are sea animals (fish, shellfish). Dietary requirements for arsenic have not been established, although 12 to 15 micrograms daily is probably sufficient.

What Does Arsenic Do in the Body?

Although arsenic has long been regarded as an unwanted substance, it may be an essential component after all. Although its involvement has not been clearly identified, arsenic is most likely important in the metabolism of two amino acids, methionine and arginine.

What Happens in Arsenic Deficiency and Toxicity?

Arsenic deficiencies have resulted in a reduced growth rate in animals. Arsenic deficiency may also reduce conception rates and increase the likelihood of death in newborns. Perhaps no other constituent of the body conjures a stronger notion of toxicity than arsenic. It certainly is the only nutrient that can be fatal in milligram amounts. Arsenic, in the form of arsenic trioxide, can be fatal at doses greater than 0.76 to 1.95 milligrams.

Silicon (Si)

What Foods Provide Silicon?

Not much is really known about the silicon content of various foods. Plant sources, including high-fiber cereal grains and root vegetables, seem to be better sources than animal sources. The RDA for silicon has yet to be established.

What Does Silicon Do in the Body?

Silicon, in the form of quartz, is one of the most abundant minerals on the planet. However, silicon makes only a minuscule contribution to human body weight. Silicon seems to be involved in the health of connective tissue. In bone, silicon seems to improve the rates of both bone mineralization and growth. The manufacturing of collagen, a predominant protein found in connective tissue, relies upon an adequate supply of the nonessential amino acid proline and a slightly modified form of proline called hydroxyproline. Silicon is probably required for the optimal production of both proline and hydroxyproline. Silicon is also important for the manufacturing of other proteins and substances vital to proper connective tissue.

What Happens in Silicon Deficiency and Toxicity?

Silicon deficiency can result in poor growth and development of bone, including decreased mineralization. Not much is known at this time regarding silicon toxicity.

FAQ Highlight

Zinc and Vitamin C and the Common Cold

Can Zinc Supplements Cure the Common Cold?

Although zinc supplements cannot cure the common cold, some evidence suggests that timely zinc supplements may reduce the severity and duration of a cold. The results of some clinical studies, but not all, have suggested that when people with a cold were provided zinc supplements their symptoms were less severe and they recovered more quickly than people not receiving the supplements. Most of the zinc tested was in the form of zinc gluconate lozenges; currently nasal sprays are also available.

Zinc might bind to the virus that causes the cold and decrease its ability to infiltrate cells. Because a virus is not a living thing in order for it to make new copies of itself, it must break into a living cell and use that cell's protein-making machinery to manufacture multiple copies of itself. This large-scale production of the virus allows it to spread. When the immune system catches up and the rate of destruction of the virus exceeds production, the virus is eliminated. This can take a week or so and the symptoms can be significant, as we all know.

It should be recognized that zinc supplements will not necessarily keep people from "catching a cold," and they should not be used preventively. Furthermore, not everyone will respond to zinc supplements so talking to a physician is recommended. Furthermore, zinc supplements exceeding the RDA are not suggested as this can lead to a reduction in copper absorption.

11 Exercise and Sports Nutrition

To move around is a fundamental part of human existence. Humans move to gather and prepare food, protect themselves, and to reproduce. This type of functional movement is called physical activity. Meanwhile, exercise is a planned act of moving at specific speeds and for a given duration and/or against a resistance. In this chapter we will answer questions about exercise and how to plan an exercise program to achieve a desired outcome such as muscle development, better performance, and body sculpting.

Exercise Basics

Why Do or Should We Exercise?

To the public, the terms *exercise* and *workout* are synonymous. Regular exercise can provide numerous benefits. Depending upon the type of exercise, these benefits can include:

- improved cardiovascular health,
- a tool for weight management,
- improved body composition,
- a positive impact on bone density,
- a vehicle for relaxation and social interaction, and
- improved self-image.

What Is Exercise Training?

When we exercise regularly the muscles that are involved can adapt to be more efficient in performing the exercise task. This is a "training effect" or "adaptation" that is visually obvious for weight trainers as the targeted muscles enlarge to provide more strength and power. Their exercises will involve near maximal or maximal intensity for very short durations. Meanwhile, during regular exercise, consisting of lower intensity tasks performed for longer durations, muscle will adapt to become more inclined to aerobic energy metabolism, as will be explained shortly.

What Are the Most Important Concepts in Exercise Training?

The most important aspects of training are the *intensity* and *duration* of the exercise. The relationship between these factors is what determines the nature of the associated adaptation. Aspects of genetic predisposition also will influence the degree of adaptation as well as the inclination toward a certain type of training. More on the genetics of training and achievement in sports soon enough.

What Does Exercise Intensity Mean?

Exercise *intensity* refers to the level of exertion. For instance, lifting a weight that results in muscular fatigue after just a few repetitions or "reps" of an exercise is pretty high with respect to intensity. So too would be an all-out running or cycling sprint where fatigue occurs in a minute or so. Basically, the higher the intensity, the shorter the possible duration of the exercise. To reach such a high level of intensity, exercise often includes resistance against an otherwise simple movement of a muscle group or related groups. Examples of resistance training include weight training or running on an incline (for example, running on hills or a graded treadmill) or cycling (for example, cycling uphill or an exercise bike with variable resistance). It is the level of the resistance that dictates the level of intensity. Higher intensity and muscular fatigue will be associated with muscle adaptations that will allow for greater strength and power. In this case, muscles can enlarge or "hypertrophy."

What Is the Difference Between Work, Strength, and Power?

Work relates the amount of force necessary to move something (for example, a weight) a certain distance—hence the term "workout." Strength then refers to the amount of force that can produced by someone to perform work. Further still, power is concerned with how long it takes to perform the work. The faster the work can be performed the more powerful the effort. Mathematically:

Work = Force × Distance

and

Power = Work × Time

What Does Exercise Duration Mean?

Duration refers to how long an exercise is performed continuously. Activities like running and cycling are performed at a lower or moderate intensity and tend to last for a half to one hour or longer. Sustained exercise for longer durations is often called *endurance* training. It is also referred to as *cardiovascular* training as adaptations can include the development of a more powerful heart and more blood vessels in our heart and skeletal muscle.

> Intensity and duration are the most important factors in determining if an exercise is resistance or endurance or both.

How Does Exercise Change Our Body?

It is the intensity level of an exercise that will be the primary determinant of the range of adaptation. This means that although some sports are associated with a certain type of adaptation, it is not an absolute. For instance, weight training can be more aerobic and cardiovascular if the weights (resistance) are not heavy enough and the number of reps is very high. Running and biking are often associated with more aerobic and cardiovascular adaptations but it is easy for runners or cyclists to train for greater strength and power by including more resistance in their training.

Muscle Is Fueled Primarily by Carbohydrates and Fat

What Fuels Muscle Activity?

Muscle contraction is fueled by ATP, which is generated by both anaerobic and aerobic energy metabolism. Because ATP is found in low concentrations in all cells of the body, these ATP-generating mechanisms must be increased with the onset of activity in an attempt to meet ATP demands of working muscle cells. This means that muscle cells need to stoke up those chemical reaction pathways that break down carbohydrate and fat for ATP generation (see Figure 2.8). Muscle cells have a little stored carbohydrate (glycogen) and fat and also receive glucose and fatty acids from the blood. So increased blood delivery to the exercising muscle delivers not only needed oxygen but also fuel.

What Is Creatine?

Another power source for working muscle is creatine phosphate. Creatine is a substance found mostly in skeletal muscle cells, but it is also found in heart muscle cells and brain. When ATP is abundant in these cells, such as

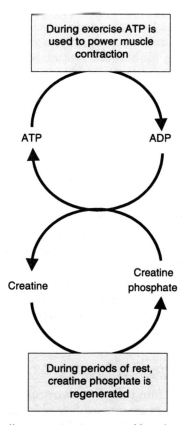

Figure 11.1 Muscle cell contraction is powered by adenosine triphosphate (ATP). The energy released by ATP allows myosin to pull actin filaments towards the center of the sarcomere. The net effect of all the sarcomere contraction results in the shortening of the whole muscle cell. Carbohydrate and fat are mostly used to regenerate ATP as it is being used.

when muscle is not active (at rest), phosphate is transferred to creatine. This forms creatine phosphate, which is a rapid ATP-regenerating source (Figure 11.1). When ATP is used to power muscle contractions, the phosphate of creatine phosphate can be transferred to ADP to regenerate ATP. This involves only one chemical reaction and can happen very rapidly.

How Does Creatine Power Skeletal Muscle Efforts During Exercise?

The regeneration of ATP from creatine phosphate is especially important for quick-burst activities such as sprinting and weight training. However, this system is extremely limited and will last only a few seconds. Yet this operation helps muscle cells bridge the gap between the rapid deple-tion of ATP at the onset of exercise and the point when a muscle cell's other ATP-generating operations are appropriately stoked up. Then when the muscle cell is resting (in-between sets or between sprints) creatine phosphate is regenerated to prepare for the next exercise effort. Later in this chapter supplementation practices involving creatine will be discussed.

Muscle Cells Are Not All the Same

Are There Different Types of Muscle Fibers?

Researchers refer to skeletal muscle cells as fibers because they are thin and long. In fact, some muscle fibers can extend the entire length of a muscle, such as in the biceps. That is several inches! In addition to their unique design, skeletal muscle cells are not all the same. In fact, humans are blessed with more than one type of skeletal muscle cell, which vary in performance and metabolic properties (Table 11.1). This allows our body to efficiently perform a broad range of activities or sports that vary in nature. This includes sports that are longer duration/lower intensity and short duration/higher intensity.

What Are the Different Classes of Muscle Cells?

Muscle cells are grouped into two general categories or "types" (Type I and II). Type II muscle fibers are often subclassified as IIa, IIb, and IIc. For this book, it is enough to only distinguish between the two main types. Skeletal muscle is actually bundles of a mixture of Type I and II muscle fibers. In fact, the average person will tend to have about a 50/50 mixture of Types I and II muscle fibers. Meanwhile, highly successful athletes tend to have a significant imbalance one way or the other which, as will soon be discussed, will allow them to excel at a particular sport.

Table 11.1 Performance and Metabolic Properties of Muscle Fibers

Type I Muscle Fibers	Type II Muscle Fibers
Develop force more slowly than Type II muscle fibers	Develop force more quickly (more powerful)
Have more mitochondria and capillaries and thus are more aerobic	Have fewer mitochondria and capillaries and thus are more anaerobic
Generate very little lactic acid (lactate)	Generate more lactate
Do not fatigue quickly	Fatigue quickly

Type I muscle fibers are more aerobic and can perform longer than Type II muscle fibers.

What Are Type I Muscle Cells?

Type I fibers (sometimes called slow-twitch or slow-oxidative fibers) are better designed for prolonged exercise performed at a lower intensity. In comparison to Type II fibers, Type I fibers will have more mitochondria and rely more heavily on the aerobic generation of ATP. The primary energy molecules used to generate ATP in these muscle cells will be fatty acids and glucose. Since ATP production in mitochondria requires oxygen, proper function of these muscle fibers is very dependent upon oxygen supply via the blood. Luckily, Type I muscle cells always seem to have many capillaries around them to deliver oxygen-endowed blood. In addition, Type I fibers contain a substance called myoglobin. As mentioned in Chapter 10, myoglobin is an iron-containing protein that binds oxygen and serves as an oxygen reserve for these cells during exercise.

What Are Type II Muscle Cells?

Type II muscle fibers (sometimes called fast-twitch or fast-glycolytic fibers) can execute a much faster speed of contraction than Type I muscle fibers. This is to say that Type II muscle fibers are designed to generate force more rapidly, thereby allowing them to be more powerful. This will allow a job to be performed in a shorter amount of time. Meanwhile, Type II muscle fibers are relatively limited in their ability to generate ATP by aerobic means. So, when these cells break down glucose to pyruvate and generate a couple ATP in the process, much of the pyruvate that is formed will then be converted to lactic acid (lactate). This is because these muscle cells have less mitochondria and receive less oxygen as they are served by fewer blood vessels (see Table 11.1 and Figure 8.3).

How Does the Brain Know Which Type of Muscle Cells to Use for Different Sports?

This is a no-brainer for the brain! This is because the brain will always call upon Type I muscle fibers first and then Type II. The major factor will be the required force to perform the exercise. For instance, when an exercise requires less force (for example, jogging, fast walking, casual cycling) the brain will for the most part call upon Type I muscle fibers (Figure 11.2). However, as the necessary force to perform an exercise increases (such as running, cycling fast, weightlifting), the brain will also

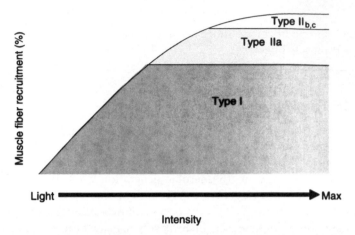

Figure 11.2 The order of recruitment of muscle fibers begins with our Type I fibers for lower intensity exercise (such as walking, casual cycling). As more force is needed, Type II fibers are also called upon (for example, in weight training, sprinting).

call upon Type II muscle fibers to generate force to support the force generated by Type I fibers.

How Does Recruiting Different Muscle Fibers Relate to Performance?

Calling upon Type II fibers is sort of a win/lose situation for performance. It is a winner in that it will allow us to generate a lot more force to perform an exercise. However, it is a loser in that the exercise will become fatiguing as more lactic acid is generated in Type II fibers. This is why 5K runners cannot sprint the entire race. What they will do instead is run at the highest level they are able to, but that also keeps them from fatiguing before the end of the race. Their brains will call upon enough Type II muscle fibers to generate the force that allows them to run faster but not, however, enough Type II muscle fibers to generate critical levels of lactic acid and other factors that would result in fatigue before they cross the finish line.

Do Successful Athletes Have an Imbalance of Muscle Fiber Type?

Successful athletes seem to have an imbalance in muscle fiber types that favors excelling in a sport. For instance, successful sprinters often have a higher percentage of Type II fibers, allowing them to generate more force in a very brief period of time. This then allows them to be more powerful, generate more speed, and complete a sprint distance more quickly. Conversely, successful endurance athletes tend to have a greater percentage of Type I muscle fibers. This allows them to generate more force through aerobic energy systems in muscle cells. They can perform at a higher intensity before they generate critical amounts of lactic acid.

> People who excel at certain sports tend to have a genetic predisposition based on predominance of muscle fiber type.

Are Athletes Born or Developed?

Often the question is asked whether top athletes are born or bred. The answer is both, but probably more of the former than the latter. Most very successful athletes are born (genetics) with the propensity to excel physically at a particular sport. Training can then improve that potential. This is mostly true for sports that are endurance based or involve extreme power, as mentioned. An athlete's genes direct the formation of more Type I or Type muscle cells and body design and potential for skill development to excel at one or more sports. Then, to truly excel at a sport, the athlete must train and practice to optimize that performance.

Can Training Allow Muscle Fibers to Change Type?

We do know that training results in changes in muscle metabolism, which may make us think that it is possible for Type I fibers to change into Type II fibers and vice versa. However, this probably is not the case. For instance, endurance training can lead to changes associated with Type II muscle fibers that will make them more aerobic. The fibers will adapt to have an increased ability to generate ATP by using oxygen. However, they don't adapt to the point where we would classify them as Type I. Oppositely, we all know that resistance training (for example, weight lifting) improves the strength and power of a muscle group. Although it would be logical to think that half of this effect might be related to adaptations in Type I muscle fibers—as though they are being transformed into Type II muscle fibers—surprisingly this is not the case either. In fact, as the muscle group grows in size, most of the growth is related to enlargement (hypertrophy) of Type II fibers.

Resistance Training Is Hard Work

What Are the Benefits of Resistance Exercise?

Although weight lifting has long been associated with bodybuilding and power sports such as football and field events (shot put, discus, etc.), it is more popular with the general population than ever before. Clearly, resistance training can favorably influence bone density and increase the amount of muscle attached to the skeleton. Thus resistance training can reduce the risk of bone-related disorders such as osteoporosis and improve energy expenditure, reduce body fat content, and improve self-image.

What Are Options for Resistance Exercise?

Today there are numerous options for resistance training beyond free weights and weight machines. Many people use pulley machines and resilient resistance materials such as bows (for example, Bowflex®) and elastic bands (such as Soloflex®). Of course, in a pinch, gravity alone may provide enough resistance for a positive impact. For instance, people accustomed to a regular workout will often do a few sets of push-ups on the floor if no gym equipment is available.

How Does Weight Lifting Increase Muscle Mass?

The goal of most weight lifters is to increase the size of the muscles that are targeted. Muscle mass development through weight training hinges on the "overload" principle. The use of weights places a greater than normal stress (load) upon the challenged muscle fibers. The overload stimulates the muscle to grow primarily by increasing the size (hypertrophy) of the overloaded muscle fibers. This means that the muscle cells get thicker as well as get stronger. Therefore, as a biceps muscle enlarges from doing dumbbell curls it is really a reflection of an increase in size of the overloaded muscle fibers within that muscle. Although growth may occur in both Type I and Type II fibers, as mentioned, it is believed to be more significant in the challenged Type II fibers. Table 11.2 provides more detail to how the muscle cells get bigger.

> Weight lifting and other resistance exercise overloads muscle causing it to adapt to get stronger and thus bigger.

Table 11.2 Processes Associated With Adaptation After Resistance Training

- Building of more protein for myofibrils
- An increase in number of mitochondria
- An increase in enzymes specific to the task
- Making more connective tissue for sheathing around muscle fibers and bundles
- A slight increase in glycogen stores

How Do You Know How Much Resistance to Use to Promote Muscle Development?

To overload a muscle, three sets of six to ten repetitions is probably adequate to stimulate growth. More sets will certainly provide a greater rate of hypertrophy, within reason. To begin, you need to estimate your "one-repetition maximum" (1-RM). This will be the maximum weight you can overcome to complete one repetition. Certainly it is not recommended that you try to determine your 1-RM by experimenting with heavy weights if you are just getting started. You can experiment with light weights and determine the best weight for an exercise (for example, shoulder press, bench press, curls) with which you are able to do about five to ten repetitions. This should be about 80 to 85 percent of your 1-RM. Your goal for muscle development is to do three to four sets of 8 to 12 repetitions before experiencing muscle fatigue.

Should You Increase Resistance over Time?

As you continue to train that muscle, over time you will find it necessary to increase the level of resistance to continue to make progress. This is evident as the number of repetitions you can do before fatiguing exceeds the recommended range for muscle development and is an indicator that your muscle is adapting and getting stronger. Initially, some of this adaptation is merely your muscle becoming more efficient in the exercise. However, overall most of the improvement in performance will be because the muscle is developing more contraction machinery and as a result getting bigger. Try increasing the amount of resistance by 10 percent and determine if that puts you back in the muscle development repetition range.

How Much Rest Do You Need In-Between Sets Within the Same Workouts?

When you engage in resistance training you are making great demands on your muscles. Therefore, the worked muscle should be given adequate time to rest and recover after a set of repetitions. Depending on the intensity of the set, muscle will need about 1 to 3 minutes to rest between sets to recover. During a set the limited stores of ATP and creatine phosphate are rapidly depleted. Giving muscle a break between sets allows for regeneration of ATP and creatine phosphate. The period of rest between sets also allows for the blood to bring more nutrients and oxygen and remove waste and at the same time also. As muscle contracts it temporarily pinches blood vessels and hinders blood flow within that muscle. This not only decreases nutrient and oxygen delivery to working muscle fibers but also decreases the removal of waste such as lactate and carbon dioxide.

How Much Rest Do You Need Between Workouts?

If a muscle is trained hard it is generally recommended to rest a muscle for at least 48 hours before working the same muscle again. This allows muscle to recover and adapt. Often people will train the same muscles on Mondays, Wednesdays, and Fridays or Tuesdays, Thursdays, and Saturdays and rest the muscle in-between. If a muscle is trained very hard in a given workout by doing extra sets, that individual may train that muscle only two times a week or every 5 days or even once a week.

Rest is necessary between resistance exercise to allow muscle to repair, recover, and adapt.

What Does It Take for Muscle to Recover and Repair After a Workout?

Recovery and repair processes include those that prepare muscle to perform efficiently again. This includes: reducing the lactate level of the muscle fibers worked, which may not take that long; repleting glycogen stores, which can take hours; and repairing cellular damage in the trained muscle fibers, which can also take hours or even a day or so. Adaptation, on the other hand, refers to those processes designed to allow muscle to be better prepared to work again. This will include a net production of muscle proteins that will support contraction the next time around. As muscle cells accumulate more protein, they will also accumulate more water. Therefore, much of muscle hypertrophy is protein and water. In addition, connective tissue providing integrity and support to the overloaded muscle will be enhanced as well.

Does Our Energy Expenditure Increase Due to Weight Training?

The increased energy demand of weight training depends on the intensity level and duration of a workout coupled with the energy needed for recovery and adaptation. The energy needed for a workout may be along the order of 5 to 10 calories per minute while recovery and adaptation may demand 100 to 300 calories over the next day. This additional energy expended should be calculated into your total energy expenditure (see Chapter 8).

The predominant fuel powering weight training is carbohydrate, derived mostly from muscle glycogen stores and secondarily fat from fat tissue and within muscle tissue itself. One of the strongest influences will be epinephrine, which is released from the adrenal glands during intense training. Epinephrine will promote the breakdown of glycogen and fat stores, making those energy sources available to working muscle. On the other hand, both fat and carbohydrate fuel adaptive processes over the next few hours up to the next day or so. The most important factors dictating fuel preference will be meals and corresponding fluctuations in insulin and glucagon levels.

How Much Energy Should Be Eaten to Make the Body More Lean and Muscular?

To become more muscular and lean, people combine weight training with dietary control. In addition, integrating aerobic training will certainly be beneficial. It's not important not to drastically restrict energy intake, if at all. Drastic energy restriction can place an extra demand upon skeletal muscle to provide amino acids for energy, thus counteracting resistance training to some degree. Thus drastic energy restriction and weight training may create a futile cycle as muscle breakdown contradicts muscle hypertrophy.

If you are at a fairly comfortable body size but you want to increase your muscularity and leanness, you will be best served by eating enough energy to meet your expenditure. That would include the energy expended due to exercise training while also choosing foods higher in healthier carbohydrates and protein versus fat. The major thrust of your efforts should focus on the change in body composition, not necessarily body weight. In fact, as you add skeletal muscle, it is possible that you will gain weight.

For heavier people with a higher percentage of body fat who wish to become leaner, they can begin by estimating their daily calorie needs (see Chapter 8) and then restrict energy intake by 10 to 20 percent. This is easily done by substituting foods with a greater percentage of energy from carbohydrate and protein versus fat. Furthermore, engaging in regular aerobic activities will be of benefit, as discussed shortly.

How Much Protein Is Needed During Weight Training?

Protein is the major nonwater component of skeletal muscle accounting for more than 20 percent of its total weight and more than 80 percent of water-free weight. Logically, if you want to build more muscle, you need to eat more protein beyond the needs for normal maintenance. People who engage in serious weight-training athletes may benefit most from a protein intake of 1.4 to 1.75 grams per kilogram of their body weight or more. This translates to about 1.75 to 2.25 times the RDA for protein. Several research studies using protein intakes above this level have failed to show additional benefit (more muscle gain). Furthermore, the intensity and extent to which individuals train will dictate where they may fall within these ranges for protein recommendations.

Serious weight training can double daily protein requirements in order to repair and adapt muscle tissue.

Is the Timing of Protein Consumption Important to Developing Muscle Size and Strength?

The importance of protein to muscle development has been known for decades. However, recently "protein timing" has become of greater interest. Sophisticated research techniques have allowed for an understanding of the importance of consuming protein around a workout to maximize gains in muscle development. As discussed above, a resistance training sessions results in a simultaneous increase in protein synthesis and breakdown. Consuming protein either just before or immediately after a workout helps maximize muscle protein synthesis and along with carbohydrate to minimize muscle protein breakdown, which combined will lead to better results. Furthermore, protein is needed throughout the day to support on-going repair and adaptation, which can last as long as a day.

Are Certain Proteins Better Than Others for Building Muscle Size and Strength?

Protein from animals is rich in essential amino acids and in particular branched-chained amino acids. This includes red meat, poultry (meat and eggs), fish, and milk (dairy). Soy is also a good source of essential amino acids. Any or combinations of these protein sources consumed before or after a workout will support muscle development. On the other hand, supplement manufacturers target single-protein ingredients such as whey protein isolate or a blend of protein ingredients to create a more strategic muscle development food. Furthermore, protein fractions from milk namely, whey protein isolate, whey protein concentrate, and casein can be used strategically as whey is more rapidly digested and absorbed than casein. This has led to the idea of "fast" and "slow" protein, which is like a time-release system. Whey also seems to be a little more advantageous in supporting muscle development processes than soy, which is one reason why whey is the principal protein ingredient in many bars and shakes and soy is either absent or contributes less to the formulation.

Nutrition Supplements for Strength and Muscle Building

What Are the Most Prominent Supplements Touted to Increase Muscle Strength and Development?

Sport supplements have evolved into a multibillion dollar industry, yet their evolutionary process really has not been that long. Today there are numerous supplements available to people looking to improve their muscle mass or leanness. While many of them are well known, not all are known to really make a difference. Among the more efficacious supplements are protein (level and timing), creatine, HMB (β-hydroxy β-methylbutyrate), carnitine and β-alanine. In this next section we will discuss only the most prominent and promising of supplements on the market today.

Can Creatine Supplementation Enhance Muscle and Strength Development?

Creatine is naturally made by the human body and has become one of the most studied sport supplements. As discussed, in muscle and other tissue, ATP is used to transfer energy and a phosphate group to creatine, forming creatine phosphate. This substance then becomes a readily available means of regenerating ATP when it is in demand. For muscle, this would be during the early stage of an exercise. In the brain, it can help to maintain ATP levels during brief periods of poor oxygen supply. The brain relies on aerobic ATP production so periods of decreased oxygen availability are extremely critical. ATP can be regenerated from creatine phosphate in a single chemical reaction, which does not require oxygen.

> Creatine supplementation can enhance muscle strength and size, and positively affect body composition.

Creatine is made in the body using three amino acids (methionine, glycine, and arginine) and two organs (liver and kidneys). Creatine is also found in animal foods, primarily the muscle part of animals. Therefore, meat eaters tend to consume 1 to 2 grams of creatine in their diets. The practice of supplementing creatine became extremely popular in the 1990s as several scientific studies showed that muscle creatine levels could be increased with supplementation. This change was often associated with increases in total body mass, lean body mass, strength, and power. Creatine is mostly supplemented as creatine monohydrate, but other forms do exist such as polyethylene glycol, ethyl ester, fumarate, malate, etc. While these other forms are often marketed to be more effective than monohydrate, they remain unproved to be so in a head-to-head study. It can be purchased as a powder to dissolve in a drink, or as a concentrated liquid to be administered orally via a dropper.

A few years ago it was more popular for individuals to begin creatine supplementation by way of a "loading" phase. In this phase, roughly 20 to 25 grams of creatine may have been ingested for 5 to 7 days, followed by a longer "maintenance" phase involving about 3 to 5 grams daily. What scientists found was that when young men were provided 20 grams of creatine monohydrate daily for about a week they developed a 20 percent increase in muscle creatine levels. Furthermore, this increased muscle content of creatine could be maintained when the loading phase was followed by a maintenance dose of only 2 grams daily. Interestingly, researchers also found that you could get to the same level of muscle creatine after 4 weeks by starting off and maintaining a supplement dose of 3 to 5 grams daily, which offers a more economically and practical alternative. At this time creatine supplementation is believed to be generally safe when users follow the recommended levels.

Can Arginine and Lysine Increase Growth Hormone Levels?

Growth hormone is linked to muscle protein production. Interest in possible athletic benefits from supplementing with individual amino acids was raised after researchers realized that when certain amino acids, such as arginine, are infused directly into the bloodstream of hospital patients with burns, there was a corresponding rise in growth hormone levels in their blood. Some researchers have found that taking arginine and lysine supplements can increase growth hormone levels in healthy young men as well. However other research studies did not show this and some research has suggested that even if arginine does transiently increase growth hormone levels, the raise is not greater than what normally happen in response to resistance exercise. So from a practical standpoint arginine would need to be taken several hours before or after exercise. Because it takes several grams of these amino acids to produce a growth hormone response, some participants of the studies complained of intestinal discomfort. Researchers at this time are not really convinced that this happens or would happen in everyone.

Can Arginine Increase Nitric Oxide and Enhance Blood Delivery to Working Muscle?

Nitric oxide (NO) is a powerful vasodilator. It is produced by cells lining blood vessels and arginine is used by the enzyme nitric oxide synthase (NOS) to make NO. The idea is that arginine supplementation is able to increase NO production and increase blood delivery and thus amino acids and other nutrients to muscle cells during and after exercise. These nutrients could in turn strengthen the processes that build muscle in response to resistance exercise. In addition to the positive benefits of arginine in this manner, researchers have also indicated that citrulline might also be beneficial, as it can be used to make arginine. One reason is that a lot of the arginine that is consumed is metabolized by the intestinal bacteria and arginase in the small intestine wall and liver, and never makes it to the blood vessels of muscle. On the other hand, citrulline is not metabolized in such a manner. And, on a related note, polyphenolic compounds in grapes and extracts might serve to optimize NOS activity.

> Arginine is used to make nitric oxide, which can dilate blood vessels leading to muscle tissue.

Can Ornithine or OKG Enhance Muscle Mass?

Ornithine and its derivative ornithine-α-ketoglutarate (OKG) have received considerable interest from weight-training athletes more so than in the past. Ornithine is an amino acid not found in our proteins. However, it does exist independently in our body and is fundamentally involved in the formation of urea. Like arginine, supplemental ornithine was popularized after scientists reported that when ornithine was infused into blood there was a corresponding increase in growth hormone. Some researchers have also reported that oral supplementation of ornithine also increases circulating growth hormone in a respectable percentage of participants. However, the needed dose translates to as much as 170 milligrams of ornithine per kilogram body weight, which amounts to 14 grams of supplemental ornithine daily for a 180-pound male. Ornithine dosages of this size are usually associated with intestinal discomfort and diarrhea; again, it has not been determined whether the potentially induced increase in growth hormone leads to increased muscle gain. On the other hand, other researchers have not found that OKG raises growth hormone levels, and no one has found increases in muscle mass with supplementation.

Can Glutamine Slow Muscle Breakdown?

Glutamine is a nonessential amino acid that has become a popular supplement for weight lifters and bodybuilders. It has been touted as a supplement that causes a net gain of muscle protein and thus muscle mass. From the discussion of proteins, you will recall that body proteins are broken down and rebuilt on a daily basis. This is called *protein turnover* and it reflects the dynamic efforts of our cells to adapt to metabolic conditions that change minute by minute, hour by hour, and day by day.

In muscle tissue, protein turnover reflects demands placed on muscle itself. In response to a weight-lifting session there will be an increase in the breakdown of muscle proteins as well as production (synthesis) of muscle proteins. Together these seemingly counteractive processes drive muscle repair and adaptation and can endure for several hours to a day or more. When protein production exceeds breakdown, there will be a net growth of muscle tissue as seen in weight training. It is a matter of simple algebra.

Glutamine is often purported to limit these breakdowns, which results in greater net gains of muscle protein. Interestingly, there are several review articles related to glutamine and muscle protein turnover and the potential application to athletes. However, the review articles outnumber the research efforts actually testing glutamine and showing it to be effective. Therefore, at this time, there is limited information with regard to the efficacy of glutamine supplementation to enhance muscle development associated with resistance training.

Can HMB Improve Muscle Development?

HMB is the abbreviation for β-hydroxy β-methylbutyrate, which is a derivative of the essential amino acid leucine. HMB is a fairly popular supplement with weight trainers at this time and it also added to some sport bars. HMB may also be found in limited amounts in citrus and catfish. There are several research articles that suggest that HMB supplementation (1.5 or 3 grams of HMB daily) for a couple of weeks can improve strength and lean body mass of previously untrained men. However, other researchers have not found such an effect. Therefore, questions still linger as to whether HMB supplementation can have a positive effect on muscle protein turnover and the development of greater lean body mass and strength.

Can β-Alanine Improve Performance?

β-Alanine is naturally found in meats and is a little different structurally from alanine and the other amino acids that can be used to make proteins. However, β-alanine can be combined with histidine to make carnosine. Carnosine, which is an important acid buffer in muscle cells, especially Type II. However, ingested carnosine is broken down in the blood and thus supplementation of carnosine does not effectively increase muscle carnosine levels. Meanwhile β-alanine can enter muscle cells and be used to make carnosine. Researchers are finding that supplemental β-alanine is indeed effective in raising muscle carnosine levels as well as improving the muscle acid buffering abilities during high intensity activities such as sprinting and weight training. This in turn is related to improvements in performance.

β-Alanine is an important acid buffer in muscle and supplementation has been shown to improve exercise performance.

Can Carnitine Help People Burn More Fat to Become Leaner and More Muscular?

The role of carnitine in fat burning has been known for decades. Basically, carnitine helps shuttle the principle fatty acids used for energy into mitochondria, the part of cells that breaks them down for energy. Despite this vital role in burning fat, supplementation of carnitine has generally failed to demonstrate increased fat burning. Recently, however, researchers have shown that carnitine combined with a special form of carbohydrate is able to enhance carnitine uptake into muscle and potentially increase fat burning. Time will tell how successful this novel carnitine delivery system will be.

Can Chromium and Chromium Picolinate Cause Muscle Development?

Chromium, especially in the form of chromium picolinate, has drawn the attention of some athletes. Because chromium appears to potentiate insulin activity, it has been theorized that supplemental chromium may increase amino acid uptake in skeletal muscle and promote muscle protein synthesis. This could lead to the building of more muscle. Picolinate is simply a molecule that, when bound to chromium, is touted to enhance the efficiency of chromium absorption.

Earlier reports by some researchers stated that participants taking chromium picolinate for 40 days in conjunction with weight-training programs increased their body weight. Furthermore, most of the increase in weight was attributed to lean body mass. Another research study described a slight weight reduction in chromium-picolinate supplemented football players. It was reported that these athletes became leaner as a result of a decrease in their body fat. However, other scientists challenged these studies because the methods used in these studies suffered from flaws that easily cast doubt upon the credibility of the results. More recent and better designed studies, including those published in the highly reputable research journals, failed to show beneficial effects of chromium supplementation. Furthermore, studies exploring the potential toxic effects of long-term chromium supplementation have not been completed. Some scientists also speculate that picolinate itself may unfavorably alter brain neurotransmitter levels. So at this time chromium supplementation is not recommended for muscle mass development in otherwise healthy and well nourished athletes.

Can Vanadium and Vanadyl Sulfate Lead to Muscle Mass Gains?

Like chromium, vanadium as vanadyl sulfate has also received a fair amount of attention from weight-training individuals. However, contrary to the attention, there has been very little research performed regarding the possibility of vanadium as a mass-enhancing supplement. Like chromium, the potentially toxic effects of vanadium supplementation are not known, and many nutritionists caution against supplementation until more research is completed in this area.

Can Boron Raise Testosterone Levels?

When boron supplements led to elevated levels of testosterone in post-menopausal women, boron supplements became somewhat popular for weight trainers and bodybuilders, as it was believed that boron could increase testosterone levels. However, researchers have not been able to prove that boron supplementation increases testosterone levels, strength, and muscle mass in weight trainers. At this time, boron supplementation does not appear to be beneficial for weight-training athletes.

Can DHEA and Androstenedione Enhance Testosterone Levels?

DHEA and androstenedione are prohormone molecules. When the body makes sex hormones such as testosterone and estrogens, they are actually constructed during several chemical reactions beginning with cholesterol. In the gonads (ovaries for females and testes for males) cholesterol can be completely converted to testosterone and estrogens and released into the blood. Two molecules along the way to the sex hormones are *DHEA* (dehydroepiandrosterone) and *androstenedione*, with the former coming just prior to the latter (Figure 11.3). Androstenedione is just one chemical reaction shy of testosterone which is one of the most significant factors that evokes muscle protein production and promotes growth.

In order for androstenedione and DHEA to raise testosterone levels they must be absorbed from the digestive tract, circulate, and be converted to testosterone by enzymes in organs such as the liver and testes. Interestingly, skeletal muscle lacks the enzymes needed to convert DHEA and androstenedione to testosterone. It should also be mentioned that both androstenedione and DHEA can be converted to estrogen molecules as well. To counter this, some supplement manufacturers recommend taking substances such as diadzein or chysin (flavonoids) in an attempt to block this undesirable conversion.

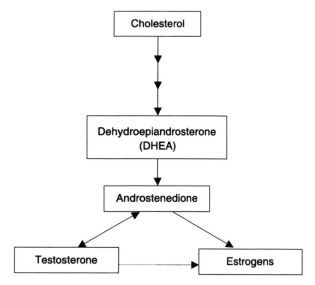

Figure 11.3 Potential reaction pathway for the production of popular steroid substances (dehydroepiandrosterone (DHEA) and androstenedione) and derived hormones (testosterone and estrogens).

In general, researchers have failed to show that androstenedione and DHEA supplements do indeed increase testosterone levels in the blood when dosages mimicked manufacturer recommendations (100 milligrams of androstenedione and 25 to 50 milligrams of DHEA). However, in a research study, when three times the recommended dosage for androstenedione was tested, testosterone levels did increase by 24 percent but estrogen levels also increased by 128 percent. Furthermore, another research study revealed that when men with more body fat were provided androstenedione supplements they were more efficient in converting androstenedione to estrogen than leaner men. This makes sense, as adipose tissue contains the enzymes necessary to convert androstenedione to estrogens.

Both DHEA and androstenedione can be used by our body to make testosterone (and estrogen) and use is banned in some sports.

Androstenedione and DHEA are considered nutrition supplements as they are naturally found in foods such as meats (muscle and organ). Recently the FDA demanded that supplement companies stop selling supplements with androstenedione because of health risks. It should be mentioned that both of these substances are among the list of so-called sport doping agents banned by the International Olympic Committee, National Football League, and the National Collegiate Athletic Association.

Can Inosine Enhance Strength and Mass Development?

The molecule adenosine triphosphate (ATP) provides the energy that directly powers muscle contraction. Logic would have us believe that if we provide the building blocks of ATP in supplements, muscle cells would have more ATP available and exercise performance would be enhanced. The adenosine in ATP can be made from the molecule inosine. However, adenosine concentrations in the cells seem to be tightly controlled and supplemented inosine is not efficiently converted to adenosine. Furthermore, it has been suggested that the processes necessary to break down the excessive inosine may generate free radicals. In addition, inosine is broken down to uric acid, which is involved in the formation of certain types of kidney stones and gout if not proficiently removed from the blood

Aerobic Exercise Is Good for Your Heart and Metabolism

In the late 1970s and early 1980s, the aerobic boom took place and gyms and health clubs around the United States began to include aerobic classes and early forms of cardiovascular equipment. Today, health clubs are often evaluated on the content and variety of their cardiovascular equipment, classes, and programs. Equipment now includes precision bikes, treadmills, steppers, gliders, and classes that are hybrids between classic aerobics and martial arts and weight training.

What Is Aerobic (Cardiovascular) Exercise?

Many people engage in regular aerobic exercise such as running, cross country skiing, bicycling, rowing, fast walking, roller blading (in-line skating), distance swimming, and health club aerobic programs. During these activities the resistance against movement is not as great as weight training and the activity is sustained for 15 minutes or longer. Because muscle energy is generated by burning fat and carbohydrate in oxygen required processes mostly, these forms of exercise are termed aerobic. And, because the heart and blood vessels are responsible for delivering the oxygen-endowed blood to muscle, these types of activity are also called cardiovascular exercise.

What Are the Training Adaptations That Occur From Aerobic Exercise?

Because the resistance to muscle movement is much lower than resistance exercise, muscle enlargement (hypertrophy) is much less pronounced, if at all. However, muscle will adapt in another amazing way. Here the adaptation allows the trained muscle to have greater endurance by increasing its aerobic ATP generative capacity. In doing so there is an increase in the number of mitochondria in the trained muscle cells. Furthermore, the trained muscle develops more capillaries to deliver blood. The increase in the number of capillaries provides more oxygen and energy nutrients during exercise. The heart grows a little as well to provide a more powerful *stroke* and greater cardiac output (blood delivery) to working muscles. A greater heart stroke is often reflected by a slower heart rate when not exercising. Some top endurance athletes have resting heart rates as low as 40 to 45 beats per minute whereas inactive people tend to have heart rates between 60 and 75 beats per minute.

Regular aerobic exercise can strengthen the heart and increase muscles' ability to store and burn fat.

Which Type of Muscle Fibers Are Used in Aerobic Exercise?

During sustained lower intensity efforts (for example, brisk walking, slow swim) the brain will call upon primarily Type I muscle fibers. Here the intensity is low so epinephrine levels will only be slightly elevated. In a fasting state, working muscle cells will be primarily fueled by fatty acids, with the majority coming from the blood (Figure 11.4 and see Figure 5.4). However, as the intensity of the effort increases so too will epinephrine in the blood and as a result the breakdown of glycogen in working muscle. As this occurs, glucose from glycogen stores starts to become a bigger contributor of fuel. As the intensity level continues to increase, so too will the reliance on glucose. One reason for this is that as the intensity level is increased the brain will support Type I muscle fiber efforts with more and more Type II muscle fibers. Type II muscle fibers tend to use more glucose.

Fat and Carbohydrate Are the Principal Fuels of Aerobic Exercise

What Factors Determine What Muscle Uses for Fuel During Aerobic Exercise?

The primary fuel for aerobic and endurance activity depends on both the intensity and duration of the effort. The relative contribution of the different energy nutrients fueling the working muscle will vary depending upon whether exercise lasts for 15 minutes, 30 minutes, 1 hour, or 2 hours. Furthermore, the mixture of fuel will be different at these time

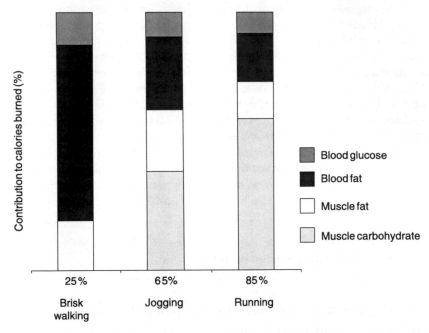

Figure 11.4a Approximate percentage contribution of carbohydrate and fat after 30 minutes of aerobic exercise (cycling) at either lower (walking), moderate (jogging) or higher (running) intensities. While the lower intensity will allow for a greater percentage of fat use, the moderate intensity will allow for a greater quantity of fat used.

intervals when they are performed at different intensities. Another important factor is when and what a person last ate and whether or not they are using sport drinks during activity. Whether it is exercise intensity or timing and composition of last meal, hormones will direct the fuel use during exercise. Nutrient availability from sport drinks or pre-exercise food and beverages will also influence the relative amounts of fuel used.

What Neurotransmitter and Hormones Are Involved in Aerobic Exercise Fuel Use?

At low intensities such as walking, the brain sends a signal through nerves to fat tissue to breakdown fat. The fat can then circulate to muscle and be used as fuel. As the intensity of an aerobic effort increases the level of circulating epinephrine will increase, while the level of insulin will decrease. The brain is mostly responsible for doing this by sending signals to the adrenal glands to release epinephrine and to the pancreas to limit the release of insulin. This is important since epinephrine will promote the breakdown of glycogen in muscle and liver as well as fat in fat cells. Meanwhile, insulin promotes the building of these stores, which is

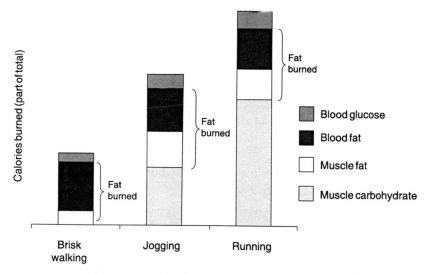

Figure 11.4b Approximate percentage contribution of carbohydrate and fat at 30 minutes of different aerobic exercises (walking, jogging, running). While the lower intensity will allow for a greater percentage of fat use, the moderate intensity will allow for a greater quantity of fat used.

opposite of what you want. Therefore, as exercise intensity increases, more glucose is available in muscle cells and more fatty acids are circulating to and available within muscle cells.

What Is the Relative Breakdown of Fuel During Aerobic Exercise?

A general rule is that for durations longer than 20 minutes, the percentage of fat utilized climbs as the intensity level decreases. For instance, an unfed person performing lower intensity activities, such as brisk walking, bicycling (13 to 15 mph), jogging, and light roller blading, will burn a higher percentage of fat (60 to 70 percent). However, at more moderate intensity activities, such as bicycling (16 to 20 mph) or running (8 to 9 mph), the reliance upon fat for fuel decreases to about 50 percent. Further, as even higher levels of intensity are performed, such as by professional marathon runners and endurance cyclists, carbohydrate is the primary fuel followed by fat and then amino acids.

How Do We Burn the Most Fat During Cardiovascular Exercise?

The amount of fat used as an energy source is greatest at a moderate intensity as displayed in Figure 11.4. So even though fat accounts for a lesser percentage of total energy expended compared to lower intensity, there is more total energy used at the moderate intensity. This leads to greater amounts of fat used. Think of it this way. Which would you rather have—60 percent of $100.00 or 40 percent of $200.00? This is one reason why cardiovascular exercise equipment often has a graphic on the display indicating the "fat burning zone." Here the fat burning zone rate is associated with the moderate level of intensity in Figure 11.4, or the level of intensity in which you are burning the greatest amount of fat.

> Moderate-intensity aerobic exercise will burn more total fat per minute than lower or higher intensity efforts.

Is More Fat Burned as Exercise Is Extended?

Another important factor in fat burning is exercise duration. Cardiovascular exercise is always encouraged to last at least 20 minutes and preferably 30 to 45 minutes for most people. The reason for this is that it seems to take a little time for all the needed events for optimal fat utilization to come on line. This includes everything from mobilizing fatty acids from fat stores to increasing the delivery of oxygen to working muscle. There are a few other biochemical reasons for this as well, but they are beyond the scope of this text. The important thing is that it takes a while, often 12 to 20 minutes, to reach optimal fat burning efficiency. So be patient and include a period of lower intensity warm-up as well.

What Causes Muscle Exhaustion in Endurance Activities?

A principal factor associated with exhaustion during endurance exercise is the availability of carbohydrates to working muscle. Quite simply, when muscle glycogen stores are depleted, muscle exhaustion ensues shortly thereafter. The depletion of muscle glycogen along with dehydration are the most significant contributors to exhaustion or what endurance athletes call "hitting the wall" or "bonking." From this it is easy to see why sport drinks such as PowerAde®, Gatorade®, and Accelerade® are so popular. Electrolyte imbalances may also lead to fatigue, but this might occur only during very long efforts in which only water is provided. Today, with the popularity of sport drinks and endurance foods the risk of an electrolyte imbalance is often reduced.

Can Diet Affect the Onset of Exhaustion?

Stored carbohydrate in the form of muscle and liver glycogen reflects dietary carbohydrate intake. During training or competition, researchers have shown that athletes can significantly increase their training time or time till exhaustion by eating a high carbohydrate diet. For instance, one athlete on a low carbohydrate diet will reach muscle exhaustion long before another athlete on a high carbohydrate diet (more than 60 percent carbohydrate).

A high carbohydrate diet allows the body to replenish glycogen stores in-between training sessions. Contrary to what many people think, it actually takes a while to rebuild muscle glycogen stores that have been used during exercise. In fact, if an endurance athlete reduces his or her muscle glycogen to nadir levels during training or competition; it can take an entire day to rebuild them. This means that the athlete should eat carbohydrates immediately after completing a training session and throughout that day to provide the needed glucose to rebuild those stores.

What Is Carbo-Loading?

Some athletes preparing for a big event will attempt to *carbohydrate load* or *carbo load*. These events include marathons, triathlons, bicycle centuries or longer, and long-distance swimming. The desired outcome is achieving the highest possible level of muscle glycogen just prior to the onset of the competition by coordinating a high carbohydrate intake (over 60 percent) for at least a week prior to competition while at the same time tapering both the intensity and duration of training sessions.

Theoretically, if you start out with more glycogen you should be able to perform longer. A more common method of carbo-loading is explained next and would be most beneficial when an event is to last more than an hour. Carbo-loading would not be beneficial for shorter endurance efforts or sports involving only brief efforts (for example, power lifting, velodrome cycling, or most track and field events). However, intermittent sport athletes such as soccer, football, and field and ice hockey players might benefit; however, the practice and game schedule would make carbo-loading unrealistic in some cases.

How Do You Carbo-Load?

Carbo loading can be successfully performed with common high-carbohydrate foods such as pasta, grains, fruits, and vegetables. The preferred method of carbo-loading involves maintaining a high carbohydrate diet (over 65 percent total calories) during the week prior to the event. During the same period of time exercise is pretty much halved every 2 days in duration and intensity and halted a day prior to the event (Table 11.3).

Table 11.3 Example protocol for Glycogen Loading

Prior to Competition	Training Protocol	Diet Protocol
6 days	90 minutes at intensity approximating 75% VO$_2$max	50% energy as carbohydrate and hydrate
5 days	40 minutes at intensity approximating 75% VO$_2$max	50% energy as carbohydrate and hydrate
4 days	40 minutes at intensity approximating 75% VO$_2$max	50% energy as carbohydrate and hydrate
3 days	20 minutes at intensity approximating 75% VO$_2$max. Rest muscle	70% energy or 10 g carbohydrate/kg body weight and hydrate
2 days	20 minutes at intensity approximating 75% VO$_2$max. Rest muscle	70% energy or 10 g carbohydrate/kg body weight and hydrate copiously
1 day (day before)	Rest muscle as much as possible	70% energy or 10 g carbohydrate/kg body weight and hydrate copiously
Competition	Rest prior to event	Eat carbohydrate-based meal >2–3 hours if possible; ingest carbohydrate 15–30 minutes prior. Hydrate appropriately

VO$_2$max = maximal oxygen consumption.

Protein Needs Are Increased for Endurance Athletes

Do We Use Body Protein for Energy During Endurance Exercise?

Depending on the duration of exercise, amino acids may be counted on to generate as much as 6 to 10 percent of the fuel with the remainder split between fat and carbohydrate. The use of amino acids for energy is mostly a consideration for higher-level endurance athletes. This would include people who train seriously several times a week for extended periods such as a couple of hours. This is one reason why marathoners often look very lean but not as muscular as sprinters or milers, for example. One of the most significant reasons that more and more amino acids are used for energy is because cortisol levels in the blood are increased as the higher intensity activity is endured. Cortisol can cause the breakdown of muscle protein and the freed amino acids can be used for energy. Some amino acids will be used directly by muscle to make ATP, while others will circulate to the liver and be converted to glucose.

What Are Protein Recommendations for Endurance Athletes?

Bodybuilders, power lifters, and football players recognize high protein intakes as an avenue to achieve and maintain enhanced muscle mass. Contrarily, endurance athletes recognize a relatively higher protein (total grams) intake as a means of replacing the body protein used for fuel during training, competition, and recovery and adaptation. Although individual protein requirements will vary with the level of intensity and duration of the activity, some sport nutritionists recognize that 1.4 to 1.75 grams of protein per kilogram body weight will provide adequate protein along with a little extra padding. This is pretty much the same recommendation discussed previously for weight trainers; however, because of differences in body weight the resulting protein quantity is lower for endurance athletes.

> Protein requirements are increased for people who seriously engage in regular aerobic exercise.

Do Endurance Athletes Need a Protein Supplement?

Before traveling to the local nutritional supplement supplier for a protein supplement, first estimate current protein intake. Since many people, especially males, already eat 100 to 130 grams of protein daily (about two times the RDA) only small if any dietary adjustments may be needed. Furthermore, endurance athletes tend to eat more energy than more sedentary people, so more protein is probably, but not definitely, included. This is because many endurance athletes, especially runners, may eat more plant-based foods including pastas, breads, rice, etc. Thus, even though they may be eating more energy, more of it is coming from carbohydrate-rich sources. Endurance athletes should assess their diet prior to spending their money.

Can Fat Loading Improve Aerobic Performance?

Fat loading is a dietary attempt to enhance fat utilization during exercise, thereby decreasing carbohydrate usage and thus slowing glycogen breakdown. The most important considerations with this protocol are timing and practicality as it will take about a week or so for this adaptation to occur and a high fat diet may not be tolerable for many athletes.

Eating more fat and less carbohydrate will not build the same glycogen depth prior to competition. So even though they may use less carbohydrate during competition they might have less available to spend during exercise anyway. This may be okay for a marathoner running a slower pace (for example, 8 minutes per mile), however, for a runner competing at a higher intensity such as 5 or 6 minutes per mile, this could be disastrous. This is something that an athlete would have to experiment with and become comfortable with prior to competition.

Several Supplements Target Endurance Athletes

Can Caffeine Enhance Endurance Performance?

Caffeine has long been considered a stimulant and is used by many individuals in normal daily life as well as by athletes. Caffeine and related substances are found naturally in foods and beverages, such as coffee, teas, and chocolate; and as part of recipes, such as in various soft drinks. Coffee contains caffeine whereas tea contains theophylline and chocolate contains theobromine. These factors are considered stimulants as they impact the central nervous system and increase alertness, which alone can improve the enjoyment of exercise and help some people perform at a higher level. Caffeine and related substances also enhance and prolong the effects of certain hormones such as glucagon and epinephrine in fat tissue. If fat release is increased and made more available to muscle then more fat might be used during aerobic exercise and improve performance and help lean the body.

Several studies have reported that the beneficial effects of caffeine on performance are negated in people who use caffeine daily (in coffee, soft drinks, etc). However, by going caffeine free for several days prior to an event, caffeine may enhance performance. Recent studies have shown that caffeine ingestion can indeed enhance endurance performance. Based on the current research, 3 to 6 milligrams of caffeine per kilogram body weight prior to training or competition might enhance endurance performance. Meanwhile levels exceeding 9 milligrams of caffeine per kilogram body weight might decrease performance.

> Caffeine can enhance aerobic performance for some people but too much can be problematic.

Caffeine seems to enhance mental alertness in smaller doses (200 milligrams), although many individuals complain of nervousness and anxiety when larger doses are used (over 400 milligrams). A cup of coffee contains 100 to 150 milligrams of caffeine while a cup of tea and cola contain 25 to 60 milligrams. The over-the-counter stimulant Vivarin contains 200 milligrams of caffeine per tablet. Caffeine is metabolized and removed from the body fairly slowly. It may take several hours for the caffeine in one cup of coffee to be completely removed in the urine.

Can Glycerol Support Better Hydration for Athletes?

Glycerol has long been considered a candidate for supplementation during endurance events. One reason is based upon glycerol's potential to be converted to glucose in the liver. The glucose could then circulate to muscle and support muscle operations during exercise. Theoretically, this could decrease the rate of breakdown of glycogen stores. However, it seems that the torpid rate of converting glycerol to glucose seriously decreases its candidacy.

Alternatively, glycerol supplementation in conjunction with water consumption may be of benefit to endurance athletes preparing to perform in warmer environments. It is proposed that glycerol can enhance water retention prior to an event and thus may allow more sweat to be lost prior to any reductions in performance due to dehydration. Scientists have also reported that glycerol supplementation prior to an event increases heat tolerance during competition in warmer environments. This could potentially aid athletes training or competing in warmer environments without ample opportunity to drink fluids. One example of this type of competition is soccer. However, glycerol may lead to digestive tract discomfort so athletes will have to experiment here as well.

Should Endurance Athletes Use Antioxidants Supplements?

Oxygen-based free radicals are normally produced by aerobic energy metabolism. During aerobic activities even more free radicals are created as energy expenditure increases several fold. In response, muscle produces and maintains greater levels of antioxidants. In addition, antioxidants from foods can incorporate into muscle and help keep free radicals at bay. Food-derived antioxidents include carotenoids, polyphenolics, vitamin C and E, lipoic acid, and coenzyme Q. However, supplementing excessively large levels of these nutrients is not recommended.

Can Endurance Performance Be Improved with Coenzyme Q?

Coenzyme Q, also known as CoQ10 and *ubiquinone*, can be found in the cells as a key component of the electron-transport chain. It also functions as an antioxidant and it has been used as a supplement by many individuals who are taking statin drugs. Some of the earlier studies regarding the effects of supplemental CoQ10 on athletic performance were positive; however, more recent and better designed studies have failed to show a significant performance benefit of CoQ10 supplementation. However, CoQ10 might be a desirable supplement for antioxidant protection for athletes.

Can Lipoic Acid Enhance Performance?

Lipoic acid (α lipoic acid) is a naturally occurring substance in cells and is a key factor in the metabolism of energy nutrients. In addition, lipoic acid also functions as a muscle antioxidant. At this time researchers have not found that lipoic acid supplements provide performance benefits to athletes. However, lipoic acid might be a desirable supplement for anti-oxidant protection for athletes.

Can Medium-Chain Triglycerides Increase Performance?

Medium-chain triglycerides (MCTs) contain fatty acids, which are both saturated and are only six to twelve carbons in length. The shortness of these fatty acids gives them unique properties, including the ability to:

- be absorbed from the digestive tract into the blood (portal vein) and not be generally incorporated in chylomicrons
- provide a rapid energy source for the liver and muscle
- possibly increase fat mobilization from fat cells

These properties make MCTs a possible candidate for supplementation during endurance events. Theoretically, MCTs can slow glycogen break-down and decrease some muscle protein breakdown during endurance exercise by providing a readily available energy source for liver and muscle. Researchers have indeed found that supplemented MCTs are used during endurance exercise, however, they seem to substitute for other fat and do not slow the rate of glycogen breakdown nor do they improve athletic performance.

Should Choline Be Supplemented to Enhance Performance?

Choline is a component of acetylcholine, which is a neurotransmitter of great importance to skeletal muscle activity. First, nerve cells reaching skeletal muscle cells release acetylcholine, which then stimulates muscle cells to contract. Furthermore, choline is a component of phosphotidyl-choline which is a structural component of muscle cell membranes. Choline, along with *betaine (trimethylglycine [TMG]), dimethylglycine, sarcosine (N-methylglycine), methionine,* and *S-adenylsyl methionine,* is involved in some of the processes that build several molecules which may be important for muscle performance, such as creatine and nucleic acids. Choline supplementation for the purposes of enhancing athletic performance (with and without other substances) requires further study.

FAQ Highlight

Sport Drinks Are Liquid Performance

Sport drinks were pioneered in the 1960s when a scientist at the University of Florida (home of the Gators) developed a product designed to provide fluid, energy, and electrolytes to athletes. The product became known as Gatorade®, and a multibillion-dollar industry was born.

What Is Sweat?

As discussed in Chapter 7, sweat is a combination of mostly water and electrolytes. Water is needed to help remove the excessive heat generated from the body during exercise. One liter of sweat allows for the removal of 580 calories of heat from the body. So, if an activity such as running for 2 hours generates about 900 calories of heat, then theoretically about 1.5 liters of sweat may have been lost. The primary electrolytes lost from the body in sweat are sodium and chloride. However, their concentration in sweat is lower than in the plasma of the blood. Thus, sweat is dilute compared to blood. Even when someone is sweating profusely, the sodium and chloride content may be only about one-half of the concentration of human blood plasma.

What Is the Composition of Sport Drinks?

Sport drinks provide fluid, energy, and electrolytes and possibly other nutrients such as protein, amino acids, calcium, magnesium, B-complex vitamins, and antioxidants. The energy in sport drinks is provided largely in the form of carbohydrates such as glucose, sucrose, fructose, corn syrup, maltodextrins, and glucose polymers. Maltodextrins and glucose polymers are mostly cornstarch that is partially broken down. Glucose and fructose are monosaccharides, whereas corn syrup is derived from cornstarch, which has been partially broken down to short, branching chains of glucose. Maltodextrin is just a few glucose molecules linked together with a branching point. Glucose polymers may just be short chains of glucose. Carbohydrates usually make up about 6 to 8 percent of the sport drink. Recently protein and amino acids have been formulated into sports drinks with research suggesting better hydration, performance, and recovery. Time will tell whether these ingredients provide more benefit and are tolerated well.

How Does the Carbohydrate in Sport Drink Help
Sustain Performance?

One of the principal factors involved in the onset of exhaustion or fatigue is a depletion of muscle glycogen stores. The carbohydrate in sport drinks becomes an available source of glucose to working muscle. It was once thought that the carbohydrate in a sport drink might slow the rate of glycogen breakdown and thus prolong endurance exercise. However, research has shown that the carbohydrate in a sport drink actually becomes an increasingly more important carbohydrate source for working muscle as glycogen stores wane. This contribution seems to be significant enough to push back the onset of fatigue. This could be the difference in finishing strongly during a marathon or fatiguing in the last couple of miles.

Who Would Benefit from a Sport Drink?

For a well nourished and hydrated weight-training athlete, there is probably no need for a sport drink unless he or she is training for longer periods and sweating profusely. The need for sport drinks for endurance athletes largely depends on the duration of exercise and the environmental conditions. Generally, for single shorter events such as 5-kilometer runs and half-hour aerobic sessions there isn't a need. However, as an event or training session becomes longer, the need increases. For bouts lasting an hour or more, water replacement is certainly necessary and performance can be enhanced by a sport drink.

Even athletes competing in intermittent action sports such as soccer, ice hockey, and football can benefit from a sport drink. These sports are powered by muscle glycogen and a sport drink can improve performance in repeated sprinting efforts. Plus for sports such as ice hockey and football uniforms and gear can increase sweating and thus the need for fluid to maintain optimal hydration becomes more important.

Can Fortified Water/Fitness Water Help Performance?

Over the past few years numerous enriched waters or fitness waters such as Propel® and Option®. These beverages tend to be low calorie (for example, 10 calories per 8 to 10 ounces) and include electrolytes with or without calcium, magnesium and B-vitamins. While these beverages are not advantageous for more strenuous and/or prolonged athletic efforts they are good options for maintaining optimal hydration especially in the heat (for example, walking or a half hour or so on the elliptical or weight lifting).

12 Nutrition Throughout Life

The life of a human typically spans 80 years, longer in some countries and shorter in others. It is a remarkable process that begins at conception and features the development of highly specialized cells, tissues, and organs to create a functional synergy and a unique appearance. During that time the brain develops and matures yielding the thought-processing and personality that will further distinguish each individual among billions of peers. In this chapter we will discuss many of the key happenings and conditions of the human lifespan and how nutrition plays a key role.

Making a Baby Is Complicated

How Does Conception Occur?

A female ovulates once a month during her reproductive years. Ovulation culminates in the liberation of an egg, which then settles in one of the fallopian tubes. There the egg sits and plays a waiting game, as it has but 24 hours or so to become fertilized by a sperm. Semen from a male counterpart is a mixture of sperm (produced by the testes) and nourishing and supporting fluids from various accessory reproductive glands, such as the prostate and Cowper's gland. Ejaculation produces about one-half teaspoon of semen, which will contain millions of sperm. This high number of sperm is very important because the task at hand is so great. Ultimately, however, only one sperm will fertilize the egg and initiate the genesis of human life.

What Happens Early on in Pregnancy?

The fertilized egg now develops into a *zygote*, which is the very basis of human life. All humans begin their lives as a single cell. This single cell now has combined the genetic information (DNA) from the mother and father and can develop into a complex cell orchestration of metabolism, movement, and mentality. All the zygote needs is a nourishing place to develop, namely the mother's uterus. Within a brief time after conception, the zygote divides into two cells, which then divide into four cells, which then divide into eight cells, and so on. From conception to 2 weeks is referred to as the *pre-embryonic* period, while from week 2 to the closure of week 8 marks the embryonic period. By the end of the embryonic period the embryo will show small but fairly developed organs and begin to take on a more recognizable human form. The commencement of week 9 to the moment of birth marks the *fetal* period. During this time the fetus will show remarkable growth and maturation of organs and appendages. At approximately 13 weeks, the heart begins to beat, even though the fetus still weighs but a few ounces.

> At conception, human life begins with a single cell called a zygote.

How Long Does Pregnancy Last?

Normal pregnancy lasts approximately 40 weeks and is typically broken into three equal time periods called trimesters. It is desirable to deliver after at least 37 weeks of pregnancy with the newborn weighing greater than 2.5 kilograms or about 5.5 pounds. Infants born prior to the 37th week are referred to as premature, while those born weighing less than 2.5 kilograms are called low birth weight infants. Premature and low birth weight infants find life more challenging in the days, weeks, and months that follow as they are at greater risk for medical complications. Premature infants are often introduced into the real world before their organs, especially their lungs, are fully developed and capable of coping with the new environment. On the other hand, babies cannot stay in the womb much longer than 40 weeks. Babies must be born before the skull becomes too large to pass through the birth canal. From a developmental standpoint, babies probably should stay in the mother's womb for a few more weeks.

Weight Gain Is a Must During Pregnancy

How Much Weight Should a Woman Gain During Pregnancy?

During pregnancy the energy needs of a woman are increased to allow for a healthy gain in body weight. The mother's energy needs are slightly increased during the first trimester, while on the average an extra 300 calories/day are needed during the second and third trimesters. A weight gain of roughly a pound per month during the first trimester is generally recommended. Then, during the second and third trimesters, a three-quarter to a pound per week weight gain is considered healthy. This allows for a total pregnancy weight gain of 25 to 35 pounds.

How Much Weight Should an Overweight or Underweight Woman Gain During Pregnancy?

If a woman is underweight at the onset of pregnancy, a 28 to 40-pound weight gain is often recommended. On the other hand, if a woman is overweight or obese at the onset of pregnancy, a weight gain of 15 to 25 pounds is considered safer. It is important to recognize that pregnancy is not the time to try to lose weight. A healthy weight gain for the mother translates into a healthy growth for the unborn infant. Weight loss is never encouraged during pregnancy.

What Should a Woman Do If She Gains Too Much Weight During Pregnancy?

If during early pregnancy a woman experiences an excessive weight gain, she should not be encouraged to lose weight. However, she should be encouraged to be more careful and try not to exceed the 1 pound per week in the remaining weeks. In contrast, if a pregnant woman fails to gain the recommended weight during early pregnancy, she should be encouraged to gain at least a pound per week for the remaining weeks, while not dramatically overcompensating. She can divide her recommended weight gain by the number of remaining weeks and use that figure as a guide.

What Contributes to Weight Gain During Pregnancy?

As a female gains weight during pregnancy, usually about 7 to 8 pounds is attributable to the weight of the infant at birth. The rest of the weight is distributed throughout the mother in various tissues developed during pregnancy. These tissue include the placenta, amniotic fluid, increased breast tissue, expanded blood volume, and fat storage and muscle. These all help support the mother and fetus during pregnancy and after birth. Even the mother's bones will become a little denser during pregnancy.

Weight gain during pregnancy is attributable to baby weight as well as supportive tissue for the mother.

Certain Nutrients Play a Special Role During Pregnancy

How Much Protein Does a Mother Need During Pregnancy?

Protein requirements are increased during pregnancy to allow for adequate protein production in the mother and developing baby. An increase of 25 grams of protein per day above the RDA is recommended for pregnant teens and women, going from 46 to 71 grams daily. The use of a protein supplement is probably not necessary for most women as their typical protein intake is typically greater than requirements during pregnancy or is accounted for through increased energy intake during pregnancy. Vegetarian females should be particularly careful of their protein intake, especially vegans or fruitarians.

Are Vitamin Needs Increased During Pregnancy?

Vitamin needs are generally increased during pregnancy with special consideration for folate and vitamin D. Since the manufacturing of DNA requires folate, and the unborn infant is composed of rapidly reproducing cells, the need for extra folate is very important. The extra folate (50 percent above the nonpregnant RDA) also supports red blood cell formation as the mother's blood volume expands. A woman can increase her folate intake by choosing folate-rich foods such as orange juice and many fruits and vegetables.

Vitamin D is also especially important during pregnancy. A pregnant woman's RDA is the same as a nonpregnant woman, but good status is crucial. Vitamin D is necessary to aid in calcium metabolism and fetal bone formation. Regular sunlight exposure as well as choosing vitamin D-fortified milk and dairy products can help meet vitamin D requirements. However, excessive direct sunlight (or tanning beds) is not recommended during pregnancy because fetal tissue is very sensitive to damage by UV light.

Why Is Folate So Important During Pregnancy?

During pregnancy the need for the proper production of DNA and RNA, which folate is critically involved, is incredible. During the first few weeks of pregnancy the neural tube that extends from the brain and runs the length of the upper body develops rapidly. Defects to the neural tube tend to occur early in pregnancy, typically around the third and fourth week, and are often irreversible. These abnormalities, including *spina bifida*, are devastating and possibly fatal. Prior to the federal government making it mandatory to fortify grain products with folate, the incidence of neural tube defects in the United States was 1 in 1,000. Today, that incidence is drastically reduced. Furthermore, researchers have determined that folate supplementation just prior to and early in pregnancy can lower the risk of neural tube defects by at least 60 percent. Good reason indeed for starting a prenatal supplement prior to conception and being sure to take it early in pregnancy.

Are Minerals Needed in Greater Amounts During Pregnancy?

As with vitamins, the need for many essential minerals increases during pregnancy. For instance, the RDA for iron increases from 18 to 27 milligrams daily. Iron is needed by the mother to form new hemoglobin for her expanding blood volume and by the fetus to meet new tissue needs. Calcium is especially important during fetal bone and teeth development. Fluoride also helps teeth and bone develop. Although the RDA for calcium for pregnant women is the same as nonpregnant women (1,000 to 1,300 milligrams), it is of the utmost importance to eat adequate quantities of this nutrient. Zinc requirements are increased by roughly 25 percent during pregnancy due to its general involvement in fetal growth and development.

> Women are encouraged to begin taking a prenatal supplement prior to conception.

Should Pregnant Women Take Prenatal Vitamin/Mineral Supplements?

Prenatal vitamin/mineral supplements are recommended by many physicians and nutritionists. An easy argument for the use of prenatal vitamin and mineral supplements is supported by the occurrence of unusual eating patterns experienced by some women during pregnancy. Even the most nutrition-conscious women will admit to some unusual preferences, cravings, or eating patterns during pregnancy. Typically, prenatal vitamin and mineral supplements include folate, vitamin D, iron, zinc, and calcium along with other key nutrients such as omega-3 fats.

Do Pregnant Women Need to Take Omega-3 Fatty Acid Supplements?

The mother is the sole source of nutrition for the developing fetus and for omega-3 fatty acids, namely EPA and DHA (eicosapentaenoic and docosahexaenoic acids) these fats come mostly from the diet or supplementation. Since many women avoid fish during pregnancy for fear of heavy metals such as lead, diet can become a poor provider of omega-3 fatty acids. Meanwhile, although some DHA and EPA can be made in the body from another omega-3 fat, found in higher amounts in flax, the conversion is fairly low. There is reason to believe that pregnant women who get these nutrients, especially DHA, in adequate amounts during pregnancy can support a healthier length of pregnancy. In addition, getting adequate intake levels during preganancy and lactation have been linked to better cognitive development as assessed at 4 years of age. In general, pregnant and lactating women are encouraged to get at least 200 milligrams of DHA daily. Vegetarian women wanting a supplement containing DHA can get an algal source with vegetarian pill coating.

Can We Get Too Much of Certain Vitamins During Pregnancy?

It is important to realize that excessive vitamin A supplementation during pregnancy can result in birth defects. Furthermore, a vitamin A derivative is the active ingredient in Accutane (isotretinoin), which is used to treat cystic acne. The use of this product should be discontinued during pregnancy, as well as when attempting to become pregnant. In fact, since this drug is metabolized slowly it can take several weeks to a couple of months before it is safe for a woman to become pregnant after discontinuing its use. If she becomes pregnant while using Accutane, the mother should discuss this with her physician immediately, as the risk of birth defects is exceptionally high.

Certain Factors Can Affect the Health of a Fetus

What Factors Can Affect the Healthy Growth of an Unborn Infant?

Other dietary and behavioral factors that can impact the proper growth and development of an unborn infant include caffeine, alcohol, and smoking. It should be understood that throughout pregnancy, the unborn infant is vulnerable to the effects of nutritional deficiency and toxicity as well as to the impact of harmful substances. However, this is especially true during the embryonic period. Proper nutritional, behavioral, and environmental care should be taken throughout pregnancy to increase the likelihood of a healthy offspring.

Is Smoking an Issue During Pregnancy?

There may not be a greater common voluntary insult upon human health than cigarette smoke, which certainly holds true for unborn infants, although it is an involuntary insult to them. Pregnant mothers who smoke are at greater risk of delivering low birth weight and premature infants. Some research suggests that these infants are also more prone to childhood cancers and sudden infant death. A pregnant woman's body should be a smoke-free environment.

Factors such as smoking, alcohol, and drugs place an unborn child at risk of developmental abnormalities.

What Impact Does Alcohol Have on a Pregnancy?

The effects of abusive alcohol consumption during pregnancy are substantial. Fetal alcohol syndrome (FAS) is a group of abnormal characteristics common to children born to mothers who drank too much during pregnancy. These characteristics include low birth weight, physical deformities, and poor mental development. It is estimated that more than 7,500 infants are born in the United States each year with FAS, while another thirty to forty thousand show milder signs of FAS. Although many physicians believe that there may be a safe level of alcohol consumption during pregnancy (for example, a glass of wine with dinner occasionally), it is not clear at this time where the threshold lies. It is therefore difficult to make general recommendations. Because of this difficulty it seems much more logical for most women to abstain completely from alcohol consumption during pregnancy.

Is Caffeine a Problem During Pregnancy?

Caffeine consumption during pregnancy and its potential effect upon the unborn infant has raised concern over the past couple of decades. Researchers have reported that there is probably a greater risk of spontaneous fetal abortion and low birth weight in pregnant women consuming the caffeine equivalent of greater than twelve cups of coffee per day. Many scientists believe that caffeine has a safety threshold, much like alcohol, and that daily caffeine intake below the threshold is not detrimental. However, many women choose to abstain completely from caffeine and caffeine-like substances (theophylline in tea and theobromine in chocolate) during pregnancy until more is known in this area.

Should a Pregnant Women Exercise During Pregnancy?

Historically, many women have given up activity during pregnancy fearing adverse effects upon the growth and development of the fetus. However, times have changed, and regular exercise does not seem to affect growth or development of the unborn infant. In fact, newer research suggests that regular exercise may provide some benefits at delivery, such as a shorter delivery time and perceived discomfort and pain. Some caution should be applied, however, to the type of activity a pregnant woman chooses. Contact sports and movements involving rapid directional changes and jarring motions should be avoided. Exercise such as low impact aerobics, walking, and swimming is considered safe during pregnancy. However, a female must pay particular attention to her energy consumption and monitor her body weight and hydration status.

> Low-impact exercise such as walking and swimming is recommended during pregnancy.

Babies Must Work Their Way Up to Adult Food

How Much Do Humans Grow During Infancy?

Infancy is the time period between birth and a baby's first birthday. At no other time in life are nutritional needs higher based on body weight. Infants will usually double their birth weight by the time they are halfway through their first year of life. Additionally, they can easily triple their birth weight by their first birthday. At the same time, an infant will increase its length by roughly 50 percent by his or her first birthday. Furthermore, the head is relatively huge at birth, roughly accounting for one-third to one-quarter of the infant's length. Since an adult's head is only one-eighth of his or her height it is no wonder an infant cannot support the weight of its head for a month or so after being born. Pediatricians and parents, checking indicators of normal growth patterns, follow changes in weight, length, and head circumference. Generally, breast milk or formula meets an infant's nutritional needs during the first 4 to 6 months. Thereafter, the introduction of solid foods allows them to become a strong nutrient contributor.

What Is Lactation?

One of the changes that occur in a female during pregnancy is an enhancement of breast tissue and the maturing of the mammary glands. This occurs due to hormonal changes during pregnancy. *Lactation* is a period of time when a woman is producing breast milk in her mammary glands. Increases in the level of the hormone *prolactin* in a female stimulates her mammary glands to produce milk. The suckling of an infant helps signal her pituitary gland to release more prolactin into her blood and is required for continued lactation.

Breast milk is not a single substance, as it changes in composition not only with time after birth but also during a single feeding. In the first few days after birth, mothers produce a very sophisticated form of breast milk called *colostrum*. Over the next 2 weeks or so of lactation, breast milk slowly loses many of the characteristics of colostrum and gains those of mature breast milk.

What Is Colostrum?

Colostrum is a yellowish, viscous solution that contains more than nutrients; it also contains immune factors. These immune factors include antibodies and other factors that can help boost an infant's developing immune capabilities. Since the infant's digestive tract is unused during pregnancy, it is relatively immature at birth and will take the first few months after birth to develop. Many of the immune factors present in colostrum pass through the infant's immature digestive tract wall intact and enter the blood. The immune factors in colostrum are believed to contribute to the fewer lung and intestinal infections observed in breast-fed infants than formula-fed infants. Further, factors in breast milk seem to promote the formation of a healthy colon bacteria population, since an infant's digestive tract is also born sterile (without bacteria).

> Colostrum is produced during the first days post-birth and is rich in nutrient for early immunity.

What Is Breast Milk?

Mature breast milk is a thinner and almost translucent solution. It is not uncommon for it to present a slightly bluish tinge. Mature breast milk contains a greater ratio of whey to casein protein than cow's milk. Infants digest whey protein more easily, whereas casein tends to form a curd during digestion. Mature breast milk also contains a protein called *lactof-errin*, which can bind iron and potentially reduce bacterial infections. This is because bacteria require iron to reproduce. In addition, the amino acid called taurine is also present in breast milk. Taurine is not used to make proteins, but it is necessary for proper bile formation and visual processes.

The fat content of mature breast milk increases during a single feeding. This is an excellent reason to encourage an infant to feed for longer periods of time (more than 10 minutes). Infants need this energy-dense liquid available later in a feeding to help meet their needs for growth and development. Further, mature human breast milk contains linoleic acid and cholesterol, both of which are necessary for the proper growth of an infant's brain and other nervous tissue.

Lactose is the major carbohydrate in mature breast milk. You will remember that lactose is a disaccharide made up of the monosaccharides glucose and galactose. Beyond providing energy, galactose also seems to be important for the development of the insulating wrapping around nerve cells. Only small amounts of vitamin D are present in mature breast milk, so a supplement may be necessary, especially if an infant has minimal exposure to sunlight. Furthermore, because the iron composition is also very low in breast milk, infants may benefit from a supplement by their second to third month.

How Much Energy (Calories) Does an Infant Need?

An infant requires about 45 to 50 calories per pound of body weight. This need is about twice as high as for adults when we look at it relative to body weight. This makes sense because of the rapid growth of infants, while during adulthood increases in height and the normal growth of the skeleton and organs has ceased. Breast milk or most formulas will provide about 700 calories per quart or liter. The addition of solid foods in the latter half of infancy makes a significant energy contribution.

How Much Protein Does an Infant Need?

Protein needs are also much higher for infants than for adults. Infants require about 1.5 to 2 grams of protein/kilograms body weight (0.7 to 1.0 grams of protein per pound). Furthermore, at least 40 percent of the protein should come from more complete protein sources. In general, protein should contribute 20 percent or a little less to an infant's energy intake, with fat (30 to 50 percent) and carbohydrate (30 to 50 percent) making up the remainder. The energy in mature breast milk is composed of about 17 percent protein, 54 percent fat, and 40 percent carbohydrate. Cow's milk formulas approximate these percentages, although they are slightly higher in protein (18 percent) and lower in fat (43 percent). Fat recommendations are higher for infants than for adults because of their high energy need versus their relatively small food intake. Do not worry about their blood lipids yet as their growth and development are more important. In fact, recommendations by the American Heart Association for eating a lower fat diet do not begin until after they have reached 2 years of age.

Are Vitamin and Mineral Needs Greater During Infancy?

Relative to body weight, vitamin and mineral needs are also higher during infancy versus adulthood. Because the vitamin K content of breast milk is low and an infant's digestive tract will not develop a healthy bacteria population for a few months, vitamin K is often administered to infants. Vitamin D supplementation may be necessary for breast-fed infants who receive minimal exposure to sunlight or who have darker skin.

Complementing breast-feeding with a vitamin D-fortified infant formula can assist in meeting an infant's needs. Because the iron content of breast milk is relatively low, the introduction to solid foods between ages 4 to 6 months becomes very important in supplying this nutrient. Iron-fortified cereals are very good choices. Many pediatricians will recommend an iron supplement for infants during their first few months of life. Again, complementing breast-feeding with an iron-fortified infant formula can assist in meeting an infant's needs. Furthermore, infants fed a vegan or other meat-restrictive diets would need a vitamin B_{12} supplement.

What Are Infant Formulas?

Cow's milk-based infant formulas offer a nutritious complement to breast-feeding and can be used in place of it. These formulas, such as Similac®, Enfamil®, and Good Start® (Nestlé), are different from breast milk in that they are taken from cow's milk and also do not contain all of the beneficial immune factors and certain other nutrients. However, manufacturers are constantly modifying these formulas to more closely match breast milk. Cow's milk-based formulas generally contain casein as a protein source, which has been partially digested by heat treatment. This improves infant digestion of this protein and drastically decreases the likelihood of the formation of a discomforting curd in the digestive tract. Some formulas include only whey protein that is partially digested to ease digestive complications.

Soy protein-based infant formulas, such as ProSobee®, Isomil®, and Alsoy®, are an option for formula-fed infants who do not tolerate the cow's milk-based formulas or for vegetarian families. The American Academy of Pediatrics advises mothers not to feed their infants plain cow's milk, especially skim milk, versus other options during the first year of the infants' lives. The composition is not compatible with an infant's needs and may be detrimental to the baby's health.

Beyond Calories and Protein, What Special Nutrients Are in Infant Formulas?

In addition to providing energy and protein, many infant formulas are iron fortified and contain a complement of vitamins and minerals to improve their composition. Recently, DHA and ARA (arachidonic acid) have been included to some infant formulations. These fatty acids are richly found in the brain and other neurological tissue and are believed to be important for proper neurological and cognitive development. Additionally, some formulas contain antioxidants as well as bacterial strains such as bifidobacteria, which are important for properly functioning digestive tract.

> DHA is important for infants and children to support proper development of the brain.

When Should an Infant Advance to Solid Foods?

The transition to solid foods (Table 12.1) should begin when the infant is ready, not necessarily when the parent is ready. An infant will let you know through physical signs when they are prepared for solid foods. One of these signs is a relaxation of the gag reflex. The gag reflex propels undesirable items forward and out of the mouth. This reflex is strongest in infants and is still maintained to some degree throughout our life. Relaxation of the gag reflex allows an infant to swallow foods of a more solid consistency, such as cereals and purees. The ability of infants to form their mouths around spoons is another sign that solid foods are becoming more appropriate.

What Changes Can You Expect as an Infant Transitions to Solid Foods?

Early in the transition to solid foods, infants will not have the hand dexterity and hand-to-mouth coordination to feed themselves. However, within the ensuing months they develop these capabilities. During this time, teeth begin to appear, and an infant may begin to take small sips from a cup. Usually by age 9 months, infants are able to participate in a meal as they begin to play with plates, cups, and perhaps help support a cup when drinking. By 10 months, many infant will be feeding themselves finger foods and drinking from a cup; however, a thorough cleaning of the infant and the surrounding area usually is necessary following these feats.

Table 12.1 Recommended Progression of Feeding During Infancy

0–4 months	Breast milk or formula
4–6 months	Iron-fortified cereals when infant is ready while still breast or formula feeding
6–9 months	Strained vegetables, fruits, and meats are added to cereals while still breast or formula feeding
9–12 months	Gradual introduction to cut and mashed table foods, meats should be well cooked to minimize chewing, juice by a small cup becomes appropriate; breast or formula feeding continues

What Are Food Allergies?

Food allergies are immune responses to food components. Six to eight percent of children have food allergies and two percent of adults have them. The most common food allergies in adults are shellfish, peanuts, tree nuts, sesame seeds, fish, and eggs, and the most common food allergies present in children are milk, eggs, and peanuts. Signs and symptoms of food allergies include swelling of lips, tongue, and airway (wheezing), itching, hives, eczema and, if severe enough, anaphylaxis. Since there is no cure for food allergies at this time, the allergic person has to avoid any and all forms of the food to which they are allergic.

How Do Food Allergies Develop?

There are a couple of theories for how food allergies develop. One involves exposure to partially digestive proteins in early life. Although the digestive tract is rapidly developing during the first few months of infancy, there remains the potential for complete or semicomplete food proteins to cross the wall of the digestive tract and enter the body. When this occurs, an infant's immune system recognizes this substance as foreign and destroys it. At the same time an infant develops "immune memory" of that substance for future reference. This immune memory includes a routine production of antibodies that specifically recognize that substance. These antibodies allow the body to develop a very rapid and potent immune response when exposed to that substance again in the future. This response causes the release of chemicals in the body (for example, histamine and serotonin), which may cause any number of the following actions: itchiness, swelling, vomiting, asthma, diarrhea, headache, skin reactions, or a runny nose.

Even in the mature digestive tract of children and adults there still remains a chance that fragments of intact substances are absorbed. When this occurs, an allergic reaction ensues. Many factors in the diet may elicit the characteristics of a food allergy or intolerance. Some of the more common foods containing these substances include those food items listed in Table 12.2. Sometimes a food allergy is difficult to identify. Physicians who specialize in this area (allergists) may have the allergic

Table 12.2 Food Items Suspect in Many Food Allergies

Fish and other seafood	Oats and oatmeal	Nuts (especially peanuts)
Oranges and citrus fruits	Legumes	Mustard
Eggs	Tomatoes	Milk
Garlic	Wheat	Rye
Chocolate	Cucumbers	Corn
Various colorants and flavorants		

patient eat a very plain diet and then introduce foods that are suspect one at a time until the culprit food is identified.

Are Food Intolerances Different from Allergies?

Food intolerance is often confused with allergies. However, the major difference is that the symptoms of food intolerance are mostly experienced in the digestive tract and include cramping, bloating, and diarrhea. The symptoms of a food allergy are said to be systemic, which means throughout the body and can include the digestive tract. The most common food intolerance is lactose intolerance, as described in Chapter 4.

Kids Grow Fast!

How Are Eating Behaviors Affected During Childhood and Adolescence?

The progression from infancy to childhood and then adolescence brings many new eating situations and experiences. During early childhood if not well before, children are weaned from breast milk or formula completely and have also made the transition from infant foods to regular foods. Eating develops into a very social and impressionable time in our lives. The number of meals children eat in a day will decrease and many food likes/dislikes and eating behaviors are formed in childhood. Children watch others at the table and also respond to moods and changes in the environment at the table. During childhood, television, radio, and interaction with peers at day care, camps, and grade school impact the development of children's likes and dislikes, and eating behaviors. Many of these characteristics remain throughout life, while others are phases.

How Much Growth Can Be Expected During Childhood and Adolescence?

The rapid pace of growth of infancy slows during early childhood, and a typical weight gain for the second year is only 5 pounds. During this time, though, body composition is changing slightly as fat percentage decreases and lean tissue increases. Within the next few years the rate of gain in both height and weight further slows. Then, sometime around age 7, the rate of weight gain escalates and does not begin to taper off until the mid-teen years. The rate of height growth tapers until a growth spurt is recognized sometime around 10 to 12 for girls and 11 to 14 for boys (Figure 12.1).

During infancy, the status of height, weight, and head circumference, relative to other infants of the same age and gender, can be used to

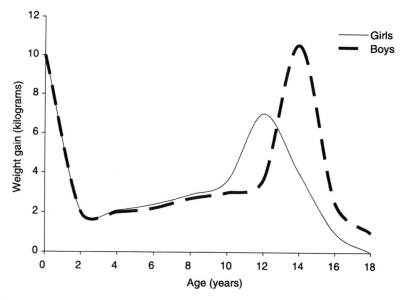

Figure 12.1 Average annual weight gain of boys and girls.

gauge growth and ability to thrive. This assessment can be continued throughout childhood and adolescence as well, although only height and weight are used during this time. These measurements are used for placement at a certain percentile in reference to other children.

What If a Child Refuses to Eat Certain Foods?

The number of meals and relative food intake decreases during child-hood. Therefore it is important to provide a variety of nutrient-dense foods, including meats (if applicable), fruits, and vegetables. Children should be encouraged but not necessarily forced to eat a variety of foods. Since many children avoid or refuse to eat vegetables, what should a concerned parent do? First, be sure that you and others at the table set a positive example. Second, a policy of taking "one bite" of every item on the plate may help a child overcome an aversion to a food over time. Furthermore, children may become more comfortable with a food if they participate in its preparation or serving. Perhaps even naming the dish after the child may increase interest.

Does Sugar Cause Hyperactivity in Children?

For many years researchers tried to link hyperactivity in children to a high-sugar diet. Much of the work completed in this area failed to show that a relationship exists. Hyperactivity or attention deficit hyperactivity disorder (ADHD) is currently believed to stem from a deficit in an individual's inhibitory processes in the brain. Although millions of children have been diagnosed with ADHD, many researchers believe that a significant percentage of those individuals did not actually have ADHD. Current treatment involves psychological treatment and/or taking an amphetamine-like substance called Ritalin (methylphenidate).

Do Sugary Foods Cause Acne?

High-sugar foods do not seem to contribute to acne development. Acne appears to be more related to hormones circulating in the blood. In many situations, acne results from a clogging of pores that connect oil-releasing glands to the surface of our skin. When pores become clogged, they may eventually become infected, inflamed, and rise up. Many dermatologists recommend keeping the face clean without overwashing. Overwashing can irritate and dry the skin. Dry, tight skin from excessive washing may narrow or close pore openings, doing more harm than good.

Do Sugary Foods Cause Cavities in Teeth?

It appears that perhaps the only direct cause-and-effect relationship between dietary sugar and disease is tooth decay. The warm and moist mouth is also exposed to the outside environment and is the entry point for food. Thus, the mouth becomes a natural home for bacteria. When sugary foods adhere to the teeth, bacteria can break down the sugar and produce acids that erode the outer layer of teeth, creating cavities. Brushing the teeth physically removes the sugar and much of the bacteria adhered to them. Furthermore, some toothpastes contain baking soda, which, as a base, may help neutralize the acid produced by bacteria.

Is Childhood and Adolescent Obesity an Issue?

At presence as much as 15 percent of children in the United States are considered obese and that number has increased over the past few decades. What's more, similar trends are occurring in other leading industrialized countries such as Australia and England. It appears that the combination of reduced activity, more television and computer time, and the increased availability of foods (especially calorie dense foods), have rendered youth heavier than ever before.

Childhood obesity is a growing problem and can lead to medical issues that continue though life.

Are There Medical and Social Concerns with Childhood Obesity?

Overweight children are fraught with many of the same concerns as adults. Socially, overweight and obese kids are subject to teasing and other negative peer interactions leaving them prone to feeling isolated. Medically, the incidence of Type 2 diabetes mellitus in overweight children continues to climb along with the diagnosis of hypercholesterolemia and hypertension. Sadly, about 40 percent of obese children and 70 percent of obese adolescents maintain their obese status into adulthood. In addition, obese children who achieve a healthier weight before becoming adults are more prone to obesity during adulthood than children who never were obese. This is a huge concern as we are all aware of the low success rates of weight reduction and maintenance in adults.

What Can Be Done to Reduce Childhood Obesity?

The key to lowering the number of obese children includes increasing their activity level and increasing nutrition and health awareness. Getting children as active as possible early in life is vital since they are forming many behaviors that will be with them throughout their lives. This is the responsibility of the parents at home and they should also be involved in planning and monitoring activity at day care centers and schools. Furthermore, parents should model an active lifestyle for their children to see and participate.

Furthermore, establishing healthier food choices and eating behaviors early in life is crucial. Again parents must model good choices and healthy behaviors. This can be a challenge as the television blitz of high-fat food commercials, such as cookies and snack chips, during child and teen programming seems to be very effective in boosting product sales along with the body fat of the targeted audience. Furthermore, food has never been so available to children and adolescents as they are today. On almost every child's walk to school or across town they encounter a convenience store, supermarket, cookie shop, pizza joint, or ice cream/yogurt parlor. Furthermore, parents should be involved in what foods are available in schools, whether it is vending or food service.

What Is Anorexia Nervosa?

Teens become a lot more involved in their self-image. A distorted body image for a teen, or an adult, may result in an eating disorder such as *anorexia nervosa*. Anorexia nervosa is more common in teenage, white middle-class females who engage in chronic energy restriction to accommodate their fear of being "fat." Even when their body weight is below ideal standards, they still consider themselves "fat" and continue the energy restriction. Combined with reductions in body weight from fat stores are also reductions in body protein. As the ritual continues, the reduction in body protein ultimately affects heart muscle and other vital organs and tissue. Thus, these individuals jeopardize their very existence. Anorexics are obsessed with food and may play with their food when dining with family. They may also have memorized the energy and fat content of most foods.

What Is Bulimia?

Bulimia is similar to anorexia nervosa in that individuals have a distorted self-image. However they will binge on food only to purge it shortly thereafter. It is not uncommon for a bulimic person to ingest several thousand calories of food in an hour or two. Usually the choice of food during this time includes snack chips, cookies, ice cream, pizza, candy, and other fast food. Self-induced vomiting and an engrossment in guilt shortly follow the eating binge. Bulimia is a self-perpetuating behavioral disorder, as the next food binge becomes a coping vehicle for guilt from the previous binge/purge episode. Physical signs of bulimia may include a discoloration of teeth from frequent vomiting and also cuts to fingers and knuckles from frequent induction of vomiting.

Can Someone Be Both Anorexic and Bulimic?

Often an individual will have disorder characteristics of both anorexia nervosa and bulimia, often called *bulimiarexia*. Both anorexia nervosa and bulimia are psychological disorders, which makes them somewhat difficult to treat. Typically treatment will include the efforts of an eating disorders counselor and a dietitian who specializes in eating disorders. Usually there is a root psychological issue that needs to be addressed. Today, many professionals are characterizing some patterns of overeating, leading to obesity, as an eating disorder as well. Here, food is used as a coping or comforting tool. Again, there are probably psychological issues at work here too.

Adults Are Faced with a New Set of Nutrition Concerns

What Nutrition-Based Issues Do Adults Face?

The threshold for adulthood is arbitrary and depends on whom you are asking. Some may define it based upon age, such as 18 years of age and greater. Others may take a more physiological approach and define it as the point at which one's greatest stature is reached. However, this latter explanation becomes problematic as some humans may reach their maximal stature in their teen years while others may not obtain their peak stature until their early twenties. While much of this book has discussed nutrition applicable to younger adults, most of the following discussion will focus upon older adults. However, alcohol consumption will first be addressed as the legal drinking age in the United States is 21. Also addressed will be the importance of young adulthood with regard to osteoporosis prevention. And in the next chapter the importance of the younger years of life to preventing heart disease and cancer will be discussed. Young to middle adulthood years are probably the most important years with regard to preventing the most significant diseases plaguing older adults, namely heart disease, cancer, and osteoporosis.

Is Alcohol Good or Bad for Our Health?

This may be one of the few books that even considers calling alcohol a nutrient. However, it does nourish our body by providing energy, and research has suggested that ingesting small amounts of alcoholic beverages daily is associated with a lower occurrence of heart disease. Alcoholic beverages contain antioxidants and other health-promoting nutrients. For instance, wine contains many polyphenolics substances such as EGCG (epigallocatechin gallate) as well as resveratrol that function as antioxidants and in other ways have a positive impact on aspects of health. This notion serves as the basis of the French Paradox, whereby the French have a dramatically lower incidence of heart disease despite eating and activity patterns that aren't that much different from Americans. The major difference appears to be based on the greater wine consumption.

What Is Alcohol and How Does the Body Metabolize It?

Alcohol is a substance called ethanol or ethyl alcohol. Alcohol is not made in the body, thus alcohol circulating in the blood has been derived from drinking alcohol-containing beverages. Many tissues throughout the body can break down alcohol, but the liver handles the majority of the task by far. In liver cells, alcohol can be used to make a substance called acetate (a short-chain fatty acid), which then leaves the liver and circulates to other tissue for further energy production.

Can Alcohol Consumption Affect the Metabolism of Other Energy Nutrients?

When alcohol is in the blood it is broken down in the liver preferentially before other energy nutrients. When alcohol is consumed in higher amounts, its metabolism can disrupt normal liver cell operations, especially those that generate glucose when blood glucose levels begin to fall. Therefore, it is not uncommon for blood glucose levels to fall below normal several hours after heavy drinking without eating food. This isn't a big concern when enjoying a glass of wine or two with dinner occasionally or having a couple of beers during the ball game. However, when the quantity and frequency of alcohol consumption increases this can eventually lead to complications.

What Are Some Concerns with Chronic over Consumption of Alcohol?

Long-term alcohol abuse also results in excessive accumulation of lipids and disease in liver cells (fatty liver) as well as other cells throughout the body. Alcohol-related liver disease is the sixth leading killer in the United States. Luckily, the most important liver cells (hepatocytes) can regenerate themselves if the damage is not too severe and the alcohol abuse ceases.

Other direct or indirect effects of alcohol abuse include impaired drug metabolism and elevated blood uric acid levels. The latter can lead to gout and kidney stones. Barbiturates, which are sedative drugs (pentothal, pentobarbital, seconal), are metabolized and inactivated by one of the same mechanisms that metabolizes alcohol. Since the metabolism of alcohol is given higher priority than the inactivation of barbiturates, these drugs stay active longer and build up in the body. Barbiturates depress the CNS, breathing, and heart activity. Therefore, combining barbiturates with alcohol can be a lethal combination.

How Does Metabolism Change as We Get Older?

As humans progress through life, many changes occur with regard to body function. One such change is a decrease in resting metabolic rate (RMR). Typically, daily calorie expenditure will generally not be as high as during younger years. Regular exercise can help minimize this reduction by slowing the loss of muscle tissue. In fact, when researchers studied the effects of weight training in older adults they found that their muscularity increased, as did their metabolic rate. So keep up the resistance training!

Daily caloric expenditure tends to decrease during aging largely because of changes in activity and body composition.

Researchers have also realized that levels of certain hormones may also decrease with age. We are all familiar with estrogen and menopause for women. Men too seem to experience reductions in testosterone as they age. In fact, physician-prescription testosterone for aging men has been called the hormone replacement therapy of the twenty-first century. Not every man's testosterone level decreases as they age, so the best thing to do is monitor the levels regularly. Also, adults of an even more advanced age tend to experience reduced digestive capabilities and decreased senses of taste, smell, and thirst—all of which can certainly impact their nutritional status.

How Does the Need for Vitamins and Minerals Change in Older Individuals?

Recent research studies have reported that people 51 years of age and older can maintain adequate vitamin A status on intakes approximating the RDA level for this group. Contrarily, the requirement for vitamin D in this population is increased dramatically based on a reduced ability to make vitamin D in the skin as we get older. Furthermore, there may be reductions in the ability to properly metabolize vitamin D in the organs, especially in the liver and kidneys. In accordance the AI for vitamin D for people over 50 is double that of younger adults and the recommendation is tripled for those over the age of 70. In addition, some research suggests that these levels of intake for older populations might still under serve their needs.

Some researchers believe that the RDA and AIs for other vitamins such as vitamin B_6 and B_{12} and riboflavin are also too low for older people. Increased vitamin E consumption may also be helpful in the prevention of heart disease. Furthermore, the reports of some scientific studies suggest that the 1200 milligrams recommendation for calcium may still be inadequate for people 51 years of age or older. For these and other reasons, a multivitamin and mineral supplement would benefit most adults over the age of 50.

Osteoporosis Is Bones with Holes

How Big of a Problem Is Osteoporosis?

Osteoporosis is a reduction in the density of bone. The remaining bone is then compromised in strength and resistance against fracture. The National Osteoporosis Foundation estimates that forty-four million Americans or about 55 percent of the people (including all races) age 50 and older will be affected by osteoporosis, which occurs six to eight times more frequently in women than in men. It is estimated that ten million adults already have osteoporosis, eight million of which are women, and as many as thirty-four million are estimated to have low bone mass (called osteopenia). In fact as many as a million and a half new fractures are attributable to osteoporosis in the United States each year. Sadly, many of these fractures result in permanent immobility.

Osteoporosis is a reduction in the density of bone, which includes reductions in minerals as well as proteins.

How Is Osteoporosis Diagnosed?

The World Health Organization (WHO) has set guidelines for characterizing the degree of bone loss. In order to do so, bone density must be compared with what is typically seen in younger people. *Osteopenia* is a level of bone density reduction that places a person at greater risk of fracture. It is said to be a measured bone density that is 1 to 2.5 standard deviations (a measure of statistical variability) below an average (or statistical mean) for a younger person of the same gender. Osteoporosis is more severe, whereby the reduction of bone density is greater than 2.5 standard deviations below the average. Individuals should talk to their physicians about where they are relative to others and X-ray measurements such as DXA (dual energy X-ray absorptiometry, see Chapter 8) are used in the diagnosis. Generally, osteoporosis develops without symptoms. It is usually not until a person fractures a bone or complains of severe back pain that an X-ray diagnosis is made.

What Is the Composition of Bone?

There are 206 bones in the human body and the entire skeleton represents about 12 percent and 15 percent of young adult women's and men's body weight, respectively. That is roughly 5.5 kilograms (15 pounds) for a woman and 11 kilograms (23 pounds) for a man. Typically, when we think of bone, we think of minerals such as calcium and phosphorus, but minerals make up only 30 to 40 percent of bone weight. Beyond minerals, bone is also composed of bone cells, nerves, blood vessels, collagen, and other proteins.

Is Bone Actively Modified?

Bone is often considered dead or at least inactive tissue. Maybe this comes from images of skeletons at Halloween or the bone fossils of animals that lived long ago. Whatever the case, bone is actually fairly active. It is constantly engaged in remodeling processes by bone cells called *osteoblasts* and *osteoclasts*. The osteoblasts are responsible for making and laying down new collagen protein and other substances. The collagen provides the network for the deposition of calcium and phosphorus mineral complexes such as hydroxyapatite to cling to. This is an important and often overlooked point, because without collagen you cannot properly mineralize bone. For this reason the osteoblasts are said to be active in making new bone tissue and are often called "bone makers."

Osteoporosis is caused by a general loss of minerals and protein from bone, rending it weaker.

Osteoclasts, on the other hand, are primarily responsible for initiating the events leading to the breakdown of bone substances. For this reason they are often called "bone destroyers." Osteoclasts ooze acids that will dissolve the mineral complexes as well as enzymes (collagenase) that will dissolve collagen. The actions of osteoclasts may seem destructive, but their role in bone remodeling is pivotal. Furthermore, when osteoclasts break down bone mineral complexes, the minerals can become available to the blood. This can be important in maintaining blood calcium levels if diet levels are low.

How Is Bone Remodeled?

The activities of osteoblasts and osteoclasts are indeed antagonistic and occur simultaneously. Therefore the body is building new bone at the same time as it is breaking down older bone. This is referred to as "bone turnover" and is similar to tearing up and pouring new concrete for a street or tearing down and constructing a new wall in a building. This reconstruction allows for that street or wall to be most appropriate in its functions.

Throughout life there are periods when the activities of these cells are out of balance. This can be purposeful or pathological. The imbalance in turnover results in either a net gain or loss of bone. For example, in childhood, as bones are lengthening and growing thicker, the activities of osteoblasts will exceed those of the osteoclasts, and new bone is built. On the contrary, in later adulthood, osteoclast cell activity tends to be greater than osteoblast activity. This results in a slow loss of bone. During periods when there is neither a net loss nor gain of bone, the activities of osteoblasts and osteoclasts are in balance and coordinated to properly remodel bone.

Even though a finalized bone length and therefore adult height is realized in the late teens to early twenties, bone is constantly being remodeled. The turnover process is governed by factors such as hormones (growth hormone, PTH, estrogen, testosterone, and calcitonin) and vitamin D. Mechanical forces, such as pressure exerted upon bone during resistance exercise, also play a big role in bone turnover. These factors affect bone remodeling primarily by increasing or decreasing the activity of osteoclasts and osteoblasts.

Is There a Point in Life When Bones Peak in Density?

Throughout the first few decades of human life, and providing that adequate minerals are provided by diet, the body deposits these minerals into bone in order to strengthen it and also to serve as a future mineral reservoir. Humans typically reach peak bone mass or maximal bone density by their late twenties to very early thirties. After this time, bone density seems to decrease slowly. So from a osteoporosis prevention standpoint, maximizing peak bone mass is crucial as discussed below.

How Much Bone Is Lost as Osteoporosis Develops?

The decrease in bone density appears to be more substantial in women versus men. It has been estimated that a woman may lose 27 percent or more of her bone mineral from peak bone mass to her seventies. Bone mineral losses of up to 50 percent have been reported in women diagnosed with osteoporosis. The point should again be made that while the focus has largely been on minerals, osteoporosis is a disease resulting from loss of bone material in general. This means that protein as well as minerals are lost, and as mentioned above, some researchers believe that the key to preventing osteoporosis may actually be found in preserving (and rebuilding) the collagen foundation. Without collagen, the minerals cannot properly stick in bone. Perhaps the analogy of hanging drywall on the wooden frame of a house will help. Here the wooden frame is collagen and the drywall is hydroxyapatite. In fact, hydroxyapatite crystals resemble sheets of drywall (see Figure 10.1).

How Is Estrogen Involved in the Loss of Bone Mineral?

A reduction in blood estrogen levels, as typical after menopause (post-menopausal), is directly associated with a decrease in bone density. Thus, estrogen is a principal factor in the development of osteoporosis. Researchers have reported that osteoblasts (bone makers) have receptors for the hormone estrogen, and estrogen also appears to decrease the activity of osteoclasts (bone destroyers). Despite these findings, the exact mechanisms for how estrogen protects women against excessive bone material losses is not clear. Postmenopausal estrogen replacement therapy has proven effective in slowing the rate of postmenopausal bone mineral loss in women; however, there are other medical concerns and each women should understand these.

What Nutritional and Behavioral Factors Are Important in Preventing Osteoporosis?

Beyond reductions in circulating estrogen in postmenopausal women, other factors can increase the loss of bone mineral. These factors include poor calcium and/or vitamin D intake as well as abnormalities in metabolism. Additionally, physical activity increases the mechanical stress placed on bone and stimulates a reinforcement of bone strength. Perhaps this effect is most obvious in the absence of any weight-bearing demands upon bone. For instance, astronauts subjected to extended periods of time in space at zero gravity (weightlessness) experience decreases in bone density. On the other hand, regular weight-bearing exercise seems to help strengthen bone and also to slow the gradual loss of bone material as the body ages.

Smoking seems to exert a negative influence upon bone mineral content and the rate of bone mineral loss, especially in postmenopausal years. Smokers tend to have lower bone densities than nonsmokers. One reason for this occurrence is that smoking reduces blood estrogen levels. Smokers also seem to reach menopause at a younger age.

Can Osteoporosis Occur Earlier in Life?

Although osteoporosis is most often diagnosed in postmenopausal women, it should be noted that signs of osteoporosis have been observed in younger women as well. Younger female athletes who are excessively lean can reduce or halt their estrogen production and establish the opportunity for bone loss. In addition, the positive effects of weight-bearing exercise are not apparent in excessively lean women. The positive effects of resistance training will not balance out the negative impact of reduced estrogen levels. Anorexia nervosa, which is most common in teenage and younger adult women, is characterized by abnormally low body weight. This state can also reduce estrogen production and invoke bone demineralization.

What Are the Most Conventional Ways to Prevent Osteoporosis?

The best defense against osteoporosis is a good offense. Some weight-bearing exercise and a diet (with supplementation) providing adequate protein, vitamin D, calcium, magnesium, boron, zinc, vitamin C, copper, and iron in the years prior to peak bone mass will optimize bone density. Copper, iron, and vitamin C are important for making proper collagen. An early start and a continuation of these practices throughout adulthood in conjunction with regular medical checkups and a periodic X-ray will provide the most benefit. In fact, it seems that one of the most important times for the positive effects of activity on bone density is during the prepuberty years. Children should be encouraged to be involved in physical activities. Furthermore, women should discuss menopausal/postmenopausal hormone replacement therapy with a physician. Do not smoke and encourage others to quit as well.

> Regular exercise and adequate intake of calcium, and vitamins D and C support bone health.

Can Soy Help Prevent Osteoporosis?

Some of the most promising nutraceutical substances in the prevention of osteoporosis are isoflavones found mostly in soybeans and soy foods (tofu, tempeh, and miso). There are about twelve forms of isoflavones in soy, including genestein and daidzein. Researchers believe that these factors may have the ability to bind to estrogen receptors and that would include those in bone tissue. At this time scientists are optimistic that a positive link exists between soy or isoflavone consumption and bone health. However, it will probably take time and a few more well performed human studies to draw more specific conclusions. So at this time it would seem wise to include some soy in the diet (Table 12.3).

Table 12.3 Ways to Improve Your Soy Intake

- Eat soy nuts out of hand as you would roasted peanuts or use in party mix or chop up and use to replace other nuts in baking, scatter on your chef's salad.
- Cook fresh green soybeans (also called edamame) as you would lima beans and serve as a fresh vegetable. The fresh soybeans have a sweet taste like peas.
- Use dry soybeans as you would use other dried beans. Soak overnight, cook slowly 1 to 2 hours, then use where the recipe calls for kidney, pinto, black, or navy beans.
- Use soy milk in place of regular milk when cooking (puddings, soups, cream sauces) and baking (cakes, cookies, yeast, and quick breads).
- Replace up to one-fourth of the total flour in a baked recipe with soy flour.
- Blend softer tofu with tomato sauce or a can of cream soup.
- Use tofu in place of mayonnaise or sour cream in salad dressings or dips.
- Substitute for all or part of the cream cheese in a cheesecake.
- Use in place of cottage, ricotta, and mozzarella cheese in stuffed pasta shells, manicotti, or lasagna.
- Use firm tofu in salads, stir-frys, and soups.
- Make "egg" salad: cut tofu into small pieces, add celery, onion, salt, pepper, low-fat mayonnaise, and mustard.
- Marinate tofu cubes in teriyaki sauce. Grill on skewers with sweet peppers, cherry tomatoes, mushrooms, and zucchini.
- Use in place of beef, pork, or chicken in a stir-fry, fajita or create-a-meal dish.
- Barbecue tempeh, crumble it in chilli, stews, and soups or make it into sloppy joes.
- Cube for kabobs after marinated in teriyaki and broiling or grilling.
- Crumble it and use in recipes where you would use ground beef or small chunks of meat, like taco meat, burrito meat or spaghetti sauce.
- Top a pizza with tempeh crumbles.
- Add a couple of slices of soy cheese as you prepare macaroni and cheese.
- Use in recipes calling for cheese, baked and unbaked.

Can Caffeine or Coffee Cause Osteoporosis?

The results of a couple of studies revealed a correlation between excessive coffee consumption and a higher hip-fracture rate. However, even if there is a true effect many researchers believe that there is a safe level of consumption. It does seem that one to three cups of coffee a day probably does not factor into the development of osteoporosis.

13 Nutrition, Heart Disease, and Cancer

A little more than a century ago, infectious diseases including smallpox, tuberculosis, cholera, typhoid, and yellow fever were among the major killers of Americans. Today, advancements in medicine have controlled or nearly eliminated diseases like these. However, we are left to deal with seemingly more complicated killers, namely cardiovascular disease and cancer. When combined, these two diseases account for roughly 60 percent of the deaths of adults in the United States. In Canada and Australia heart disease and cancer are also very prominent medical problems as in other developed countries.

As prominent as cardiovascular disease and cancer are, many health professionals are convinced that these diseases are largely preventable or their critical points can be pushed back years to decades for most people. Nutritional intake has proven to be one of the most important factors with regard to the prevention and treatment of these diseases. The influence of nutrition can be both a matter of what is eaten that supports the development of these diseases or supports the prevention or slows the progression of these diseases.

> Heart disease and cancer account for more than 60 percent of deaths in the US

Information on these diseases is certainly abundant. However, the websites developed by the American Heart Association (www.americanheart.org) and the American Cancer Society (www.cancer.org) are very informative and helpful in understanding these diseases.

Cardiovascular Disease: A Matter of Plumbing Problems?

Diseases of the heart and cardiovascular system are many, but "heart disease" is the term most often used to address a condition in which atherosclerotic development in the arteries of the heart (coronary arteries) impedes blood flow within the heart itself. When blood flow through a coronary artery is inhibited, the region of the heart that it supplies suffers—in fact, when the condition becomes critical, that tissue suffocates as it doesn't get enough oxygen. This type of heart disease is called coronary heart disease, coronary artery disease, or atherosclerotic heart disease. Like many medical terms, atherosclerosis has its roots in the Greek language. *Athero* means gruel or paste and *sclerosis* means hardness.

The heart, which is largely made up of muscle cells, relies almost exclusively upon aerobic energy metabolism. Heart muscle cells die in a short period of time (minutes) if they are deprived of oxygen. When cells in a region of the heart die, it is medically known as an infarction and is realized in the form of a *heart attack*. The medical term *myocardial infarction* (MI) means death of heart muscle cells.

What Are the Major Components Involved in Atherosclerosis?

Atherosclerosis is a complex process with many players. The major players of atherosclerosis include:

- lipoproteins
- macrophages
- platelets
- smooth muscle cells
- calcium-based mineral complexes
- connective tissue proteins

What Are Macrophages?

Macrophages are derived from monocytes, which are a type of white blood cell. Remember that many white blood cells function by recognizing substances that are either foreign or no longer of use to the body and then facilitate its destruction. They are the protectors of the body, sort of "biological bodyguards" if you will.

Circulating monocytes normally leave the blood by squeezing through the wall of blood vessels and patrol the spaces in-between the cells. While patrolling, if monocytes come in contact with something that does not belong, they swell and engulf the material. These swollen, aggressive monocytes are referred to as macrophages which literally means "big eater"!

What Are Lipoproteins and What Do They Do?

As discussed several times in this book, lipoproteins are a normal component of the blood. They function to shuttle lipids, which are water-insoluble substances such as fat, cholesterol, and other nutrients throughout the body in circulation. They are in effect lipid-laden submarines. Since the cholesterol in the blood is found aboard lipoproteins, total blood cholesterol is the sum of the cholesterol being carried in the different types of lipoproteins. A clinical laboratory is able to determine the quantity of cholesterol in each lipoprotein class (for example, HDL-cholesterol or LDL-cholesterol).

Where Does Low Density Lipoprotein Come from and What Does It Do?

You will also recall that the liver packages up cholesterol and fat (triglyceride) into very low density lipoproteins (VLDLs), which are then released into the blood. As VLDLs circulate, they unload their fat cargo with most of it going to fat (adipose) tissue and other tissue such as skeletal muscle and the heart. As they lose their fat, VLDLs become LDLs, which are mostly cholesterol. As LDLs circulate they drop off cholesterol in tissue throughout the body and are eventually removed from the blood by the liver and other tissue.

Where Does High Density Lipoprotein Come from and What Does It Do?

HDLs are made by the liver and intestines. As HDLs circulate they pick up excessive cholesterol from tissue throughout the body. HDLs then transfer this cholesterol back to LDLs, which are subject to removal from the blood, or HDLs themselves are removed from the blood by the liver. In either case, much of the cholesterol that HDLs accumulate on their journey is returned to the liver. So in essence LDLs are cholesterol delivery vehicles, while HDLs go out and pick up the excess.

Where Does Atherosclerosis Happen?

Our arteries can be thought of as blood-filled tubes, the walls of which contain distinct layers. The innermost layer, or the layer closest to the blood, is called the *intima* (Figure 13.1). The middle layer is referred to as the media, as it sits in the middle of the wall. In-between the intima and the surging blood is a thin layer of cells, which is covered with a fine layer of connective tissue proteins (for example, collagen). It is within the intima that atherosclerosis develops. Damage to the cell lining and connective tissue is often referred to as "injury" and that creates the opportunity for atherosclerosis to develop. Furthermore, cells found in the media will participate in the development of atherosclerosis.

Although atherosclerosis can occur in arteries throughout the body, the most common sites are in those arteries supplying the brain and heart.

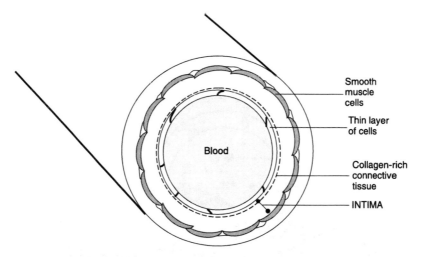

Figure 13.1 Basic anatomy of an artery. The intima is the site of atherosclerosis development.

Interestingly, atherosclerosis is much more common at branching points in arteries. This is where blood flow is more turbulent. Hindrance of blood flow within the brain and heart can result in a stroke or heart attack, respectively.

What Is Atherosclerosis?

Atherosclerosis is the process that allows for the buildup of substances within the walls of arteries. This buildup or *plaque* consists mostly of lipid, protein, and calcium in conjunction with an excessive presence of macrophages and smooth muscle cells. The lipid is mostly cholesterol derived from LDLs while the protein is largely collagen.

As the atherosclerotic plaque grows in size, it causes the wall of that artery to protrude further and further into the blood vessel. This in turn decreases the area for blood to flow through (Figure 13.2). If the narrowing becomes severe enough, it becomes an occlusion and blood flow is reduced to a critical level. Furthermore, if a blood clot develops in this location or it circulates to and gets lodged in this narrowed area, it will dam up blood flow. This is often how heart attacks occur, making them seem so sudden—heart tissue "downstream" does not receive the oxygen that it needs to survive.

How Does Atherosclerosis Occur?

Scientists believe that an initial injury must occur to the cell wall lining an artery to kick things off. Then a continual insult must occur to allow for

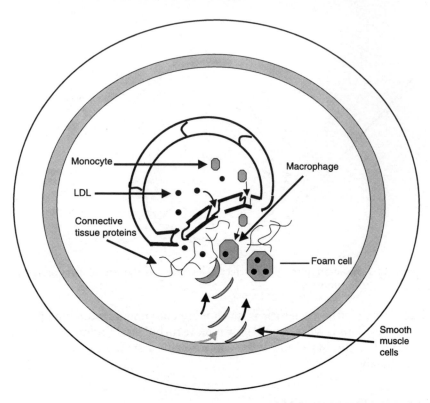

Figure 13.2 Injury to the wall of an artery allows LDLs and monocytes access to the intima. Monocytes become macrophages and smooth muscle cells also migrate into the intima. Both macrophages and smooth muscle cells engulf LDLs, especially after it is oxidized. Smooth muscle cells produce connective tissue proteins and calcium becomes deposited in the intima as well.

atherosclerosis to progress. The injury allows for monocytes to leave the blood and enter into the wall. The injured cells lining the artery release chemicals that signal monocytes to come in. Platelets arriving on the scene to patch the artery wall also release chemicals. Some of the chemicals encourage the relocation of smooth muscle cells from the media to the intima. More and more LDLs also move through the injury opening. So what we have is a mixture of stuff arriving in the intima and in excess of normal operations.

The monocytes, which are soon transformed into insatiably hungry macrophages, begin to ingest the LDLs in the intima. LDL can become modified (*oxidized LDLs*) by free radicals from cigarette smoke, environmental pollutants, foods, or produced in the body and macrophages find oxidized LDL most delicious. The ingestion of oxidized LDLs by macrophages gives them a foamy appearance when seen with a microscope and they are often referred to as *foam cells*. Furthermore, smooth muscle cells begin to release fibrous proteins into the area, and calcium-rich complexes also begin to accumulate. While all this is happening, new monocytes and LDLs continuously arrive on the scene from the blood and smooth muscle cells migrate from the media. So the process continues.

> Atherosclerosis occurs within the walls of arteries and slowly reduces blood flow.

When Does Atherosclerosis Begin?

Although the medical complications of atherosclerosis (heart attack or stroke) occur suddenly, the disease really develops over a very long stretch of time (Table 13.1). Atherosclerosis is a chronic degenerative disease, which means that the inception of atherosclerosis may be established very early in life and progresses from there to a critical point. In fact, cadavers of children have shown evidence that the foundations of atherosclerosis may be noticeable as early as 10 to 12 years of age. Therefore, it should be realized that atherosclerosis is not a disease of old age but of a lifetime. It can take decades for the blockage to reach a critical point and blood flow to become insufficient or for a blood clot to become lodged in a partially blocked vessel.

Many Factors Contribute To Heart Disease

What Are the Risk Factors Associated with Heart Disease?

Certain aspects of atherosclerosis, as well as its rate of progression, have an underlying genetic nature, meaning that family history or heredity is

Table 13.1 Warning Signs of a Heart Attack

For many people atherosclerosis may be undetected as early warning signs of a heart attack have not been experienced. Therefore when the heart attack does occur it seems unexpected and happens suddenly and without warning. In fact about half of the people in the United States who die of heart disease can be characterized as having sudden cardiac death. This means that early detection is very important.

Warning signs
- chest pain (angina)
- shortness of breath
- light headedness
- unexplainable nausea
- mild anxiety

important. Furthermore, we are greater risk of a heart attack and stroke as we get older and men seem to be at greater risk than women at least up to their postmenopausal years when the risk becomes about the same. These risk factors are often described as "uncontrollable" since we can't really do anything about our heredity, age, or gender.

Since atherosclerosis is believed to exist to some degree in most people, disease management should be practiced by everyone throughout our lifetime, beginning in childhood. Various aspects of our lifestyle that influence the development of atherosclerosis are under our control. These include:

- achieving and/or maintaining a healthy body weight
- maintaining healthy total and LDL and HDL cholesterol levels and triglycerides
- maintaining healthy blood pressure levels
- managing blood glucose levels
- not smoking
- exercising regularly, especially cardiovascular (aerobic) exercise
- minimizing saturated fat and cholesterol intake as a part of a healthy diet plan
- choosing more whole grains and fruits and vegetables
- having regular health check ups

How Important Are Blood Lipids in Determining the Risk of Heart Disease and Stroke?

LDLs are a major player in the development of atherosclerosis. Because elevations in LDL-cholesterol are associated with increased risk of heart disease and stroke, it is often deemed the "bad cholesterol." Although it may not be this simple, higher LDL-cholesterol levels means that there are more LDLs in the blood, which in turn means more LDLs that can participate in atherosclerosis.

On the other hand, HDL-cholesterol seems to decreases the risk of heart disease and it is often referred to as the "good cholesterol." Researchers believe that the virtuous nature of HDLs is due to their ability to gather some of the cholesterol associated with atherosclerotic plaque. This could slow the progression of atherosclerosis. In addition, HDLs carry antioxidants which can reduce LDL oxidation.

> Higher levels of LDL cholesterol are linked to greater risk of heart disease.

What Are Recommendations for Blood Lipids?

A blood lipid profile can help to assess an individual's risk. Among the several telling indicators are elevated total and LDL-cholesterol levels, reduced HDL-cholesterol levels, and elevated ratios of total cholesterol to HDL-cholesterol and LDL-cholesterol to HDL-cholesterol levels. However the American Heart Association suggests that physicians and individuals pay closer attention to the individual measurements versus the ratios. Table 13.2 provides the association's goals for blood cholesterol and triglyceride levels.

What Factors Raise Total and LDL Cholesterol?

LDL is called bad cholesterol because as its level increases in the blood, so does the risk of heart disease. As mentioned above, the more LDL in the blood, the more LDL can move into the artery walls and participate in atherosclerosis. The primary factors that seem to raise total and LDL cholesterol levels are:

- smoking
- inactive lifestyle
- obesity
- high saturated fat intake

Table 13.2 Standard Levels for Blood Lipids and Cardiovascular Risk

	Classification and Consideration
Total Cholesterol	
<200	Considered a desirable level for total cholesterol
200 to 239	This is a borderline high level
≥ 240	This is high total cholesterol as it is associated with more than two times greater risk of developing coronary heart disease compared with a total cholesterol is less than 200 milligrams per deciliter.
LDL Cholesterol	
<100	Considered a very desirable level for LDL cholesterol
100 to 129	This is a desirable level for LDL cholesterol to borderline high level
130 to 159	Considered a borderline high LDL cholesterol level
160 to 189	High LDL cholesterol level
≥ 190	Very high LDL cholesterol
HDL Cholesterol	
<40 (men) and <50 (women)	Considered low HDL cholesterol
≥60 mg/ 100 ml	This is a desirable level for HDL cholesterol
Triglycerides	
<150	Considered a very desirable level for triglycerides
150 to 200	This is borderline high triglycerides level
>200	Considered high triglycerides level

Hypertension Hurts the Heart and Blood Vessels

What Is Hypertension?

Hypertension is a disorder of circulation in which elevated blood pressure results in increased tension in the walls of the blood vessels. Since it is impossible to routinely measure blood vessel wall tension, hypertension is assessed indirectly by measuring blood pressure. Thus, high blood pressure and hypertension are used to describe the same condition. Almost one in three adults in the United States and Australia and one in five Canadian adults have high blood pressure. In addition, there is higher incidence in African-American adults than Caucasian or Hispanic-American adults. However, no one is safe.

Despite such high occurrence, many people (perhaps 30 percent) with high blood pressure don't even realize their blood pressure is elevated. This is because they have not really experienced significant symptoms or have not had a physical examination in a long time. For these reasons, high blood pressure is often referred to as the "silent killer."

How Is High Blood Pressure Diagnosed?

Typically, a resting blood pressure greater than 140/90 (read as "140 over 90") is regarded as high blood pressure or hypertension. Here, 140 is the *systolic* blood pressure (measured in millimeters of mercury) or the pressure in large arteries when the heart contracts. In contrast, the 90 refers to *diastolic* blood pressure or the pressure in large arteries when the heart relaxes. Many physicians consider blood pressure measures under 120/80 to be healthier. That means that a systolic of 120 or higher but below 140 and a diastolic of 80 or higher but below 90 mmHg is considered borderline high blood pressure.

Why Is Hypertension Deleterious?

Chronic hypertension is a medical problem for at least two reasons. First, if the pressure in the arteries is elevated, as occurs in hypertension, the heart has to work harder to generate more pressure to keep the blood flowing. This extra work causes the heart muscle to become overworked and become enlarged (hypertrophy). Over time an enlarging heart from high blood pressure can become dysfunction and eventually fail. The second complication associated with chronic hypertension is that the elevated pressure can traumatize blood vessel walls, which leaves them more susceptible to atherosclerotic development, as explained previously. Hypertension can result in other medical complications such as damage to nephrons, the tiny blood processing units of the kidneys.

High blood pressure physical damages artery walls thereby promoting atherosclerosis.

What Factors Are Associated with Hypertension?

Obesity is associated with the development of hypertension. In many obese people, reductions in blood pressure go hand in hand with reductions in body fat. In addition, if exercise is incorporated into the weight-reduction program, blood pressure is reduced beyond that which can be accounted for by weight loss alone. Stress reduction has also been shown to lower elevated blood pressure significantly. Furthermore, individual diet components such as high-fat and high-saturated-fat foods as well as high-sodium foods have been associated with the development of hypertension.

The relationship between diets high in sodium and hypertension does not seem to exist in everyone and will be realized in only about 10 percent of people with high blood pressure. These people are sometimes labeled "salt sensitive." This means that their blood pressure can be reduced by following a low-sodium diet (2 grams of sodium/day or less). Finally, smoking and/or chronic and excessive alcohol consumption is also associated with hypertension.

How Is High Blood Pressure Treated?

Ideally, the treatment of high blood pressure begins with nonpharmaceutical intervention, meaning no drugs. If a person is overweight, weight reduction is encouraged; heavy drinkers are encouraged to cut down their intake. Regular cardiovascular exercise and stress management is strongly encouraged. If these practices are not successful in reducing the hypertension, then the next step usually includes medication in conjunction with dietary and behavior modifications.

What Kinds of Drugs Are Used to Treat High Blood Pressure?

Drugs collectively known as *antihypertensives* are used to treat high blood pressure (Table 13.3). These drugs generally fall into a few categories which are:

- *Calcium antagonists* (Ca channel blockers)—These drugs slow heart rate and relax blood vessels. Therefore they may decrease blood pressure by addressing both cardiac output and circulation resistance.

Table 13.3 Common Drugs (Trade Name) Used to Treat Hypertension

Beta-blockers	Calcium antagonists	ACE inhibitors
Propanolol (Inderal)	Verapamil (Calan, Isoptin,	Captopril (Capoten)
Nadolo (Corgard)	Verelan)	Enalapril (Vasotec)
Timolol (Blocadren)	Felodipine (Plendil,	Lisinopril (Prinivil,
Atenolol (Tenormin)	Renedil)	Zestril)
Metoprolol (Betaloc,	Diltiazem (Cardzem)	Ramipril (Altace)
Lopressor)	Nimodipine (Nimptop)	Qunapril (Accupril)
Acebutolol (Sectral)	Nifedipine (Adalat)	Fosinopril (Monopril)
Oxprenolol (Trasicor)		Amlodipine (Norvasc)
Pindolol (Visken)		Nicardipine (Cardene)
Labetalol (Trandate)		

- *ACE inhibitors*—These drugs act by decreasing the activity of an enzyme in the blood called angiotensin converting enzyme (ACE). Angiotensin loosely translates to vascular tension. This enzyme is responsible for activating a hormone called angiotensin to its active form. Active angiotensin (angiotensin II) is a potent constrictor of blood vessels and also increases aldosterone levels in the blood. Aldosterone in turn can increase the volume of the blood by decreasing the loss of sodium in the urine. The extra sodium in the blood attracts water, which thus swells blood volume. This in turn may increase blood pressure by increasing the resistance of blood flow through blood vessels. Other drugs act to decrease the potency of angiotensin by interfering with its ability to interact with its receptors.
- *Beta-blockers*—These drugs work by decreasing heart rate and stroke volume by decreasing the potency of norepinephrine (noradrenaline). To do so the beta-blockers "block" the ability of norepinephrine to interact with receptors called beta-adrenergic receptors.
- *Diuretics*—These drugs work by increasing water loss in urine, which in turn can decrease blood volume, which then may decrease blood pressure.

Foods, Nutrients, and Heart Disease

How Does Food Cholesterol Impact the Development of Heart Disease?

One of the earliest recommendations for reducing blood cholesterol levels was to follow a low cholesterol diet. However, it soon became apparent that blood cholesterol levels are influenced more by how much saturated fat is eaten rather than cholesterol. Cholesterol is derived from animal foods; as a general rule, animal foods that are higher in saturated fat usually contain cholesterol. Focusing on reducing the level of saturated fat in the diet usually results in a reduction in diet cholesterol as well.

About 500 to 1,000 milligrams of cholesterol is made in the body daily, with the liver producing the most. What's more, the level of production in the liver can be affected by diet levels, meaning as diet consumption goes up, production goes down and vice versa. Thus, the negative impact of eating more cholesterol may not be as significant as we think. For instance, the impact of eating a diet containing 400 milligrams of cholesterol versus 300 milligrams of cholesterol a day results in an increase of only a couple of milligrams of total blood cholesterol.

How Does Saturated Fat Influence Risk Factors for Heart Disease?

Eating a diet higher in saturated fat seems to increase total and LDL-cholesterol levels. Most, but not all saturated fatty acids seem to have the ability to raise blood cholesterol levels. These saturated fatty acids may impact blood cholesterol levels by slowing the mechanisms that remove circulating LDL from the blood and potentially increasing production of cholesterol in the liver. As a result, there is a general increase in LDL and total cholesterol levels.

How Can Saturated Fatty Acids Slow the Removal of Cholesterol from the Blood?

The types of fatty acids eaten will be reflected by the fatty acid composition in the plasma membranes (phospholipid fatty acids). When more of the fatty acids are saturated, and thus fairly straight, neighboring molecules can get closer making the membrane more crowded and less dynamic (fluid). When LDL receptors surface on the plasma membrane, they actually must migrate to anchoring sites (Figure 13.3). Once they are anchored they can then bind circulating LDLs and bring it into that cell. The LDL is then broken down and the cholesterol is available to that cell. Meanwhile the receptor is then able to resurface on the plasma membrane and migrate to the anchoring site. This process is often called LDL receptor cycling and the rate-limiting step is the LDL receptor migration from its surfacing site to its anchoring site. Therefore if the migration takes longer, the whole cycle takes longer and less LDL is removed from the blood throughout the day.

How Do Unsaturated Fatty Acids Affect Cholesterol Levels?

Regarding unsaturated fatty acids, neither monounsaturated fatty acids (MUFAs) nor polyunsaturated fatty acids (PUFAs) have a

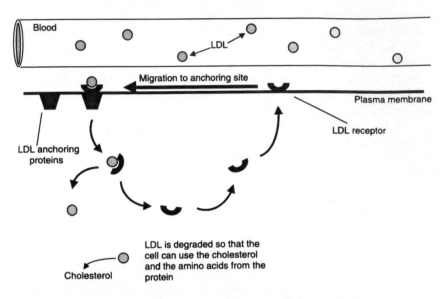

Figure 13.3 LDL receptors surface at one point in the plasma membrane and then must migrate to anchoring proteins. Once anchored, LDL can interact with the LDL receptor and the LDL/LDL receptor complex enters our cell. The LDL receptor then dumps the LDL and resurfaces on the plasma membrane. Meanwhile the LDL is degraded so that the cholesterol can be used by that cell.

cholesterol-elevating impact. In fact, if they are used to replace saturated fatty acids in the diet, total cholesterol will probably be lowered. This is especially true for people whose blood cholesterol levels were elevated well above recommended levels. This is one reason why populations consuming higher fat intakes, with less of the fat via saturated fat sources, enjoy lower rates of heart disease.

How Does Olive Oil and Oleic Acid Impact Heart Disease?

Much interest in MUFA, namely oleic acid, was generated when studies of heart disease in various populations around the world revealed that certain Mediterranean countries enjoyed a relatively lower incidence of heart disease despite eating a diet that would be considered rich in fat. Further evaluation revealed that these people ingested much of their fat in the form of olive oil, which has a high percentage (77 percent) of the MUFA oleic acid. This resulted in several research studies which determined that when oleic acid replaced palmitic acid in a diet, blood cholesterol levels were lowered by decreasing the amount of LDL-cholesterol in the blood. Researchers also determined that while this significantly impacted heart disease risk it didn't explain all of the cardioprotective effects of olive oil consumption. Olive oil contains antioxidants such as phenolic compounds (for example, hydroxytyrosol, tyrosol, oleuropein) and other nutraceuticals that can promote a healthier cardiovascular system.

Olive oil doesn't raise cholesterol levels and contains antioxidants that can protect arteries.

How Does Linoleic Acid (Omega-6 PUFA) Impact Heart Disease?

When saturated fat is replaced in the diet with polyunsaturated fat, total and LDL-cholesterol levels are reduced, particularly in people with elevated levels. In fact, linoleic acid, an omega-6 fatty acid, is likely to be the most potent fatty acid when it comes to lowering blood cholesterol levels in this manner. By lowering total and LDL cholesterol, heart disease risk is lowered. Linoleic acid can be found in safflower, sunflower, corn, soybean, and canola oils. So replacing animal fat with plant fat (oil) could be helpful in preventing heart disease. However, one important consideration is that the level of omega-6 fatty acids should be in a healthy ratio with omega-3 fatty acids as explained below.

How Do Omega-3 Fatty Acids Impact Heart Disease?

Omega-3 PUFAs, such as linolenic acid and DHA (docosahexaenoic acid) and EPA (eicosapentaenoic acid) can have a favorable impact, lowering the risk of cardiovascular disease. However, since omega-3 fatty acids have not been shown to lower blood cholesterol levels in a consistent manner in research studies, the cardioprotective effects must extend beyond that mechanism. For instance, omega-3 fatty acid intake is associated with:

- decreased risk of arrhythmias that can lead to sudden cardiac death
- decreased risk of blood clots (thrombosis) that can lead to heart attacks or stokes
- lower serum triglyceride levels
- slowing the growth of atherosclerosis process (plaque formation)
- improving the function of blood vessel walls
- decreasing inflammation

Thus the positive impact of omega-3 fatty acids extends well beyond simply reducing LDL and total cholesterol. It is more likely that much of the cardioprotective benefits of omega-3 fats is based on the formation of particular eicosanoid factors as discussed below. EPA and DHA are found in Atlantic and Pacific herring, Atlantic halibut and salmon, coho, albacore tuna, bluefish, lake trout, and pink and king salmons. It is probably a good idea to include these fish in a regular diet a couple of times a week. Linolenic acid, which can be converted to DHA and EPA is found in canola oil and soybean oil, and in even smaller amounts in corn oil, beef fat, and lard.

Is the Ratio of Omega-6 to Omega-3 Important and What Ratio Is Best?

At this time, linoleic (18:2 omega-6) and alpha-linolenic acid (18:3 omega-3) are considered the dietary essential fatty acids. These fatty acids can be used to make a family of hormone-like substances called eicosanoids (thromboxanes, prostaglandins, prostacyclins, and leukotrienes) as shown in Figure 5.11. In addition, EPA (eicosapentaenoic acid) and DHA (docosahexaenoic acid) are omega-3 PUFAs in fish and other sea animals and can substitute for linolenic acid. In fact, EPA is the starting omega-3 fatty acid for derived eicosanoids, and the omega-6 fatty acids arachidonic and dihomogamma linolenic acid are used to make the eicosanoids derived from omega-6.

Many of the eicosanoids made from omega-3 fatty acids reduce some of the key operations involved in atherosclerosis and heart attacks. For instance, one prostaglandin called prostacyclin or PGI_2 is very potent inhibitor of blood clotting. This seems to be very significant as many heart attacks occur because blood clots form or become lodged in a narrowed coronary artery. Other omega-3 fatty acid based eicosanoids reduce inflammation, a key process in atherosclerosis and promote vasodilation to allow for better blood flow through heart arteries. This helps us understand why individuals who eat diets higher in omega-3 fatty acids, such as certain Eskimo populations, show a lower incidence of heart disease. In general a ratio of around 4 to 1 (omega-6 to omega-3) is recommended.

A healthy balance of omega-6 to omega-3 fatty acids supports a healthy heart.

Should Fish Oil Supplements Be Used to Promote a Healthy Cardiovascular System?

At this time there is enough supporting research to suggest that anyone not consuming ample fish or other seafood should take a fish oil supplement to derive the beneficial omega-3 fatty acids—DHA and EPA. In fact, many people are avoiding fish and other seafood today because of concerns related to the level of heavy metals such as mercury in seafood. Furthermore, the conversation of alpha-linolenic acid to EPA and DHA might not be as efficient as needed for optimal health, especially during certain situations such as in older people.

People with high blood cholesterol (total and LDL) and triglyceride levels who take fish oil supplements might experience reductions in one or both, particularly the latter. In addition, fish oil supplementation has also been suggested to lower blood pressure in people with high blood pressure as well as improving glucose tolerance in Type 2 diabetes. For many people, fish oil supplementation can modestly reduce blood pressure and with regard to improving glucose levels in people with Type 2 diabetes, more research is needed to better understand whether or not there is benefit.

Do Trans *Fatty Acids Increase the Risk of Heart Disease?*

Trans fatty acids are naturally found in low percentages in most animal fats, including milk and dairy products. These fatty acids are made by bacteria in the stomachs of cows and other grazing animals, by converting *cis* unsaturated fatty acids in grass and leaves to *trans* (see Chapter 5). Furthermore, when vegetable oils are hydrogenated, some of the points of unsaturation are converted from a *cis* to a *trans* design. It does appear that *trans* fatty acids impact blood lipids in many people by raising total and LDL-cholesterol when compared with oils containing unsaturated fatty acids. In addition, HDL-cholesterol levels may also be reduced. Thus the important message is that *trans* fatty acids can have an unhealthy effect similar to saturated fatty acids. Thus, one of the most potent ways to lower your total and LDL cholesterol is to limit saturated fat and *trans* fatty acid levels in your diet.

> *Trans* fatty acids promote heart disease in a manner similar to saturated fat.

What Other Dietary Factors Influence the Development of Heart Disease?

Beyond fat and cholesterol, other dietary factors appear to impact the development of atherosclerosis. Studies investigating different diets and the incidence of heart disease have shown that diets richer in fruits and vegetables, fiber, and possibly other diet-derived factors, such as garlic, are associated with a lower incidence of the disease. Fruits and vegetables probably exert a beneficial effect in several ways. First, they can replace fat- or cholesterol-rich foods and also provide more essential nutrients compared with less nutrient-dense foods. Second, fruits, vegetables, and whole grains are sources of health-promoting factors called nutraceuticals which will be discussed next. In addition, smoking has a negative impact by introducing numerous free-radical compounds as well as possibly raising blood pressure. On the other hand, regular exercise can promote cardiovascular health by improving circulation, increasing HDLs, and lowering triglycerides and improving body weight/composition and glucose tolerance.

Does Supplemental Vitamin C Help Deter Atherosclerotic Development?

Vitamin C is a water-soluble antioxidant and several research studies suggest that people with higher intakes (over 300 milligrams/day) by way of food and supplementation can have a positive impact on cardiovascular health. Meanwhile, other research suggests that maximal status of vitamin C can be achieved at levels approximating 400 milligrams daily. This provides a good level of recommendation for adults (non-smokers) to help prevent heart disease.

Can Vitamin E Help Prevent Heart Disease?

Vitamin E provides some protection against heart disease as it circulates throughout the body aboard lipoproteins. As discussed, one of the primary factors associated with atherosclerotic development is the oxidation of fatty acids and proteins in LDL to form oxidized LDL. Vitamin E may provide some antioxidant protection for these molecules. Several large population research studies indicate that people with higher intake levels had a lower incidence of heart attacks and death related to heart disease. Supplementation of 200 International Units of vitamin E daily is recommended in addition to food sources.

Do β-Carotene and Other Carotenoids Decrease the Risk of Heart Disease?

Fruit and vegetables are endowed with carotenoids, many of which provide antioxidant support in the fight against heart disease. Being fat-soluble, carotenoids circulate throughout the body aboard lipoproteins and provide protection against oxidation (which promotes atherosclerosis). Several large population studies have reported that the incidence of heart disease is lower in people who eat a diet rich in these substances and have higher levels in the blood. However, which carotenoids are more potent or whether they act in tandem and with other factors found in fruits and vegetables remains to be determined. Along this line of thought it is still unknown whether there is additional benefit of supplementation for individuals eating a diet already rich in carotenoids.

Can Garlic Help Prevent Heart Disease?

Garlic has sulfur-containing substances including allicin and its breakdown products diallyl sulfides, which are purported to have medicinal properties. There are several reasons to believe that garlic can play a role in preventing heart disease. First, garlic-derived compounds lessens the activity of the key enzyme in cholesterol formation. However, garlic supplementation has not consistently been shown to lower blood cholesterol levels. Researchers have determined that garlic might be an inhibitor of blood clot formation, which is a principal cause of heart attacks, as well as having anti-inflammatory and antioxidant properties. Considered together there is strong reason to believe that garlic can play a contributing role in promoting a healthy cardiovascular system.

What Role Do Folate and Vitamins B_6 and B_{12} Play in Relation to Heart Disease?

Recently it was determined that higher levels of homocysteine in the blood can increase heart disease risk possibly by negatively influencing blood clotting and vasodilation. Homocysteine is naturally produced in the cells as they go about their molecule-making business. As displayed in Figure 9.3, homocysteine can be converted to the amino acid methionine via the assistance of folate and vitamins B_6 and B_{12}. Thus having adequate levels of these vitamins can help manage the level of homocysteine. Over the next few years ongoing research should shed more light on the exact role homocysteine plays in heart disease development and the best way to apply folate and vitamin B_6 and B_{12}.

Folate and vitamins B_6 and B_{12} can support a healthy heart by supporting homocysteine metabolism.

Can Fiber Impact Heart Disease Prevention?

Dietary fiber, especially soluble fiber found in oats, barley, and legumes (for example, beans, peas and lentils), and psyllium can have a positive impact on blood cholesterol levels. The relationship between fiber (namely beta-glucans) from these food sources and cholesterol lowering has lead to the development of health claims that food manufacturers can use on packaging such as the one below. In order for the claim to be used in a food product, one serving must contain either 0.75 grams of oat or barley fiber or 1.7 grams psyllium fiber.

> Soluble fiber from foods such as (name of soluble fiber source or product), as part of a diet low in saturated fat and cholesterol, may reduce the risk of heart disease. A serving of [name of food product] supplies x grams of the [necessary daily dietary intake for the benefit] soluble fiber from [name of soluble fiber source] necessary per day to have this effect.

Soluble fibers from these sources influence blood cholesterol levels by interacting with cholesterol digestive tract and decreasing its absorption. These fibers may also undergo breakdown by bacteria in the colon and the byproducts have been noted to potentially reduce cholesterol production in the liver.

How Can Plant Sterols Help Lower Heart Disease Risk?

Plants make sterol molecules that are very similar to cholesterol that human and other animals produce. In fact, many of us might have a hard time telling the difference between these plant sterols and animal cholesterol (Figure 13.4). Research by scientists in the United States and around the globe (such as in Finland) has suggested that sterols such as

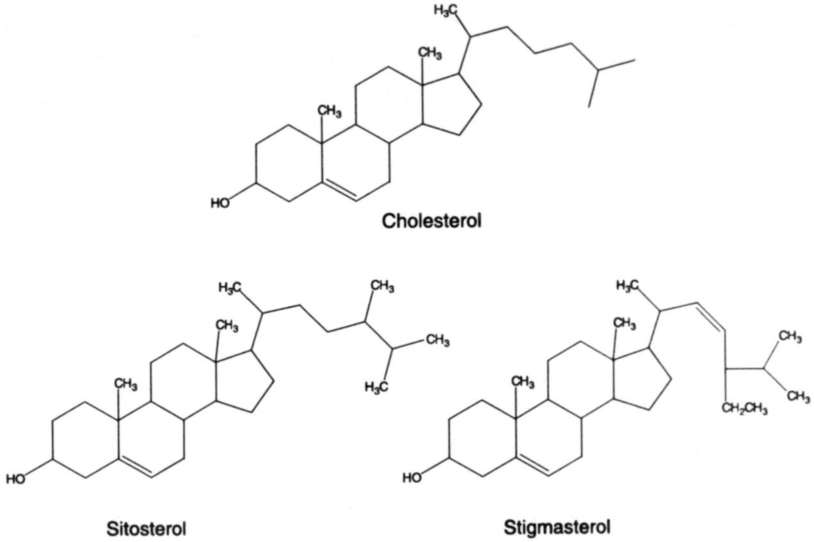

Figure 13.4 Cholesterol (animal sterol) and the structure of two plant sterols.

sitosterol, stigmasterol, campesterol, and sitostanol can lower blood cholesterol levels. Phytosterols appear to block the absorption of cholesterol in the digestive tract, which in turn lowers the level of total and LDL cholesterol in the blood. As these sterols are found in plant oils (especially unrefined oils), this may help explain some of the cholesterol-reducing properties of those oils. Phytosterols are also found in nuts, seeds, whole grains, and legumes. Commercially available spreads such as Take Control® and Benecol® are produced with phytosterols to be used by people trying to lower their cholesterol.

Can Eating More Flavonoids Lower the Risk of Heart Disease?

In short, probably. However, the details and recommendations are still a little out of reach at this point. Flavonoids (isoflavones or isoflavonoids, flavones, flavonols, catechins, and anthocyanins) are a class of chemicals produced by plants and are often called polyphenolic compounds with respect to their molecular structure. Onions, citrus, some teas, and red grapes (red wine) contain a flavonoid called quercetin which is a potent antioxidant and seems to favorably impact blood pressure.

Researchers in the United States, Finland, and around the world have determined that people who eat or drink less of flavonoids have a higher death rate from heart disease. Some of these flavonoids may act to decrease the level of total and LDL-cholesterol in the blood, while others may decrease free-radical activities, thereby protecting LDL from oxidation as well as helping to protect the walls of the arteries. So again, eat more fruits, vegetables, and whole grains and, if you like, enjoy a glass or two of red wine daily or a few times a week.

Can Drinking Wine Decrease the Risk of Heart Disease?

A few years back it was recognized that there was a decreased incidence of heart disease in France despite the consumption of a high fat diet, a phenomenon referred to as the "French Paradox." Since it was well known that this population and others such as Denmark also drink a lot of red wine, scientists began to investigate the potential benefits of red wine. The consumption of wine in these regions is chronic yet only moderate—one to four glasses daily. Red wine consumption has been recognized to reduce the incidence of heart disease by perhaps helping keep blood pressure lower, reducing blood clot formation, and reducing LDL oxidation. It is also likely that substances found in red wine, such as quercetin, resveratrol, and similar molecules, provide much of the benefit. Interestingly, the prophylactic effects of alcohol are not limited only to red wine. Researchers have determined that alcohol in a variety of forms (that is, liquor, wine, and beer) consumed chronically but in smaller quantities is associated with reduced risk of heart disease, however not to the same extent as red wine.

Wine contains nutrients such as quercetin and resveratrol that can support a healthy heart.

What Drugs Are Prescribed to Reduce Blood Cholesterol?

The drugs commonly prescribed to treat hypercholesterolemia include those that either decrease cholesterol synthesis in the liver, decrease VLDL production, or decrease dietary cholesterol absorption. Drugs such as lovostatin are known to reduce the manufacturing of cholesterol by the liver, although the benefits of this medication may also include increased LDL removal from the blood. Cholestyramine or colestipol will bind cholesterol in the digestive tract and render it unavailable for absorption. Gram doses of nicotinic acid, a form of niacin, seem to decrease the production of VLDL in the liver. It is believed that nicotinic acid impedes fat mobilization from the fat cells, which ultimately decreases fatty acids returning to the liver. If fewer fatty acids are in the liver, then less VLDL will be made.

Is Iron Status in the Body Related to Heart Disease?

A few years ago research reported that a relationship may exist between heart attacks and higher levels of an iron-storing protein that can be found in our blood. The protein, ferritin, is typically found in tissue such as the liver and is a storage container for iron atoms. However, some ferritin can leak out of cells and circulate, which allows for it to be assessed. Researchers have noted that the risk of a heart attack is higher in individuals with higher ferritin levels in conjunction with a higher LDL-cholesterol level (greater than 193 milligrams per 100 milliliters of blood). Other researchers have reported that while total dietary iron intake was not associated with a greater risk of a heart attack, higher intake of heme iron was associated with a greater risk. Heme iron comes from animal sources, largely red meat. Furthermore, those men with a higher heme iron intake who took a vitamin E supplement were at a slightly lower risk for heart attack than those men without a vitamin E supplement. In addition, factors such as smoking and diabetes also placed those men with a higher heme iron intake at an even higher risk of heart attack.

Can Coenzyme Q (Ubiquinone) Be Helpful in Preventing Heart Attacks?

Coenzyme Q10 (CoQ10) is found in a variety of plants and animals, and better food sources include meats (especially organ meats such as heart and liver), sardines, mackerel, soybean oil, and peanuts. The research involving CoQ10 is difficult to assess for several reasons. Often the studies are short, not long term, or the CoQ10 is provided in addition to other drugs. CoQ10 acting as an antioxidant can be yet another protective factor against free-radical activity and thus heart disease development. Furthermore, some researchers believe that CoQ10 may decrease damage to heart muscle after it has been deprived of oxygen for a brief period of time. In this situation, when oxygen floods back into the deprived cells, there is an increased opportunity for free-radical production. Further still, many researchers have determined that the use of statin drugs for high cholesterol levels may compromise CoQ10 status in cells making CoQ10 supplementation along with statin drug use good practice.

Cancer Is When Good Cells Go Bad

Cancer is by no means a new disease, as researchers have found evidence of cancer in dinosaur fossils and mummified remains of ancient civilizations. Yet because cancer is granted so much attention today it is easy to think of cancer as a modern biological phenomenon. However, it is more likely that cancer is merely a consequence of life, one that perhaps humans have significantly potentiated. Each year more than 550,000 Americans will die as a result of cancer—more than 1,500 Americans lives a day are cut short. In fact 23 percent of all deaths in the United States is caused by cancer, making it the number two killer behind cardiovascular disease. Figure 13.5 provides a breakdown of the relative amounts of cancer (for example, breast, lung, colon, etc) in both men and women.

Where Does Cancer Come From?

Like many diseases, cancer is merely an alteration of normal biological processes. It is not "caught" like the common cold but developed in the body. The basis of the cancer is the very foundation of life itself, cell reproduction. As a rule of nature, all cells must come from existing cells. In order to make a new cell, an existing cell grows in size, makes an exact copy of its DNA, and then divides into two identical cells, each with a complete copy of DNA. These two cells can then grow in size, copy their DNA, and divide, creating four cells total, and so on (Figure 13.6).

Throughout life, all tissue in the body grows in this manner until its genetically predetermined size is realized. Thus the brain and other organs will get only so big under normal conditions. At this point there

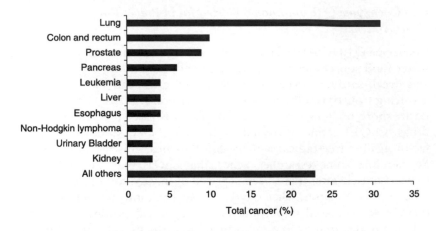

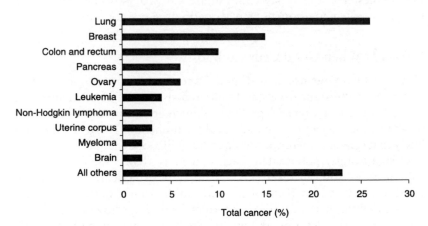

Figure 13.5 Estimation of total and type of cancer in 2006 in the United States.

are two possible scenarios. One scenario is that the current cells will exist for extremely long periods. For example, once tissue such as the brain, pancreas, and adrenals reach their intended size, their cells may exist for several decades or even throughout life. These cells simply are arrested in their ability to grow and divide.

The second scenario is that cells of a particular organ or tissue will continuously undergo turnover. The term *turnover* describes the balance between cells being broken down and those being made. New cells are constantly being made to replace cells of the same type that have a limited life span. The replaced cells are either broken down in the body, such as blood cells, or are removed from body surfaces, such as cells lining the digestive tract and skin cells. Cells that line the stomach and small intestine may have a life span of only a few days, while a red blood cell will live about 4 months.

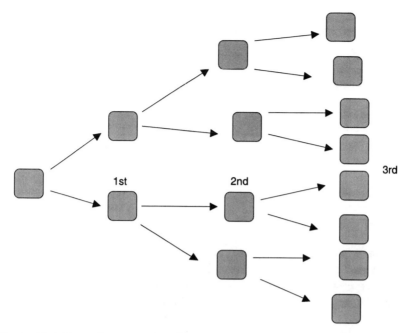

Figure 13.6 Shows how a single cell can replicate to form eight new cells in three generations.

Source: American Cancer Society.

How Does Cancer Develop?

It is important to realize that almost all of the cells in the body inherently possess the ability to grow and divide and that these functions are tightly regulated by certain proteins within these cells. These cell proteins are ultimately produced from DNA genes. Quite simply, cancer is a disruption in this fine regulation. Cells that are arrested in their ability to reproduce can begin to reproduce. Or cells that are already reproducing at a specific rate, such as in the colon, uterus, or prostate, can reproduce at a rate greater than normal, thus resulting in more cells being produced than broken down.

What Is the Difference Between a Tumor and Cancer?

Not all forms of rapid uncontrolled cell growth are cancerous. Therefore, the term tumor is more appropriately applied to any unregulated cell growth. Once the presence of a tumor is recognized, the next step is to discern whether it is benign or malignant. The characteristics of benign compared to malignant are listed in Table 13.4. It should be recognized that not all types of cancer are in the form of tumors. Leukemia is an

Table 13.4 Tumor Characteristics

Benign	Malignant (Cancer)
Usually encapsulated in a fibrous sack which may be surgically removed	Not encapsulated in a fibrous sack and therefore making it more difficult to remove surgically
Tumor growth is uniform in expansion boundaries	Cell growth is not uniform on boundaries again making accurate surgical removal difficult
Has not spread to other regions of the body	Utilizes the blood or lymphatic circulation to spread to other regions of the body
Limited blood supply (arteries and capillaries)	Development of blood vessels to support rapid growth and spread

example whereby the dangerous cells are blood cells, a fact that allows blood-based cancers to easily spread through the body.

Cancer is a disease that is in essence unregulated cell growth of a malignant nature. Thus, cancer is a malignant tumor. Because a benign tumor grows within a fibrous sack of connective tissue with uniform expansion boundaries, it can often be treated by surgical removal. However, malignant cell growth is not contained and does not show even and somewhat organized expansion. This certainly makes it more difficult to remove completely by surgery.

One deplorable characteristic of malignant cell growth is the ability of some of the cancerous cells to break away from the original tumor site. They then travel in the blood or through lymphatic circulation to find new residency and reproduce in a different region in the body. Thus the cancer is able to spread throughout the body (Figure 13.7).

What Causes a Normal Cell to Go Awry?

One way a normal cell can be converted to a tumor-producing cell is by inflicted alterations in the associated genes in DNA. These genes are very special because they contain the instructions for a cell to make the proteins involved in the reproduction of that cell. The process of altering DNA is called a *mutation* and it takes several mutations in key proteins for a cell to transition into one that could give rise to a tumor.

Cancer is caused by changes to key genes that regulate cell reproduction.

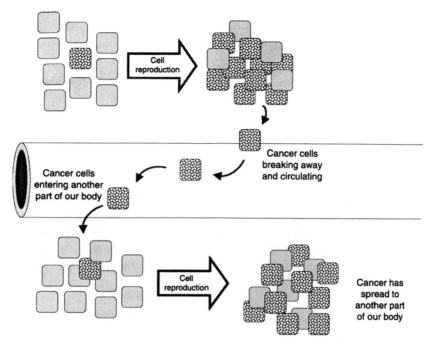

Figure 13.7 Shows cancerous cells breaking away from the original tumor site and spreading to another region of the body.

The factors that can cause mutations to genes include a variety of chemicals and ultraviolet light. Collectively, substances that can cause DNA mutations relevant to tumor production are referred to as *carcinogenic* agents. Carcinogenic means to potentially give rise to cancer.

Can We Fix Mutations Before Cancer Develops?

Fortunately, most mutations in DNA are not harmful. Researchers have estimated that the human body's cells collectively face millions of these assaults on DNA every day. In many cases the mutation does not involve the cell reproduction genes and/or DNA-repair mechanisms quickly repair the damage. DNA repair involves "proofreading enzymes," so called because they endeavor to check over the DNA, looking for abnormalities, and when found they fix them if they can. Certainly, however, by exposing ourselves to more and more carcinogenic agents we increase the likelihood of developing tumors and cancer.

How Is Cancer Treated?

The treatment of cancer typically involves one of three medical options or a combination of them: surgical removal, radiation therapy, and

Table 13.5 Complimentary Cancer Therapies

Music therapy	Prayer, spiritual practices
Aromatherapy	Biofeedback
Meditation	Art therapy
T'ai chi	Yoga

chemotherapy. These are the proven or conventional modes of treatment. In addition, several other options (Table 13.5) are available that can be used in conjunction with the conventional modes. These are often called complementary therapies.

Surgical removal of cancerous tissue is somewhat tricky. If the tumor is benign, then cutting out the tumor is somewhat like removing seeds from an apple. However, when the tumor is cancerous, it may be spreading out within an area unpredictably, which makes it difficult to remove entirely. Theoretically speaking, if even one cancerous cell remains in the body, the tumor can regrow.

How Bad Is Smoking to Human Health, and Is It Associated with Cancer?

Smoking is the most preventable cause of premature death for people. In fact, one of five deaths of Americans can be directly attributed to tobacco smoking. Almost 90 percent of all lung cancers in American men (80 percent in women) are due to smoking, and smoking is also highly associated with cancers of the mouth, pharynx, larynx, esophagus, pancreas, uterus, cervix, kidney, and bladder. When tobacco is burned and inhaled the smoke contains thousands of chemicals with dozens of them known cancer-causing agents or carcinogens. Clearly, the best thing a smoker can do for himself or herself is to stop smoking as soon as possible.

How Is Nutrition Involved in Cancer Prevention?

There are many components of the food supply or human lifestyle that have either been shown to or are at least speculated to impact cancer either by increasing or decreasing its occurrence. Those that may provide benefit include vitamins A, E, C, and folate, calcium and selenium, dietary fibers, omega-3 fatty acids, carotenoids, organosulfur compounds, and polyphenolic substances. Those that possibly increase the risk of cancer include fat, alcohol, smoking, nitrites, aflatoxin, and pesticides.

Many chemical carcinogens can be rendered powerless by optimizing normal cell defense mechanisms such as antioxidants and detoxifying enzyme systems. Optimal nutrition helps assure us of maximal defensive mechanisms. Furthermore, once cancer has established itself, optimal nutrition has been reported to slow and in some situations reverse the spread of cancerous cell growth.

Does Obesity Place Us at a Higher Risk for Cancer?

Large studies of populations have indicated that obesity is a significant risk factor for almost all types of human cancer including endometrial, colon, breast, and prostate. Quite simply, individuals who eat less energy and maintain body weights closer to their ideal body weight tend to be at a lower risk for most cancers. Whether increased body fat directly causes cancer is doubtful, but research suggests that some of the chemicals that swollen fat cells release can increase the rate of developing cancer. This is because some of these chemicals are associated with the growth of cells and tissue.

Is Dietary Fat Related to Cancer?

Eating a diet with a higher percentage of the calories derived from fat appears to place people at greater risk of many cancers. This may partly be explained by the association between a high fat diet and the development of obesity. However, some researchers believe that a high fat diet exerts an independent effect as well. In addition, diets containing higher amounts of linoleic acid, an essential omega-6 PUFA, have been reported to place people at a greater risk of various cancers.

Why Are Antioxidants Important in Cancer Prevention?

Vitamin C, carotenoids, polyphenolic compounds, vitamin E, selenium, copper, zinc, and manganese are very important factors in normal antioxidant activities. These factors then become very important in cancer prevention as many cancers begin with free-radical damage to key cell components, such as DNA. All of these factors can be found to some degree in fruits, vegetables, legumes, and whole grains, which probably is a primary reason why people eating a diet rich in these natural foods are at a lower risk of most cancers. Furthermore, people eating a diet rich in fruits, vegetables, whole grains, and legumes tend to eat less fat and exercise more frequently. Whether there is a need for antioxidant supplementation is the subject of much debate.

Antioxidants can lower the risk of cancer development by inactivating harmful free radicals.

Can Vitamin C Decrease the Incidence of Cancer?

Among all of the vitamins, perhaps vitamin C has received the most attention as an anticancer agent. Much of the research involving vitamin C and cancer in people has been correlation studies, which are used to determine an association between the two or more entities. In regard to cancer of the mouth, larynx, esophagus, and colon, as the vitamin C content of the diet increases, the risk for these cancers decreases two to three times. In more direct research studies it seems that individuals getting less than 80 milligrams daily appear to be at greater cancer risk than individuals with higher levels of intake. The true impact of higher levels of vitamin C intake is difficult to assess on an individual basis and thus a more general recommendation of 400 milligrams of vitamin C daily seems reasonable for general health promotion. One important consideration for vitamin C consumption is recognized in smokers. Researchers have reported that it may take as much as a four to six times greater vitamin C intake for smokers to achieve the same blood level of vitamin C as nonsmokers. This is especially important as cigarette smoke contains an abundant supply of free radicals and free-radical-creating substances, and appears to increase the risk for many cancers, especially lung cancer.

Is β-Carotene and Other Carotenoids Important in Cancer Prevention?

β-Carotene and other carotenoids has long been speculated as reducing the risk of cancer. In accordance, several studies of populations have suggested that when people ate more carotenoids the presence of cancer was lower. Interestingly, while β-carotene often receives the most attention other carotenoids have been shown to strong benefit as well. For example, studies involving smokers have suggested that the dietary intake of total carotenoids, lycopene, β-cryptoxanthin, lutein, and zeaxanthin have a more clear relationship to reducing lung cancer risk. Thus it makes sense to eat a diet rich in fruits and vegetables to allow for a broad variety of carotenoids and to plan a supplementation regimen along this line of thinking as well.

Is Fiber Related to Cancer Prevention?

Research suggests that as fiber increases in the diet, the risk of colon cancer and certain other cancers decreases. Dietary fiber, by increasing the rate of feces movement through the colon, decreases the time that carcinogenic agents in the digestive tract interact with cells lining the colon. Fiber may also bind carcinogenic substances in the digestive tract and decrease their absorption or interaction with colon cells. On a related note, scientists have suggested that the risk of colon cancer decreases with a healthy calcium intake.

Can Eating More Broccoli and Cauliflower Reduce the Risk of Cancer?

There is good reason to include cruciferous (or *Brassica*) vegetables in your diet arsenal to support cancer prevention. These vegetables include broccoli, Brussels sprouts, cabbage, cauliflower, collard greens, arugula, kale, kohlrabi, mustard, rutabaga, turnips, bok choy, Chinese cabbage, wasabi, horse radish, radish, and watercress. In addition to key antioxidant vitamins and minerals, cruciferous vegetables are rich sources of glucosinolates, which are the sulfur-containing compounds responsible for their pungent aromas and unique taste. Routine preparation of these vegetables by chopping as well as chewing leads to the breakdown of glucosinolates which in turn give rise to indoles and isothiocyanates which seem to help prevent cancer.

Broccoli and cauliflower contain sulfur-based nutrients that can help defend against cancer.

Can Turmeric (Curcumin) Help Prevent Cancer?

Turmeric is a spice derived that is a member of the ginger family. Curcumin is the principal polyphenolic compound in turmeric and is by itself an antioxidant and also supports the production of glutathione, another key antioxidant during times of need. In recent years researchers has revealed that turmeric can play a role in the prevention of cancer formation.

In General What Substances in Food May Be Important in Cancer Prevention?

As mentioned several times, people who eat more fruits, vegetables, legumes, and whole grains are at a lower risk for various cancers. It now appears that many other factors in these foods, beyond the established nutrients, impact the development of cancer. These substances include phenols, indole, aromatic isothiocyanates, carotenoids, fibers, terpenes, polyphenolic, and organosulphur compounds. Many of these substances have been studied in cell cultures and also in animals and appear to be very promising. Together with vitamin and mineral antioxidants such as vitamins E and C and copper, selenium, zinc, and manganese these products may account for much of the cancer risk-reducing effects associated with diets high in fruits, vegetables, legumes, and whole grains.

So, the best things to do nutritionally are:

- eat five or more servings of fruits and vegetables a day
- eat more whole grain products
- choose foods lower in fat and saturated fat
- maintain a body weight closer to your ideal body weight
- engage in regular exercise (especially aerobic) to assist in maintaining a lower body weight and reducing stress
- limit consumption of fatty red meat
- do not use alcohol excessively

Appendix A

Periodic Table of Elements

1	2	3	4	5	6	7	8	9	10	11	12	13	14	15	16	17	18
1 H Hydrogen																	2 He Helium
3 Li Lithium	4 Be Beryllium											5 B Boron	6 C Carbon	7 N Nitrogen	8 O Oxygen	9 F Fluorine	10 Ne Neon
11 Na Sodium	12 Mg Magnesium											13 Al Aluminium	14 Si Silicon	15 P Phosphorus	16 S Sulfur	17 Cl Chlorine	18 Ar Argon
19 K Potassium	20 Ca Calcium	21 Sc Scandium	22 Ti Titanium	23 V Vanadium	24 Cr Chromium	25 Mn Manganese	26 Fe Iron	27 Co Cobolt	28 Ni Nickel	29 Cu Copper	30 Zn Zinc	31 Ga Gallium	32 Ge Germanium	33 As Arsenic	34 Se Selenium	35 Br Bromine	36 Kr Kryplon
37 Rb Rhubidium	38 Sr Strontium	39 Y Yttrium	40 Zr Zirconium	41 Nb Niobium	42 Mo Molybdenum	43 Tc Technelium	44 Ru Ruthenium	45 Rh Rhodium	46 Pd Palladium	47 Ag Silver	48 Cd Codmium	49 In Indium	50 Sn Tin	51 Sb Antimony	52 Te Tellurium	53 I Iodine	54 Xe Zenon
55 Cs Cesium	56 Ba Barium	57 La Lanthanum	72 Hf Hafnium	73 Ta Tantalum	74 W Tungsten	75 Re Rhenium	76 Os Osmium	77 Ir Indium	78 Pt Platinum	79 Au Gold	80 Hg Mercury	81 Tl Thallium	82 Pb Lead	83 Bi Bismuth	84 Po Polonium	85 At Astatine	86 Rn Radon
87 Fr Francium	88 Ra Radium	89 Ac Actinium	104 Unq Unniquacium	105 Unp Unnilpentium	106 Unh Unnilhexium												

58 Ce Cerium	59 Pr Praseodymium	60 Nd Neodymium	61 Pm Promethium	62 Sm Samarium	63 Eu Europium	64 Gd Gadolinium	65 Tb Terbium	66 Dy Dysprosium	67 Ho Holmium	68 Er Erbium	69 Tm Thulium	70 Yb Ytterbium	71 Lu Lutetium
90 Th Thorium	91 Pa Protacinium	92 U Uranium	93 Np Neplunium	94 Pu Plutonium	95 Am Americium	96 Cm Curium	97 Bk Berkelium	98 Cf Californium	99 Es Einsteinium	100 Fm Fermium	101 Md Mendelevium	102 No Nobelium	103 Lr Lawrencium

☐ Component of Human Body

Index

City of Westminster College
Learning Services / Queens Park Centre

Lightning Source UK Ltd.
Milton Keynes UK
UKOW031057260612

195030UK00006BA/18/P